How to Prevent Breast Cancer

❦

Ross Pelton, R.Ph., Ph.D., and C.C.N.
Taffy Clarke Pelton, M.A.,
and Vinton C. Vint, M.D.

A Fireside Book
Published by Simon & Schuster
New York   London   Toronto   Sydney   Tokyo   Singapore

FIRESIDE

 Rockefeller Center
1230 Avenue of the Americas
New York, NY 10020

FIRESIDE and colophon are registered trademarks of Simon & Schuster Inc.

Designed by Levavi & Levavi, Inc.

Manufactured in the United States of America

10 9 8 7 6 5 4 3 2 1

Library of Congress Cataloging-in-Publication Data

Pelton, Ross.
    How to prevent breast cancer / Ross Pelton, Taffy Clarke Pelton, and Vinton C. Vint.
        p.   cm.
    "A Fireside book".
    Includes bibliographical references (p.   ).
    1. Breast—Cancer—Prevention.   I. Pelton, Taffy Clarke.
II. Vint, Vinton C.
RC280.B8P35 1995
616.99'449052—dc20   95-35251
    CIP
ISBN 0-684-80022-5

The authors are grateful for permission to utilize material from the following sources:
"Provera Brand of Medroxyprogesterone Acetate Tables," USP, by the Upjohn Company. Revised January 1992. Kalamazoo, MI 49001.

(*Continued on page 384.*)

Contents

Introduction

❦

People were often amazed when they heard we were writing a book on breast cancer prevention. "You mean, you can really prevent it?" It seems that most people believe breast cancer is a random event, a disease process beyond our control.

Twenty years ago the notion that heart disease was preventable might have stimulated the same response. Yet today, most people understand that it is a chronic degenerative disease preventable in the majority of cases by lifestyle changes, proper nutrition, exercise, and emotional well-being. With the proliferation of this information, the incidence of heart disease is decreasing.

Breast cancer, however, is increasing. Does a steady 1.8 percent increase annually since 1973 appear to be a random event? The truth is, cancer is also a chronic degenerative disease process that is largely preventable.

The current wisdom maintains that monthly breast self-examination, regular mammograms, and clinical examinations will detect cancer in time to provide a 92 percent cure rate. Such statistics suggest that breast cancer is not so bad after all, as long as we pay attention and observe the rules. But ask breast cancer patients how bad it is. They will tell you the process is a long, lonely, scary road, and most wish they had done something different to make it easier.

We hope this book will provide the knowledge to produce that "something different," along with the encouragement to take action now. We won't promise that you or your loved ones will never get breast cancer, or that it will never recur. There are many different types of cancer, many of its mechanisms are not fully understood, and it reacts differently in each individual. What we can say, however, is that we believe you have within your control the ability to significantly reduce your chances of ever hearing those terrifying words, "You have breast cancer."

We feel women can no longer afford to wait for the scientific community, with its ponderous, expensive methods, to agree on the correlation between diet and breast cancer, the impact of environmental pollutants on our health, and the role of estrogen, hormone replacement therapy, and birth control pills in breast cancer incidence. We want to tell the whole story as it is known today, so that women can begin to make new choices and diminish their chances of joining the 182,000 women who will be diagnosed with breast cancer this year. These new choices may also reduce the possibility of recurrence in breast cancer survivors.

While sharing the same vision that the breast cancer epidemic can and must be controlled, each of us brings to this book the unique perspective of varied backgrounds in medicine, psychology, and health. Dr. Ross Pelton's first experience with breast cancer was when his grandmother struggled with the disease. Since childhood he has had a vivid recollection of her scarred and burned arm and chest from a mastectomy and radiation. He remembers viewing breast cancer as a hateful enemy and being angry at its destructive power. Twenty-five years later, while working for Dr. Gerhard Schrauzer, one of the world's leading breast cancer researchers, Ross was highly influenced by the results of Schrauzer's research. He learned that trace amounts of the nutrient selenium, when added to the diets of laboratory animals prone to breast cancer, caused a

70 percent reduction in breast cancer incidence. Dr. Schrauzer often said, and Ross concurs, that if women would take selenium as a nutritional supplement daily, it would cause a major reduction in the national incidence of breast cancer.

Years later, while writing *Alternatives in Cancer Therapy* and administering an alternative cancer treatment program, Ross became convinced that there was only one way to deal with this disease: prevention. He recognized that traditional methods of treatment were not producing greater cure rates, and that pouring millions more dollars into stronger drugs and better methods of detection was not going to solve the breast cancer problem. As he gained deeper understanding of nutritional biochemistry, it became clear that the unhealthy aspects of our diets, lifestyles, and environment cause chronic degenerative diseases—diseases that are largely preventable.

Having witnessed the courageous and often poignant battle for life waged by hundreds of women with breast cancer, Ross became painfully aware that most breast cancer patients believed they were either victims of some unseen and random force or had done something wrong in thought or deed. Little, if any, information was available about prevention, and as mentioned earlier, the mere notion that breast cancer might be preventable was a novel idea to most women. Thus, the idea to write *How to Prevent Breast Cancer* was born.

Dr. Vinton C. Vint, the former head of mammography and nuclear medicine at Scripps Clinic in La Jolla, California, offers the unique perspective of a medical doctor who has completed thirty years of study in optimal health. For twenty years Dr. Vint diagnosed many women with breast cancer, monitored aspects of their treatment with follow-up mammograms and nuclear scans, then saw many of them slowly die from their disease. Many of these women had supposedly done everything "right." They were well educated, successful in marriage and/or business, did not drink or smoke to excess, and did not have a family history of breast cancer, yet they still developed breast cancer and died from the disease. Even the more than 100,000 normal mammograms Dr. Vint read were misleading;

he knew that many of these women would eventually develop breast cancer, despite modern medical care.

As a result of researching thousands of scientific studies, Dr. Vint, like Ross, realized that optimal nutrition and lifestyle changes could lessen the risk of a woman's contracting breast cancer. However, his role as a physician practicing what is known as conventional medicine deterred him from discussing preventive measures with patients. He has found it frustrating and disheartening to witness mainstream medicine's blind, ultraconservative attitude toward those preventive and health-oriented scientific findings.

How to Prevent Breast Cancer provides the long-awaited opportunity for Dr. Vint to integrate and share his knowledge from his two areas of expertise: disease prevention and the use of state-of-the-art technology to detect disease in women for whom preventive measures were not absolute. Dr. Vint wishes to offer women a medical insider's view in order to dispel the rumors and myths about the dangers of modern mammography. He also hopes to enlighten women about the best available biopsy method, which is nonsurgical. Although Dr. Vint does not believe that early detection is the primary answer to the breast cancer epidemic, he has detected many cancerous tumors before they have spread, allowing patients to enjoy high cure rates. He also possesses a well-rounded perspective on the uses of estrogen and tamoxifen, and offers herein safer treatment alternatives to help women improve overall health and lessen the chance of contracting other diseases.

Taffy Clarke Pelton brings a unique combination of professional skills and personal history to this book. With a master's degree in counseling psychology, she utilizes in private practice her training in Hakomi (mind/body therapy), group therapy, and brain wave biofeedback. Her expertise in the field of health psychology grew out of a lifetime struggle with psychosomatic symptoms coupled with an extreme fear of cancer. While counseling cancer patients in a hospital setting, Taffy had to fully confront her fears of this disease. It became clear that these fears and the sense of having no control were based largely on a lack of understanding and knowledge about health and disease. As a result, she learned how to use her fear as the motivator to implement and maintain a healthy lifestyle.

As you read this book, you, like Taffy, may find that you have been exposed to many risks to breast cancer that were not within your control at the time. She was exposed to high-dose birth control pills at an early age, radiation from X-rays, pesticides in the commercial food supply, and environmental pollutants.

Although Taffy cannot alter the unhealthy aspects of her past which may have put her at risk for breast cancer, she does focus on optimizing her existing health condition. No matter what condition your body is in, it is never too late to begin the process of becoming healthy. This attitude gives new meaning to the concept of prevention.

Prevention means acknowledging the threat of breast cancer, understanding our own personal risks, then admitting to and changing lifestyle errors. It means making new choices that may arrest or reverse a degenerative process that may already be set in motion. It could also have significant meaning for women who have already contracted breast cancer that is in remission, and seek to be proactive in avoiding recurrence.

Prevention also means that we educate the next generation. We must examine the risk factors, emotional health, and lifestyles of our daughters, *no matter how young,* and guide them in health-saving directions. Prevention also means becoming conscious of and taking action on the environmental, political, and economic issues that directly affect our ability to remain free from breast cancer.

Although we primarily address women in this book, the information within is also important for men. While few men actually contract breast cancer, they are still heavily impacted by the breast cancer that threatens the women in their lives. Besides gaining a greater understanding of what women must face, men can themselves benefit from much of the health-promoting information offered here.

Some of the information may frighten you. We believe, relative to this topic, that a little fear can be a healthy emotion, provided you use it as a "wake-up call" to motivate yourself into lifesaving action. You may also experience anger or feel victimized as you read along. We want How to Prevent Breast Cancer to serve as a call to action. We hope you will utilize your feelings and your knowledge to take personal and political action for the benefit of your own health, as well as that of other women, and, ultimately, our environment.

We wish you great health and a long life.

Ross, Taffy, Dr. Vint
1995

For information about speaking engagements, health seminars, or consultations, send correspondence to: P.O. Box 81365, San Diego, CA 92138–1365

Reader, please be advised that if quoted material is followed by a series of note numbers, the first number in the series represents the source of the quote.

Chapter 1

Fighting the Epidemic

Every three minutes a woman in the United States is diagnosed with breast cancer; every twelve minutes a woman dies from it. According to the American Cancer Society, more than 180,000 women will be diagnosed with breast cancer this year, and approximately 46,000 women will die from it.[1]

Statistics reveal the frightening truth that breast cancer is on the increase in most countries throughout the world. In the United States and many other industrialized countries, breast cancer is generating an epidemic of disease and of fear.

Breast cancer is a terrifying disease that strikes women where they feel most vulnerable. As a culture, we are overly concerned about women's breasts when it comes to image, but in denial about them when it comes to health.

In 1971, the year President Richard Nixon declared our national "war on cancer," a woman's lifetime chance of contracting breast cancer was 1 in 20. Today it is 1 in 8, and this is after twenty-four years of spending hundreds of millions of dollars fighting this disease.[2] Breast cancer has become the most commonly diagnosed female cancer. It is the second largest cause of cancer deaths among women, exceeded only by lung cancer. Furthermore, it is the leading cause of death for women between the ages of thirty-five and fifty-four and the leading cause of cancer deaths for all African-American women.[3]

The most chilling statistic yet is that since the "war on cancer" was declared, more women in the United States have died of breast cancer than the total number of American men who lost their lives in World Wars I and II, the Korean conflict, and the war in Vietnam combined!

When a disease rapidly increases in numbers, we define it as an epidemic. We conclude from the statistics that breast cancer has become a serious epidemic. However, you will not hear medical authorities publicly use this harsh and frightening terminology. An epidemic would imply that modern medicine is not only ineffective in curing breast cancer, but even more ineffective in understanding *how to prevent it.* Our purpose in this book is to examine what is actually known about breast cancer, which factors in our lives increase our risk of contracting the disease, and what can be done to decrease such risk.

❧ Is Early Detection Really Protection?

The cover of an informative pamphlet widely distributed by a California state assemblywoman states the following: "BREAST CANCER: the best prevention is early detection."[4] The latest slogan has been changed to: "The best protection is early detection." Basically, women are urged to get regular mammograms, see their doctor periodically, and do regular breast self-examinations. The rationale is that a woman has a better chance to be cured if the cancer is identified in its early stages, before it spreads to the lymph nodes and other organs in the body.

If this is a viable answer, why then is the incidence and death from breast cancer continuing to rise every year? This is a complex and multifaceted issue for which there is no simple answer. First, let us examine the problems inherent in viewing early detection as a form of prevention.

❧ *How Effective Is Mammography?*

During the past two decades the majority of funds for breast cancer have been directed toward publicizing and promoting better methods of detection and treatment. This has resulted in a significant increase in the use of mammography, a technology that enables most tumors to be detected approximately six months to three years before they are physically palpable.

If we believe that early detection increases one's chances of being cured, it would be natural to assume that an increase in the use of mammography would show a decrease in death rates. Until recently, the studies have been contradictory. Some benefit has been shown for women over the age of fifty, but there had been no conclusive evidence that mammography decreases overall mortality rates in women aged forty to forty-nine. This picture is beginning to change as new studies are being published, and as women participating in the earlier studies are being followed for an extended period of time. A recent Swedish study has demonstrated that women in their forties who received regular screening mammography had a death rate 40 percent lower than those who had no mammograms.[5,6,7]

Although mammography has been such an area of controversy and misunderstanding, we feel we are fortunate to have any technology that allows us to discover cancer as early as possible. However, because this diagnostic tool has been so heavily touted as being the first line of defense against breast cancer, we are concerned that it may trap women into the illusion that mammography can do more than it can. Mammography is not foolproof. Studies indicate that 10 percent of all cancers go undetected in this procedure even when performed properly.[8]

Until recently, when it was mandated that all facilities must be accredited, this percentage was higher. Unfortunately, millions of women do not follow recommended guidelines for annual or biannual mammograms. The most critical limitation—and this point is critical in the context of prevention—is that *a mammogram detects cancer after it has already developed.*

❧ The Problem of Metastasis

One of the possible explanations for mammography not becoming "the great new hope" is the problem of metastasis. When we say a tumor has metastasized we mean that cells from the original tumor have broken away and traveled to create a tumor in another part of the body.

Some consider that a one-centimeter tumor (the size of a pea) is "early stage." In fact, most clinicians do not detect the majority of breast cancers until they are 1.6 centimeters in diameter.[9] By this time, the cancer might have been developing for eight to ten years and already contains over 100 billion cells. During this period it is most likely that microscopic malignant cells have spread into other parts of the body. It is estimated that 50 percent of breast tumors have metastasized by the time they are large enough to be detected by mammography or palpation. The exceptions to this situation are the very early tumors that can be detected by state-of-the-art mammography equipment.

Under normal conditions a well-functioning immune system can kill these microscopic cells. However, when a tumor has had time to grow and send out more and more cells, the immune system has difficulty controlling the spread of the disease. Having cancer in the first place may be an indication that the immune system is already weakened in some way.

These disturbing facts illustrate the limitations of early detection as a form of prevention or protection. Again, we want to emphasize that the purpose of this discussion is not to discourage you from following early detection guidelines. A mammogram is appropriate for certain age and risk groups, and particularly important should you become aware of any suspicious physical signs. Breast self-examination and exams by your doctor are also strongly advocated. However, our primary point here is that early detection addresses the disease only *after* it has occurred. Early detection is meaningful primarily if the cancer is caught very early, prior to known metastasis. However, it still means that you face very difficult treatment options.

✖ Your Treatment Options

Once cancer is detected, there are basically only three types of treatment available in the United States: surgery, radiation, and chemotherapy. Often, all three are recommended. These are difficult and invasive treatments, making decisions even more burdensome, particularly during a time of physical and emotional stress. All too often, women simply walk away from treatment, feeling the cure is worse than the disease. Furthermore, as with mammograms, much controversy surrounds the efficacy of these treatments (see Chapter 20).

✖ The Lack of Breast Cancer Research

A critical part of solving the puzzle of the breast cancer epidemic is the attitude of the government and medical research community toward the disease. In twenty years the National Cancer Institute (NCI) spent $1 billion for breast cancer research. To put that number in perspective, in 1990 the NCI allocated only $81 million for breast cancer research; at the same time $248 million was spent for diabetes, $645 million for heart disease, and $1.6 *billion* for AIDS research. There were four to five times as many deaths from breast cancer as from AIDS, yet AIDS research was receiving twenty times more government spending.[10]

To address this unconscionable imbalance, the National Breast Cancer Coalition was formed in 1991. This is a grass-roots organization that includes 140 breast cancer organizations and thousands of former breast cancer patients. Using the same techniques to increase federal research allocations as AIDS activists, the coalition was successful in inciting NCI to increase breast cancer research to $93 million in 1991, $145 million in 1992, and $197 million in 1993. In addition to augmenting the NCI budget, the coalition was instrumental in persuading Congress to allocate another $210 million for breast cancer research. Ironically, these dollars came from the Department of Defense, with the mandated research to be carried out by the U.S. Army.

Approximately $400 million was being allocated for 1994, second only to the $2.1 billion designated for AIDS research. While this is great news, it is still not enough. Nineteen percent of all cancers diagnosed are breast cancer, yet it receives only 9 percent of federal research money. Furthermore, the majority of this money is spent on diagnosis and treatment, not prevention. This circumstance is not likely to change. The government and large cancer institutions are closely allied with the pharmaceutical companies; hence patentable drugs and devices guide the flow of research dollars. There is no indication that this trend will change anytime soon. Although increased research may result in dramatic improvement in the efficacy and safety of current treatments, as well as in more reliable ways to detect cancer early, *it still does not address the fundamental cause of the problem.*

Based upon what we know today about early detection and treatment options, it is obvious there is no good, clear answer to the breast cancer epidemic. There is no magic pill, nor is there a cure. The best way to put an end to this frightening problem is to look to prevention.

⊷ *Prevention*

For most women, the diagnosis of breast cancer comes as a severe shock. Their first reaction is often, "Why me?" as they struggle with the frightening implications of what seems to be a random event. Most women do not understand the many preventive factors under their control until after the crisis has occurred. The best way to dispel fear of a disease that appears to be out of control is through education. You can learn what you can do for yourself *before* being diagnosed with breast cancer. First, we will examine the probable sequence of events leading up to an actual cancer cell. Following that, we will discuss the uncontrollable and controllable risk factors.

⊷ *How Does Cancer Begin?*

A popular and highly regarded theory of cancer development involves three steps.[11] The first step is the *"two hit"* theory. This means that two "hits," insults, or bouts of damage must occur to a normal cell in order for it to become a cancer cell. The theory maintains that one insult alone could not produce such a permanent change in any cell.

The first hit is termed the *initiation* phase, and is quick and permanent. Such hits can be inherited (damaged genes) but are usually a result of environmental factors (chemicals, radiation, infections). There is evidence suggesting that if the initiated cells are detected early enough, cancer could be prevented from developing. For example, initiated cells may show up on a Pap smear as precancerous cells, allowing a woman time to avoid the development of cervical cancer.

The second hit is termed the *promotion* phase. Although it cannot occur without a prior initiation phase, it has opposite characteristics. The promotion phase happens slowly, over many years, and is reversible. Examples of the promotion phase include diet, hormones, and infection. During this phase substances such as estrogen and alcohol can promote the development of breast cancer. Fortunately, in the promotion phase, dietary supplements and modifications in diet and lifestyle can act to prevent breast cancer. For example, beta-carotenes (vitamin A precursors) have been used experimentally to reverse the promotion phase.

After the "two hits" produce a cancer cell, the next step is *progression*, the final stage before the cancer spreads. Consisting of many phases and taking ten to fifteen years, progression is dependent upon dietary factors, hormones, and the individual's immune system. The final phase of progression is invasion, in which the tumor cells have grown deeper than the lining of the organ or, as in breast cancer, the lining of the ducts or lobules.

Metastasis, in which cancer cells spread through the body by way of invasion of blood vessels or lymph ducts, is the final stage of cancer development. These cells grow into tumor masses in these distant sites, invading vital organs and eventually threatening the life of the individual.

This is a simplified, cursory view of one respected theory of cancer development. Our purpose is to give you a frame of reference with which to view cancer development, so the concept of prevention can become more meaningful. We often read that the cause and prevention of breast cancer is not known, hence the need for early detection. However, we believe it is not necessary to know all the details of the causation of breast cancer to begin appropriate and effective measures of prevention.

≈ Risk Factors

In order to know which preventive measures to take, it is important to understand your own risk factors. There are two kinds of risk factors: uncontrollable and controllable. The major risk factors categorized as uncontrollable involve gender and a woman's menstrual, reproductive, and family history.

Only 20 to 30 percent of women who have breast cancer exhibit these risk factors.

GENDER: Most breast cancers (over 99 percent) occur in women. American Cancer Society statistics from 1993 estimated that 182,000 women and 1,000 men would be diagnosed with breast cancer. During the same year approximately 46,000 women and 300 men died from breast cancer.[12]

AGE: The longer a woman lives, the more likely she is to develop breast cancer. Eighty-five percent of all breast cancer cases occur after age forty-five and 67 percent occur after the age of fifty.[13]

PREVIOUS CANCER: Women with a prior history of cancer have twice the risk of developing breast cancer. Once a woman has had breast cancer, her chances of developing it in the other breast are five times greater.[14]

FAMILY HISTORY: Geneticists suspect a gene defect when two or more first-degree relatives have developed premenopausal breast cancer. The term *first-degree* refers to parents, siblings, or children. If a woman has a first-degree relative with premenopausal breast cancer, her risk is six or seven times greater than those with no such family history. A postmenopausal relative is at much less of a risk. Postmenopausal breast cancer is not thought to be due to defective genes. Having a single blood relative with breast cancer has very little relative risk, perhaps 1.5 times greater. It is important to note that breast cancer caused by gene defects is estimated to account for only 2.5 to 7 percent of all breast cancer cases. Therefore, for the vast majority of American women, the chance of contracting breast cancer is not "set in stone." Overall, 70 to 80 percent of all breast cancer patients have no family history at all.

EARLY ONSET OF MENSTRUATION: Women who began menstruation before age twelve have a 100 percent greater risk of developing breast cancer as women who began menstruating at age thirteen or older.[15]

LATE MENOPAUSE: Women who experience menopause after age fifty have double the risk of women with earlier menopause.[16]

LATE CHILDBEARING: A woman who gives birth to her first child after age thirty has a four times greater risk of breast cancer than one who has her first child before the age of eighteen. Women who never bear children have an even greater risk.[17]

These are the risk factors generally accepted by the medical establishment. It is important for all women to be aware of these issues and to know if they are at increased risk. Understanding this is by no means the answer to the problem since approximately 70 to 80 percent of the women with breast cancer *do not* display any of these standard risk factors.[18]

CONTROLLABLE RISK FACTORS

Controllable risk factors include diet and nutrition, exercise and weight control, social ties, emotional well-being, and exposure to environmental toxins. These are the factors contributing to the disease process in approximately 70 to 80 percent of women whose cancer cannot be linked to genetic predisposition or reproductive history. It is the area of controllable factors that much of this book will address.

We are learning we have much greater control over breast cancer than one would think. In many ways the process is similar to the evolution of treatment for heart disease, the number-one killer in America. Huge sums of money have been spent on heart disease research. Highly sophisticated and expensive methods of surgery have been developed, and costly drugs have been introduced to regulate everything from blood pressure to the level of cholesterol in our bodies. We have learned how to transplant hearts, insert pacemakers, and replace diseased arteries. Yet today researchers have proven that simple lifestyle changes such as diet, exercise, and nutritional supplements are the most important factors in the development and healing of heart disease.

Clearly, breast cancer must follow a similar path as treatment becomes less desirable and more expensive, and research reveals the relationship between good health practices and the disease process. The key will be the desire and motivation to be healthy and the belief that you have a large measure of control over your well-being.

▰ Summary

It is critical that you assess your risk factors, lifestyle, environment, and emotional and psychological health, and be willing, if necessary, to implement changes that are within your control. We hope that we can provide you with an extensive education and ample inspiration so that you become one of the women who helps change the direction of this epidemic. Breast cancer incidence is on the increase in the United States and most industrialized countries throughout the world. Despite advances in technology, treatment options remain limited and mortality rates have not decreased. Breast cancer is a complex disease for which a single and absolute cause has not been determined; therefore women are led to believe that early detection is the best form of protection. Unfortunately, once detected, many breast cancers have already metastasized, thus necessitating painful and difficult treatments. Only 20 to 30 percent of women who have breast cancer display manifestations of the standard, uncontrollable risk factors, while the disease's occurrence in the remaining 70 to 80 percent can be attributed to lifestyle factors.

Chapter 2

Breast Structure, Function, and Abnormalities

This chapter will describe what breasts are made of and how they function, as well as benign and malignant breast diseases, types of cancers, and the clinical stages of breast cancer.

⮞ How Your Breasts Are Constructed

The breast is a glandular organ containing a complex network of mammary ducts, much like the branches of a tree. Ovarian estrogen stimulation in puberty is needed for its development. Each breast's fifteen to twenty mammary ducts lead to a like number of lobes, which in turn are made up of lobules. This is important because the two most common breast cancers originate in ductal and lobule cells. Within the lobules are the special cells that secrete milk; these are stimulated by the ovarian hormones estrogen and progesterone. Estrogen, especially, causes proliferation of the cells lining the ducts, especially in the smallest ducts, where the majority of the malignancy occurs. All this glandular tissue is surrounded by fibrous tissue, some of which, called ligaments, suspends the breasts from the chest wall. After multiple pregnancies, lactation, obesity, and/or aging, these ligaments become lax, and the breast starts to sag. The remainder of the breast is composed of fatty tissue. Two chest muscles are situated between the ribs and breast tissue (Figure 1).[1]

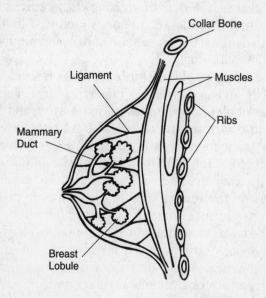

Figure 1   Structure of the Breast

❧ How Does Lactation Affect Your Breasts?

In the nonpregnant woman, the breasts contain predominantly fibrous connective tissue and fatty tissue, with little glandular tissue present. In pregnancy, the breasts go through dramatic changes. During the first trimester the breast undergoes rapid growth and maturation of both ductal and glandular tissues. During this phase the secretory cells increase in number. There is a highly intricate interplay of many hormones that initiate the production of milk. Within the first forty-eight hours after delivery, the alveoli (milk-gland sacs) become distended with milk owing to the activity of the stimulated secretory cells. Continuation of milk production is dependent upon a hormone, called prolactin, created in the brain when the nipples are stimulated. Interestingly, beta-endorphin concentrations are also elevated with nursing. (Endorphins are like internal natural narcotics, compounds produced by the brain that work to dampen the perception of pain and produce a feeling of overall well-being.)

After the cessation of breast-feeding, there is rapid shrinkage of these cells, and any remaining milk is resorbed. The alveolar cells in the lobules become smaller, some dying and being resorbed by the surrounding tissue. The relative proportion of connective tissue increases and glandular tissue decreases. The internal structures return to their resting state only after several months. Interestingly, after this regression, or "involution," is completed and the resting state has begun, even microscopic examination of breast tissue cannot easily differentiate between women who have borne children and those who have not.

Special regions on breast cell membranes, called receptor sites, can chemically bind to a woman's estrogen or progesterone, causing alveolar stimulation and growth. You can think of this as a padlock on the cell that fits only a specific key, or hormone. Postpartum, these sites are changed for up to five years or longer, possibly permanently. It is also thought these receptor sites in postpartum women are less likely to bind to the hormones, thus possibly explaining the reduced breast cancer risk in women who have their first-term pregnancy at an early age. In this situation, the "padlocks" were changed some way, so the hormone "keys" no longer fit.

Studies of the impact of breast-feeding on breast cancer reduction are many. Some have shown no beneficial effect, while many have demonstrated a significant lowering of the risk.[2,3,4]

There is no strong consensus at this time; nevertheless, it is known that there is no added risk for nursing, and there are literally dozens of excellent benefits to mother and infant for breast-feeding. One Chinese study demonstrated that if a woman nursed for a total of more than nine years throughout all her pregnancies, she would reduce her risk by 63 percent, when compared to women who nursed for a total of three years or less. Other studies, including some in North America, have confirmed these findings. These other investigations showed that both pre- and postmenopausal breast cancers were decreased in women who had breast-fed, but the added benefits of long-term breast-feeding were most important in premenopausal women. How breast-feeding tends to protect from breast cancer is unclear. It may be that changes in hormones or breast receptor sites during nursing are able to prevent tumor formation. Another possibility includes the cessation of ovulatory cycles. This itself would lower the breast's exposure to estrogen.

❧ *"Fibrocystic Disease"*

The most commonly misunderstood word regarding women's breasts is *fibrocystic*. Many women are told by their physician that they have fibrocystic breasts or fibrocystic disease. Fibrocystic should not be used in regard to the breast exam since it does not indicate any specific condition or problem. Only pathologists can make this diagnosis, and even they confuse definitions when using the term. In many women, a clinical examination often reveals a somewhat "lumpy-bumpy" consistency of the breasts, perhaps accompanied by tenderness or pain, that can vary with the menstrual cycle. By no means does this represent a disease or the presence of cysts, nor does it indicate a risk factor for breast cancer. It is a common, normal variation of breast development and should not be alarming. Many clinical physicians believe they can diagnose fibrocystic disease or changes on breast exam. This is not possible. Dr. Vint has seen hundreds of examples where radiology consultation forms were labeled fibrocystic by patients' physicians, yet the mammograms showed a completely normal breast without evidence of fibrous tissue or cysts.

❧ Benign Breast Diseases

Benign diseases or conditions of the breast are very common and they can be categorized in different ways. One classification includes benign solid tumors, dysplasia (fluid-filled cysts and nontumorous cells that are abnormal, but not malignant), inflammation (infections), and traumatic disorders. It is important to understand what these nonmalignant conditions are so that we do not confuse them with malignancy. In general, many of these benign conditions represent slight to moderate risk factors.

• *Benign tumors*

A tumor is a swelling or enlargement—a new growth of tissue forming an abnormal mass. We have known many women patients who, after being told they had a breast tumor, thought erroneously that this meant malignancy. The word *tumor* does not necessarily indicate a malignant state since there are both benign and malignant tumors (breast cancers). Benign breast tumors are the most common form of breast tumor. It may be reassuring to you to know that benign tumors do not transform or "turn into cancers." However, if you have *ever had* a benign tumor, you have a slightly increased risk of breast cancer *elsewhere in the same breast or the other breast* later in life. Having benign tumors surgically removed does not change this risk.

There are several categories of benign tumors. Fibroadenoma, which feels like a well-defined marble, is the most common benign tumor of the teens and twenties. It needs estrogen to grow and therefore rarely develops in postmenopausal women. In older women, this tumor can develop calcium deposits as it stops growing and eventually shrinks owing to decreasing estrogen levels. This calcification can be so characteristic that a radiologist can diagnose the fibroadenoma from the mammogram, without the need for a biopsy. In younger patients, however, calcification is uncharacteristic, so a biopsy is generally necessary for diagnosis. A lipoma is another benign tumor composed of fatty tissue. Often the same consistency as the rest of the breast, it can be difficult to detect by touch alone. This type of tumor can often be diagnosed with certainty from the mammogram because of its very low density. A duct papilloma is a benign tumor that grows within a mammary duct. Small and rarely detectable on clinical breast examination or mammography, it can produce a yellow or bloody nipple discharge. Cysts are a common occurrence, with most usually caused by the condition called dysplasia, which is described in the next section. Sebaceous cysts, which are formed from obstructed oil glands in the skin, can have different consistencies. They may feel like soft or hard small masses, are easily movable, and are located directly beneath the skin.

DOES DYSPLASIA INCREASE YOUR RISK OF CONTRACTING BREAST CANCER?

Dysplasia, a condition of abnormal cell development, is a type of benign breast disease that can only be diagnosed microscopically from a biopsy specimen. There have been many terms used by pathologists to describe dysplasia, including *fibroadenosis*, *fibrocystic disease,* and *chronic mastitis.* Pathologists find a multitude of breast cell types that do not fit clearly into the "definitely normal" and "definitely dysplasia" categories. Since such a broad range of classifications exists, the result is disagreement among experts attempting to diagnose dysplasia. When dysplasia is very pronounced, it may manifest itself through painful breasts, known medically as *mastalgia* or *mastodynia.* Keep in mind, however, that most painful breasts are not due to dysplasia, but rather to hormonal influences.

The form of dysplasia with the highest risk for malignancy, *epithelial atypical hyperplasia* (AH), is an *aberrant* overgrowth of cells lining the mammary ducts. Women with AH have a risk three or four times that of otherwise comparable women without the disease.[5,6] It is believed that before the ductal lining cells become malignant ductal carcinoma cells, they go through a stage of overgrowth *without* aberrance. Women in this stage share increased risk, but it is less than for AH. This disease stage then progresses to atypical hyperplasia, with its elevated risk for developing into cancer. Premenopausal women with AH are at greater risk than postmenopausal women with the disease.[7,8,9] From this atypical hyperplasia phase the cells can transform into true ductal cancer.

It has not been determined what causes the hyperplasia to sometimes progress to cancer, or what we can do to prevent the transformation. As we learned from the "two hit" theory in Chapter 1, it may be that the hyperplastic cells are the result of damage that occurred during an initiation phase and are only lacking the promotion phase before becoming cancer cells. Another way to look at this is that once a normal ductal cell is turned onto a malignant pathway by an initiator (the initiation phase), even normal levels of hormones can complete the cell's malignant transformation (the promotion phase). This implies that a normal amount of hormones may be sufficient to promote the malignant transformation of a dysplastic cell.[10] Whether or not this concept is accurate, and whether or not such hyperplastic cells can be considered to only represent a risk for breast cancer, the authors recommend following the guidelines in this book for preventing breast cancer. This advice cannot worsen the risks, and has a very good chance of helping.

ARE CYSTS TUMORS?

Another form of dysplasia produces the simple or solitary cyst, the most common benign breast tumor in the age group thirty-five to fifty-five. Cysts, which are more common than tumors, are fluid-filled structures that may be single or multiple. Tumors, by contrast, are filled with solid tissue. Cysts, which are similar to small "water balloons" and are surrounded by a thin membrane, may be firm or flaccid. Firm cysts can be felt if large enough, but are never as firm as fibroadenomas. A mammogram cannot identify a cyst with certainty since cysts may appear identical to solid tumors. If a mammogram reveals something that could be a cyst, an ultrasound exam can confirm the results. In fact, the major role of breast ultrasonography is to distinguish cysts from solid tumors. If the cyst is large and causing the patient anxiety or producing unpleasant symptoms, needle aspiration of the fluid contents may be performed. If it is small, no further treatment is needed.

CAN BREAST INFLAMMATION CAUSE BREAST CANCER?

Inflammation of the breasts is caused by various infectious processes. One of the most common is *postpartum mastitis*, where the mammary ducts become infected. If not properly treated, a breast abscess may occur. Breast inflammation is not believed to be a risk factor for breast cancer.

CAN BREAST INJURY CAUSE CANCER?

Trauma to the breasts can cause the development of nonmalignant tumors. Where there is internal bleeding, a pocket of blood known as a hematoma may accumulate. These will slowly disappear over months. Sometimes breast trauma can lead to injury of the fat cells, causing cell death (fat necrosis). In these cases, a lump that can be felt during a breast exam results. Fat necrosis may produce permanent hardening that can be diagnosed with mammography. Trauma does not cause breast cancer to develop. In the days when women did not routinely perform breast self-examinations, the only time they would palpate their breasts would be for several days after trauma. After initial swelling subsided, this palpation would sometimes result in the serendipitous detection of a preexisting cancer, so the women would ascribe the cancer to the trauma.

❧ Malignant Breast Tumors

Malignant breast disease, or breast cancer, can be classified in several ways. One method classifies the cancers into those of their cells of origin, such as duct, lobule, or connective tissue.

Each type of breast cancer can be examined for degree of "differentiation." In other words, how different from normal cells do the cancer cells appear? This can run the gamut from well differentiated to poorly differentiated. Well-differentiated cells appear much like the cells of origin. Poorly differentiated cells are bizarre, having few characteristics of the original normal cells. This description of tumor differentiation is referred to as tumor "grade." Low-grade malignancies are well differentiated, while high-grade indicate poor differentiation. Determination of tumor grade is meaningful since this is highly related to the degree of aggressiveness of the cancers and to patient survival—for example, high-grade cancers usually carry the worst prognoses.

CARCINOMA *IN SITU*

Ductal breast malignancies are the most common type of breast malignancy, accounting for 90 percent of all cases. Ductal cancers are divided into preinvasive (haven't yet invaded) and invasive forms. Preinvasive ductal cancer is called intraductal carcinoma *in situ* (Latin for "in position"). This is a very early stage of breast cancer, which, because of its minuteness, can never be detected on breast examination. Mammography is the *only* diagnostic method which can detect this *in situ* stage. In modern mammography centers, ductal carcinoma *in situ* (DCIS) composes 25 percent of all breast cancers detected by screening mammography.[11] In DCIS the ductal cancer cells remain within the ducts, with no sign of outside tissue invasion. Preinvasive carcinoma is generally recognized as a precursor to invasive carcinoma. If DCIS is not treated surgically, this cancer has the potential to evolve into invasive ductal carcinoma.[12] In fact, it is thought that ductal carcinoma *in situ* frequently progresses to the invasive form.[13] All invasive duct cancers began as noninvasive forms.

LOBULAR CARCINOMA *IN SITU*

Invasive lobular carcinomas are less common, accounting for less than 10 percent of all breast cancers. The invasive lobular malignancies are frequently associated with multiple similar lobular malignancies elsewhere within the same or opposite breast, and tend to be somewhat less aggressive than invasive ductal carcinomas.

Unlike invasive ductal carcinomas, it is now believed that lobular carcinoma *in situ* (LCIS) is *not* a precursor of invasive lobular carcinoma. The confusion exists because LCIS, while it has the word *carcinoma* in its name, does not behave as a cancer. It does not grow, form masses, transform into invasive cancer, or metastasize. Therefore, it does not represent a true malignancy. Also unlike DCIS, LCIS cannot be diagnosed on breast exam or mammogram. It is only diagnosed by accident when a breast biopsy is performed for another reason. What is confusing to many nonmedical people, and even to some physicians, is the consensus among most cancer specialists that an LCIS diagnosis is only an indicator of a high risk for *future* breast cancer development. Interestingly, when cancers do later develop in women who have been diagnosed with LCIS, the cancers found are both invasive ductal and invasive lobular carcinomas, with ductal predominating, and the cancers *do not occur in the site of the previous LCIS*. Also, the risk factor for subsequent development of such a breast cancer is the *same for either breast*.[14,15] Sometimes the confusion concerning the significance of LCIS by physicians has led to unwarranted recommendations, such as bilateral mastectomies. This is inappropriate treatment for the presence of a risk factor. Remember, if you are diagnosed with LCIS, this represents nothing more than discovering you have a moderate risk. In the future, the terminology for LCIS will likely be changed so as not to imply malignancy.

UNCOMMON MALIGNANT BREAST TUMORS

There are a few uncommon malignancies of the breasts. The first are connective tissue breast cancers, referred to as breast *sarcomas*. Second are metastases, malignancies that have spread to the breasts from a cancer in another part of the body. While metastasis to the body's organ systems is common in many cancers, metastatic tumors rarely develop in the breasts.

❧ Detecting Cancer During Breast Examination

A breast cancer has to reach a certain size to be discovered on breast examination. By this time, it is not an "early" tumor. A pea-size tumor has billions of cells and may have been developing for a year or more. Furthermore, such a tumor must be fairly close to the skin surface to be detected. If located deeper or surrounded by normal variations of benign breast lumps, it may go undetected. The time it takes for a growing tumor to double in diameter is called doubling time. With breast cancers this can vary from thirty to two hundred days, with an average doubling time at the low end of the range—about thirty days. It is estimated that in most instances, mammography can detect a breast cancer at least three years prior to clinical exam. Generally, a physician's clinical exam will detect breast cancers earlier than a properly performed breast self-examination, which in turn detects tumors earlier than BSE by an untrained woman. On breast examination, malignant tumors are usually firm and not well defined, meaning their surfaces do not feel smooth. Usually they are not painful or tender, but they might be. Invasive ductal carcinoma frequently causes a scarring reaction over its surface. This scarring—or fibrous—reaction can reach out like fine tentacles far beyond the tumor boundaries, pulling inward structures to which it attaches. For example, if there is invasion of the ligaments that support and lift the breasts, they are pulled inward, causing a dimpling of the skin where they attach. If mammary ducts are invaded, the nipple may be retracted. Sometimes subtle skin dimpling is not evident until the woman places her arms high over her head. This action pulls the deep portion of the breast's ligaments upward and inward, revealing slight dimpling. Your physician will perform this maneuver on clinical exam, and you should do likewise before a mirror, when you perform breast self-exam. In the later stages, the tumor can penetrate the skin or even the chest wall, becoming immovable and fixed. If untreated, such a tumor may lead to skin ulceration. If the tumor invades the lymph system of the breast, the skin of the breast becomes swollen and thickened, having the texture of an orange peel.

❧ *How Does Breast Cancer Spread?*

Breast cancer is able to metastasize to distant sites by two routes: blood vessels or lymph duct pathways. If the tumor invades the lymph ducts, it is carried to the armpit (axilla), where the collecting tumor cells are caught in the filtering action of the lymph nodes, causing the nodes to enlarge. They will feel like firm lumps. From these nodes the cancers can spread through other interconnecting lymph ducts to more distant nodes. Furthermore, some portions of the breast are connected via lymphatic ducts to nodes located under the breastbone (internal mammary nodes). If these are invaded and enlarge, they will not be detected on physical examination since they are within the chest cavity. Detection by CT (computerized tomography) or magnetic resonance imaging (MRI) is required. Through regional lymph nodes, malignant cells can move to the heart, lungs, or other parts of the body. Since the lymphatic ducts and blood vessels are interconnected, the prognosis is made worse when metastatic disease is detected in the regional lymph nodes. At this point, it can be assumed that cancer cell seeding throughout the body's organ systems has most likely already occurred. The first sign or symptom of breast cancer is rarely discovered as a result of problems in a distant organ. Metastatic breast cancers growing in the brain, liver, or bones can produce widely varied symptoms, depending upon the organ involved. For example, the spontaneous breaking of a bone may be the first evidence of breast cancer metastasized to bone.

❧ How Prognosis Is Related to the Clinical Stages of Breast Cancer

When designing methods of treatment, clinical staging is another way to compare patients. Each stage from 0 through IV represents an incremental worsening of overall prognosis (see the following staging chart, with associated average five-year survivals).[16] This is important in clinical trials because there must be the same number of women at each stage in both the experimental group and in the untreated control group. If researchers do not carefully balance the percentages at each stage, a trial's success could be incorrectly attributed to a new therapy, when in fact, the patient selection process caused the effect. In other words, the experimental group may have included patients with less advanced cancers and better prognoses. Clinical staging is determined by considering the size of the original tumor (T), the status of regional lymph nodes (N), and the existence of distant metastasis (M).[17]

TNM Criteria:
  T = primary tumor
          Tis = carcinoma *in situ*
          T1 = less than 2 centimeters (cm) in diameter
          T2 = between 2 and 5 cm
          T3 = more than 5 cm
          T4 = any size, but extends to skin or chest wall
  N = regional lymph nodes
          N0 = no regional node involvement
          N1 = metastasis to movable same side axillary nodes
          N2 = metastasis to fixed same side axillary nodes
          N3 = metastasis to same side internal mammary
                  nodes
  M = distant metastasis
          M0 = no distant metastasis
          M1 = distant metastasis

Clinical Staging:

	T	N	M	5-Year Survival
Stage 0	Tis	N0	M0	greater than 95%
Stage I	T1	N0	M0	overall = 85%
Stage II				overall = 66%
(Stage IIA)	T0	N1	M0	
	T1	N1	M0	
	T2	N0	M0	
(Stage IIB)	T2	N1	M0	
	T3	N0	M0	
Stage III				overall = 41%
(Stage IIIA)	T0	N2	M0	
	T1	N2	M0	
	T2	N2	M0	
	T3	N1,N2	M0	
(Stage IIIB)	T4	any N	M0	
	any T	N3	M0	
Stage IV	any T	any N	M1	overall = 10%

❧ Summary

The breast is a complex organ affected by the intricate inter-action of nerve pathways, the pituitary gland, and ovarian hor-mones. Its primary purpose is for infant feeding. Breast-feeding overall is beneficial to mother and child, and probably helps protect the mother from future breast cancer. Remember that many women have breasts with lumps and irregularities as nothing more than a variation of normal development and not fibrocystic "disease." Furthermore, recognize that there are many forms of benign breast disease, some of which are associ-ated with increased risk of developing breast cancer. When ed-ucating yourself about breast cancer, it is helpful to have a general knowledge of clinical staging and how it affects overall prognosis. Specifically, the lower the stage, the better the prog-nosis. Finally, you should know the signs of breast cancer de-tectable through breast examination, and learn to examine your own breasts (read Chapter 5: Breast Self-Examination).

Chapter 3

Mammography

Mammography, our best tool for early detection of breast cancer, has been fraught with controversy and misunderstanding. At the same time this technique has saved and extended the lives of thousands of women and remains the premier screening test for detecting early and potentially curable breast cancer.[1,2] Many women worry about the risks of mammography, are confused by the changing guidelines for screening, and are afraid to face the results. Our intention is to dispel the many myths, outline the mammogram's importance, recommend guidelines, and present the latest research. Welcome to the insider's guide to mammography.

&• Does Mammography Extend and Save Lives?

The initial recommendation of mammograms for screening purposes was based largely upon the results of a study conducted by the Health Insurance Plan (HIP) of Greater New York from 1963 to 1970. This study suggested that regular mammograms showed a decrease in mortality for women between the ages of forty and forty-nine, and an even greater benefit for women fifty to fifty-nine.[3] Since then there have been numerous studies supporting the benefit for women fifty to fifty-nine. However, no studies were able to confirm a corresponding benefit for the younger age group. In fact, the largest study (supported by the Canadian government) concluded that overall mortality rates were indistinguishable for women who had had mammograms and those who had not.[4]

The results of this study exploded in the media and the doubts and fears about mammography became magnified. Upon scrutiny, it was discovered in the early nineties that the Canadian study design was faulty, with ill-controlled study groups, outdated equipment, and poorly trained personnel.[5] In fact, major concerns were voiced in the early eighties by program consultants from the United States, with two well-respected advisors resigning in protest.[6] More recently, a National Cancer Institute biostatistician now supports criticism of the study, and recommends that the Canadian researchers reanalyze their preliminary results after eliminating key misleading data.[7] Unaware of these serious flaws, however, many women and health professionals took the findings to heart, and continue to do so today.

Recently, the mammography picture has begun to change. In 1993, Swedish researchers published the results of a study of 24,000 women aged forty to forty-nine which showed a 40 percent lower mortality rate from breast cancer among those who received regular mammograms. Other studies, such as the aforementioned HIP study, are beginning to show lower mortality rates on the younger study group of women as well, as these women are evaluated over a longer period. The most current conclusions are that screening mammography does extend and save lives in women forty through forty-nine.[8,9,10,11,12,13,14,15,16,17]

❧ What Is a Mammogram?

Mammograms are low-dose X-ray images of the breasts. Mammogram images show finer detail than any other imaging method found in a radiology department. Since mammograms can detect a fine grain of beach sand lying on a woman's breast, they can diagnose breast cancer at an earlier stage than any other test currently available. Of all breast cancers detected by screening mammography, 25 percent are in clinical Stage 0— the earliest stage—which has an overall five-year survival rate *greater* than 95 percent.[18,19] Because of this earlier detection and treatment, breast cancer mortality had *begun* to decline in 1991–92.[20]

❧ How Accurate Is a Mammogram?

In the best mammography centers using the most up-to-date equipment, with the best trained mammography technologists and the best radiologists interpreting the results, mammograms can detect 90 percent of breast cancers. Of the 10 percent undetected by mammography, most are obscured by dense surrounding breast tissue. Many times these "hidden" cancers can be felt by the woman or her physician, thus highlighting the importance of using mammography in conjunction with a physician's breast examination and breast self-examination.[21,22]

One key thing to remember is that despite mammogram results that come up negative, if you find a breast lump or mass you should seek further testing. In his experience as a radiologist, Dr. Vint cannot count the number of times that case histories were described to him in which women from other facilities were told by their doctor not to worry about a new lump in their breast because their mammograms were negative, only to have breast cancer diagnosed months later when the tumor had enlarged or metastasized.

ONE WOMAN'S PERSONAL EXPERIENCE

When a lump is found on breast exam in a woman over thirty-five, bilateral mammograms are required. The easiest way to explain why this is done is to provide a real-life example. Dr. Vint was called in to speak with Jenna (not her real name), a forty-five-year-old woman who had seen a surgeon about a small lump that had recently developed in her right breast. She had had a mammogram nine months before that came up normal. Her surgeon had ordered a *bilateral* mammogram study before carrying out further testing. Jenna was not sure she wanted *any* mammograms because the surgeon had to remove the lump anyway. She told Dr. Vint, the radiologist assigned to perform the mammogram, that she was even more certain she did not want the left mammogram because her problem was in the right breast and she had had recent mammograms less than a year earlier. Dr. Vint explained to Jenna the necessity for studying both breasts. Once she understood the reasons, she readily agreed. She was fortunate to have changed her mind. Jenna's right mammogram showed the breast lump to be a benign tumor, but the *left* mammogram demonstrated an early cancer that had not been present on the last mammogram.

There are many reasons to have mammograms when there is a palpable mass. Sometimes a mammogram shows the palpable mass to have specific characteristics of a 100 percent certain benign finding, which can be safely left alone. Other times it shows not only the mass that was felt, but also satellite masses or abnormalities separate from the original mass, or even, as in Jenna's case, cancers in the other breast that were not palpable.

❧ *The Risks of Mammography*

Is there anything in life free from risk? Probably not. Everything in life has certain benefit-to-risk ratios, from driving your car to getting out of bed in the morning. If benefits of an activity clearly go beyond risks, then this is acceptable and desirable. This is how we should look at mammography screening of women over thirty-nine.

How do we know the risks of mammography radiation of breast tissue? There has never been a scientific study of the effects of low-dose radiation on women's breasts and perhaps there never will be. To establish a study that would be considered "gold standard" (randomized, prospective) would require two groups of 10 million women each, and would take ten to twenty years to complete. The first group would receive annual screening mammography; the second group would not. Such a study, denying screening to 10 million women, could certainly present ethical and moral problems.

When conditions do not permit prospective studies, scientists will use retrospective, or past, experiences. All documented past exposures of human breasts to significant radiation (such as the atomic bomb) over the past fifty years have been examined in detail. Although no exposures studied were comparable to low-dose mammography, we learned that high-dose radiation can cause breast cancer and that breast tissue's sensitivity to radiation varies with a woman's age.

THE SENSITIVE YEARS

It takes from ten to twenty years for breast cancer to develop after exposure to radiation. Women are most sensitive to radiation exposure in adolescence, when the breast tissue is actively developing. This sensitivity begins to drop after maturity in the twenties and continues to drop to very low levels in the forties and beyond. It is postulated that this drop-off in radiation-induced breast cancer occurs because only actively growing glandular breast tissue is truly sensitive to radiation. As women mature, active glandular tissue begins to regress, becoming atrophic, and is eventually replaced by relatively radiation-insensitive fibrous, fatty, and connective tissues. Fortunately, the incidence of breast cancer in women under age forty is not common. This presents the ideal situation for mammography because in women forty years and older, sensitivity is low and breast cancers are more frequent. In other words, the benefits are great and the risks are low.

• *Benefits versus risks*

It has been estimated that the theoretical risk of screening one million forty-five-year-old women would be five unnecessary breast cancer deaths. This risk is equal to that of traveling 5,000 miles by plane or 450 miles by car, smoking three cigarettes, or simply being alive for fifteen minutes at age sixty. The benefits of screening these one million women would be 150 to 450 breast cancer deaths averted.[23,24,25] The risk of screening mammography seems small compared to the potential estimated number of lives saved.

Modern mammograms are safe. Radiation doses are much lower today than they were just ten years ago, and cancer detection is much enhanced.[26,27] Furthermore, personnel are better trained and radiologists more skilled in diagnosing early breast cancer than they were just a few short years ago.

ᴥ What Age to Start and How Often?/Should I Have a Mammogram?

There is some controversy concerning the age at which a woman should begin mammography and the frequency of the procedure.[28] For the last decade the recommendations from the American Cancer Society, the American College of Radiology, the American College of Obstetrics and Gynecology, the American Medical Women's Association, and fifteen other major health organizations have recommended and continue to recommend the following: for ages forty to forty-nine, mammograms once each year or once every two years, depending upon risk for breast cancer; and for ages fifty and over, mammograms once each year.[29,30,31]

Although the National Cancer Institute (NCI) originally agreed with these recommendations, it recently changed its policy on screening for women under fifty years of age, now recommending no screening whatsoever for this age group. This decision was based upon their review of several large-scale mammogram studies that showed no significant increase in lives saved when screening mammograms were performed on women forty to forty-nine years of age.[32,33,34,35,36] However, as previously mentioned, the studies of this age group contained significant experimental design flaws that invalidate their conclusions.[37,38,39,40,41,42,43,44,45]

THE NCI CONTROVERSY

Opponents of the NCI's decision to drop their recommendations for women under age fifty point out the power of economics to dictate policy. Basically, policymakers decided that mammography for this age group costs too much in relation to the number of cancer cases detected. They simply declared the technique ineffectual for these women, despite the fact that the NCI's National Cancer Advisory Board voted fourteen to one against dropping the recommendation.[46]

This opposition of opinions created enormous upheaval and confusion for this group of women who have relied upon mammography for peace of mind. In response to the controversy, a 1994 congressional report criticized the NCI for using a highly "flawed process" to determine its dropping of screening recommendations for women in their forties. The report, *Misused Science: The National Cancer Institute's Elimination of Mammography Guidelines for Women in Their Forties*, claims that the NCI's decision-making meetings were not scientifically run, and the NCI's scientific review of the data on mammography was inadequate. The report notes that NCI chose leaders for these meetings who were "known critics of mammography screening for women in their forties," the NCI "excluded the presentation of favorable information on mammography screening...," and "NCI failed to examine objectively all the scientific evidence on mammography." The report recommends the NCI revise its mammography statement to reflect a more balanced presentation of the evidence.[47]

WHAT IS THE IMPACT ON WOMEN IN THEIR FORTIES?

Women in this age group, while at slightly less risk than women in their fifties and sixties, generally develop cancers that are faster growing and more deadly. In addition, yearly mammograms detect faster-growing tumors when they are smaller. Biennial testing—or none at all—is a greater risk.[48] So in essence, following NCI's guidelines places a very vulnerable group of women at extreme risk.

In the United States, about 16 percent of all breast cancers will occur in women in their forties (compared with 17 percent of all breast cancers occurring in women in their fifties), but nearly 25 percent of all deaths from breast cancer occur in women in whom the cancer was diagnosed while in their forties.[49] You may recall that breast cancer is the number-one cause of death in this age group. To really bring this into focus, since this age group has a longer life expectancy than older groups, the breast cancer deaths in this group account for 41 percent of all years lost due to breast cancer.[50] We urge you to take action on this issue. If the NCI has not changed their recommendations, call and write your elected representatives in Washington, demanding their support. It's your life at stake.

OUR RECOMMENDATION FOR WOMEN IN THEIR FORTIES

Let's not gamble with the lives of this large group of women. Until a properly designed clinical trial studying women in their forties demonstrates that mammography offers *no* value, we, as do others, continue to recommend *annual* screening mammograms for *all* women over the age of thirty-nine.[51,52] Some guidelines recommend mammograms every other year for women of this age who do not have a high risk for breast cancer. Our reply is, "Show me a woman with *proven* low risk."

Since 85 percent of women who develop breast cancer have none of the traditional risk factors, we believe that no woman can be positively identified as "low-risk." Statistics back up this recommendation because if the data supporting the screening of all women aged forty to forty-nine are not acceptable to the NCI, there are *no* data that show that screening high-risk women will decrease mortality. Screening only high-risk women will not benefit the vast majority of women who develop breast cancer because the vast majority of women with breast cancer do not exhibit risk factors.[53,54]

❧ Selecting a Mammography Facility

Today the task of finding a high-quality mammography center is much easier than it was just a few years ago. In late 1994 the Mammography Quality Standards Act (MQSA) went into effect. To be in business, all mammography facilities must meet federal standards of quality, including for equipment, technologists, and radiologists. It is illegal to perform mammography without certification by the Food and Drug Administration (FDA). The FDA will choose qualified nonfederal agencies to certify the thousands of facilities.[55] One of the first agencies chosen for this task was the American College of Radiology (ACR). For the past decade it has been the only organization to set up a voluntary, but entirely thorough program of mammography accreditation. When you have your mammogram, ask to see the FDA certificate.[56,57,58]

❧ Selecting a Radiologist

The radiologist is the key to a good mammogram. Some highly respected radiologists have stated that mammograms may indeed be the most difficult X-ray examinations to interpret. Unlike a chest X-ray, which shows standard anatomy (lungs, heart, blood vessels, and bones), the mammogram reveals no consistent anatomic features. In fact, no two women have the same mammogram pattern. The nonspecific appearance of some findings adds to the difficulty of interpretation. This means that a significant number of benign and malignant "findings" (abnormal features) are not distinguishable from one another. Dr. Vint, the radiologist on our team, found that it took years of reading thousands of mammograms, as well as many textbooks, and attending dozens of conferences before he considered himself a specialist. Remember, you should always ask to have your mammograms interpreted by the radiology department's mammography specialist.

Radiologists who perform mammography as their specialty usually keep extensive records on their readings. These allow an evaluation of interpretation quality, and comparison to those of other practices. FDA certification will require such documentation of findings in the future.

CONSULTING YOUR RADIOLOGIST

Radiologists are busy physicians; however, if you have questions about your mammograms and would feel more assured discussing your study directly with the radiologist who read it, make a separate appointment at no charge. On many occasions, Dr. Vint has sat down with a patient at the view box to explain the positive or negative findings to her. It should be considered an inclusive service to provide this individual attention.

If there are suspicious findings on the mammogram, the woman may wish to have another radiologist in the mammography facility reread her study to verify the original conclusions. If a biopsy is recommended, you may wish to take your mammograms to a radiologist at another center for a second opinion. Expect to receive a bill from this radiologist for a second interpretation; however, many medical insurance companies will pay for these second opinions. Ask for the radiologist specializing in mammography.[59]

❧ *The Mammogram Procedure*

WHEN ARE SCREENING MAMMOGRAMS USED?

There are generally two reasons for having a mammogram: for screening and for diagnostic purposes. It is important to make the distinction because this can be one of the most confusing problems for patients and ordering physicians. Screening mammograms are performed to detect possible early stage tumors that cannot be felt on breast exam (nonpalpable tumors). Screening studies are not performed on women with symptomatic breasts or when there are suspicious findings on breast exam. *If a woman or her physician is aware of a mass, lump, skin changes, nipple discharge, etc., she should have a diagnostic mammogram.* Increasingly, at more facilities, the fees for screening mammograms have been reduced in keeping with our national goal of screening all eligible women in a cost-efficient manner. (A diagnostic study requires more attention and time, thus costing more than a screening study.) Screening mammograms include a minimum of two views of the breasts: a vertical view and an angled side view. These two views are necessary to produce a complete exam, displaying all regions of the breasts.

With screening mammograms, it is not necessary for a radiologist to be on-site or to view the mammograms until later in the day or perhaps the next day. This helps keep screening costs down. The radiology report should be available within twenty-four hours. If you have not received a phone report within this time, call the doctor.

WHEN ARE DIAGNOSTIC MAMMOGRAMS USED?

Diagnostic mammograms require the standard two views per breast, plus any other *additional views* determined to be necessary. The radiologist must thoroughly evaluate the breast region in question. Many times women with breast findings on clinical exam are incorrectly scheduled for screening mammography. This is not appropriate and will necessitate return visits by the patient to complete the exam. If you have localized symptoms or have a physical finding on examination by your doctor, please be sure you receive a diagnostic mammogram. During a diagnostic mammogram the radiologist may wish to perform a clinical breast exam of the area in question to correlate with the imaging study. You should have the option to discuss the findings with this radiologist the same day. Some primary physicians prefer to communicate results to their patients rather than allow the radiologist to do so. If you would rather speak directly with the radiologist, however, simply explain this to your primary physician when the exam is ordered.

❧ Why Is Breast Compression Important?

The goal of mammography is to provide the highest quality image using the lowest radiation dose. Vigorous breast compression is a vital and necessary part of a complete mammogram, but an often-discussed topic among women because of the pain it can produce. Proper breast compression is responsible for some of the largest gains in mammography benefits over the last decade. It is worthwhile, then, to go into a little detail regarding breast compression during mammography.

A compressed breast requires a lower dose of radiation because the X-rays need to penetrate less breast tissue. A compressed breast is less likely to move or shift positions, reducing the need for repeat exposures. Sometimes the beating heart of an anxious woman is enough to cause motion in the overlying breast. In the "older days" of mammography, before adequate compression became universal, a radiologist could often see that the deep tissues of the left breast were slightly blurred because the heart was only an inch or so away. Compression improves image quality, allowing sharp unblurred images and, most importantly, spreading out the overlapping breast tissue, which provides for better detection of breast cancer.

How is a breast compressed? It is gently but firmly squeezed between two flat plastic surfaces by the mammography technologist. Women differ in the degree of compression they will allow, depending upon the breast tissue characteristics and sensitivity and individual pain thresholds. Women with firmer, less fatty breasts will allow less compression, as will women with tender breasts. There is no predetermined degree of compression with a mammogram, but generally, the more compression the better. Dr. Vint would tell patients a comfortable mammogram is one that has been performed poorly. The compression should be uncomfortable, but not too painful. An informed, less anxious woman will generally experience less pain; however, some will have a painful experience regardless.[60,61,62] If your breasts are very tender at certain times during your menstrual cycle, avoid scheduling your mammograms then. It is a good rule to always schedule your yearly screening mammograms at the same time in your menstrual cycle. Occasionally, a woman with very sensitive breasts will have some degree of pain following the mammogram for a week or more. If you have sensitive breasts, inform your doctor and be aware that some discomfort is normal.

Remember, you are in control of your compression. During the exam the technologist will ask you to tell her the instant the compression is too firm. Only by offering such careful feedback can you ensure an optimal mammogram. In most cases, if you are more informed, you will have less fear of the procedure and will allow more compression. Depending on the mammography equipment available to you, you might even be able to control your compression with a remote switch.

ॐ When the Radiologist Finds Something Suspicious

What if the radiologist sees something that appears abnormal on the mammogram and recommends another test? This is quite common, occurring in about 15 percent of screening mammograms. Frequently this requires that an additional view or views be obtained, employing special techniques such as "spot compression" or magnification. These techniques involve only a portion of the breast, which allows further clarification of the area in question. If you are asked to return for some additional views, don't panic. Some women, after receiving notice that they were to return for repeat views, were so distressed that they couldn't go to work or sleep at night. It is important to remember that these "callbacks" are common, even in good facilities. In 90 percent of such instances, the original findings were benign and simply not clear as a result of overlying normal breast tissue.[63]

﹖ *What Do Radiologists Look for on a Mammogram?*

Initially, the radiologist makes certain that the mammogram technologist includes the entire breast region, that the film exposure is correct, the compression is adequate, and the image is sharp. The labeling of the woman's name, her patient number, which breast, and the exact mammogram view is checked for completeness. Next, the radiologist looks at the skin, nipple, internal breast structure, and axilla (part of the breast that extends toward the armpit). These areas are examined in two views. An important evaluation of mammogram pattern symmetry is made because some malignancies may be identified not as discrete masses, but as regions of subtle asymmetry. This is difficult to determine in many instances, as all women have some degree of mammogram asymmetry. After this initial examination, the radiologist's hunt for cancer is performed with a magnifying glass.

On mammograms, breast cancers are detected by very tiny calcifications (tiny deposits of calcium crystals the size of grains of sand), masses or lumps of all sizes, or a combination of both. Benign findings include calcifications and masses as well, some readily apparent as benign, some not easily distinguished from malignant, and some identical to malignant. Masses are examined for size, shape, texture, uniformity, contour of borders, and possible internal calcifications. A true mass, as compared to a "constructed" mass (an effect produced by overlying normal breast tissue), should be seen on both views of the breast. Calcifications are examined for number, size, shape, pattern, arrangement, density, closeness to each other, and variation from one another. If an abnormality is seen on the original mammogram, additional views will be necessary to better classify the probability of malignancy. Using all these criteria, the experienced radiologist will fairly accurately classify findings as having high, intermediate, or low probability for malignancy. In radiology terminology, any focal abnormality is called a lesion, which may be benign or malignant. If a lesion with low probability is diagnosed, no further testing or biopsies are needed, perhaps only a follow-up by mammography. If intermediate or high probability is diagnosed by the radiologist, a biopsy is required.

The primary goal of modern screening mammography is detection of cancers in their earliest stages. Our accuracy continues to improve. Thirty years ago the best screening mammography centers detected 35 percent of cancers as Stages II to IV. Currently, mammography facilities detect only 22 percent of cancers in these later stages.[64] This means that, when properly used, mammography will detect 78 percent of all breast cancers in Stages 0 and I! These are the potentially curable stages.

❧ The Importance of Prior Mammograms

When having your mammogram, it is essential to have your prior mammograms available to the radiologist. A prior mammogram, especially several exams dating back three to five years, will provide a higher level of confidence in the current interpretation. There are numerous times in which obtaining prior studies precluded the need for additional views, follow-up mammograms, or surgery, especially because a woman's personal breast pattern remains relatively constant during middle age to later life. While some suspicious patterns or findings would require follow-ups or perhaps biopsy, the presence of unchanging findings on prior mammograms can give assurance of no malignancy.[65] By law, a mammogram facility must retain all prior mammograms on that patient and have these readily available for comparison at the time of the reading. However, if your previous mammograms were performed at another facility, it is essential that you personally obtain these studies and bring them with you when you have your exam. Mailing mammograms from one facility to another is the next best option, but delays can occur, and studies are occasionally lost.

KEEPING YOUR MAMMOGRAMS AT HOME

If you tend to move frequently, it may be advantageous for you to keep all of your mammograms at home. Some facilities require the permission of your personal physician before you are allowed to take possession of your mammograms. This is due to the facility's legal responsibilities for keeping and protecting the studies. When you pay for a mammogram exam, you are legally entitled to a report of the radiologist's interpretation, not possession of the actual films. Do not accept copies of mammograms, as it is not technically feasible to make acceptable duplicates. It is, indeed, preferable for a woman to retain all her mammograms since she has the greatest interest in preserving these vital records. But with possession comes responsibility. If you fear their being misplaced or lost in a fire or similar disaster, keep them at your mammogram facility.

✿ What Other Breast-Imaging Techniques Are Available?

Other currently available breast-imaging techniques do not have the diagnostic accuracy to detect a high percentage of breast cancers and do not replace the need for mammography. They may be thought of as tests to complement a proper screening mammogram. Breast ultrasound has been found most useful in determining cystic (fluid-filled) structures. Breast CT (computerized tomography, or CAT scan) is expensive, involves high radiation dose, and is not appropriate for screening. Breast MRI (magnetic resonance imaging) is also expensive and not appropriate for screening; however, it is the method of choice for detecting small leaks in silicone gel breast implants.[66,67] (See Chapter 21: Breast Implants.) Breast thermography, which measures heat patterns emanating from the breasts, should not be used for screening. Finally, breast diaphanography, which measures light transmitted through the breast, should also not be used for screening.

❧ Summary

Despite the confusion and controversy over screening mammography, certain facts stand out. Modern low-dose mammography detects breast cancer before it can be felt and at an earlier, more curable stage. It has an excellent benefit-to-risk ratio in all women over forty. The current emphasis on breast-conserving surgery would not be possible without screening mammography and its ability to detect early disease. For the reasons documented in this chapter, we will continue to recommend annual screening mammography for all women forty years of age and older. Screening mammograms remain a vital part of each woman's health program, in addition to following the suggestion for altering lifestyle, diet, exercise, and dietary supplements that are described throughout this book.

Chapter 4

New Biopsy Options

You have been told you need a breast biopsy. You are filled with terror and anxiety, dreading the discovery of a cancer, but also fearful of a disfigured, scarred breast. You are not alone, for approximately 850,000 women had breast biopsies in 1994. What are your biopsy options? What are the nonsurgical alternatives to surgical biopsy and the advantages these newer techniques provide to you? In this chapter you will learn more about these proven, widely available, but underused techniques.

A SURGICAL SCAR: ONE WOMAN'S PERSONAL STORY

Beyond cosmetic concerns, most people wouldn't expect a surgical scar to have much impact upon a woman's life. Surgical biopsies not only leave a visible scar on the skin, but more importantly, they also leave a scar in the breast tissue. The result is that these internal surgical scars may mimic certain forms of breast cancer on mammograms and clinical exam. Some years ago Dr. Vint was asked to consult on the case of Kate (not her real name), a woman in her forties who had had a previous surgical biopsy five years earlier. He reviewed Kate's yearly mammograms dating back over the past seven years. It was Dr. Vint's opinion, after reviewing her pre- and postoperative mammograms and understanding exactly in which region of the breast the previous biopsy had taken place, that the finding, despite having an appearance of a cancer, represented only scar tissue. He advised her physicians of his interpretation. Kate chose to go to another facility, where a surgeon told her that, in his opinion, this was a cancer, and that she would die from the disease if she did not agree to surgical removal. Fearfully, she agreed to the surgery. Unfortunately, the surgeon felt the need to remove a major portion of her breast along with the "abnormality," since he believed that he was performing cancer surgery. However, the pathology report showed only old scar tissue, with no evidence of cancer. Kate was left with a deformed, asymmetric breast. She felt devastated.

Wouldn't it be a great advantage to women it there were a nonsurgical method to obtain a biopsy—a method that offered surgery's accuracy but would not leave scars. As we learned with Kate's experience, the benefits of leaving no internal scar cannot be emphasized too greatly. If this hypothetical technique were less expensive, easier for the patient, took less time, was safer, allowed immediate return to work after the procedure, and did not involve months of postoperative breast pain and discomfort, it would be in great demand. This ideal nonsurgical procedure can be found throughout the United States today, but only a small percentage of breast biopsies are performed using this technique, largely because of physician bias. Many, including the authors, feel it is the biopsy method of choice. Let's find out what it is.

✤ Breast Biopsies

Breast biopsies are performed for two reasons: either there is an abnormality on a clinical exam, or there is an abnormality on a mammogram exam. Traditionally, surgeons performed surgical biopsies in both situations. In the past decade several nonsurgical techniques for performing a diagnostic biopsy have been developed using special needles. It is important to understand who performs the biopsy and how the needles are used. We will discuss both biopsies of palpable and nonpalpable abnormalities.

✤ When You Feel a Breast Mass: Your Biopsy Options

NEEDLE BIOPSIES: FNA VERSUS CORE

Sometimes a distinct mass or new thickening is detected during physician breast examination that may or may not be visible on the mammogram. In previous years many women of all ages ended up in the operating room, where a portion of their breast was removed to diagnose a suspicious mass (surgical biopsy). Currently, the nonsurgical diagnostic methods of choice in such cases are fine needle aspiration (FNA) and gun core biopsy. These two different needle biopsy techniques are performed by many general surgeons as office procedures using local anesthetic. In the FNA technique, the physician inserts a very thin, hollow needle into the palpable mass and aspirates (withdraws cells by means of suction), using a syringe. This is done a half dozen or so times to ensure that enough cells are obtained. These cells are immediately examined microscopically by a specially trained pathologist, called a cytopathologist, and a determination is made as to whether the cells are benign or malignant.[1]

With gun core biopsy, a special high-speed gun device holds a somewhat larger hollow needle. Just as with an ear-piercing gun, the speed of the needle produces only minimal discomfort. Instead of separated and scattered individual cells produced by the FNA technique, a thin, delicate core of tissue about the size of the lead in a mechanical pencil is obtained. This is sent to the pathology lab, where standard biopsy specimen techniques are always available.

The FNA technique obtains a diagnosis more quickly, but requires the availability of a subspecializing cytopathologist (there may be none on staff), does not give a specific type of benign or malignant diagnosis, and frequently does not obtain adequate breast material with which to make a diagnosis. The core technique has no more complications than the FNA technique, is no more uncomfortable for the patient, and consistently produces adequate tissue for diagnosing the specific type of benign or malignant tumor. In addition, only core needle biopsies can determine whether or not the malignancy is invasive. Surgical pathologists, present at all medical centers, are well trained to interpret core biopsies. By contrast, cytopathologists are unavailable in many parts of the country. With either type of needle biopsy, if adequate biopsy material is obtained, the patient will not need a diagnostic open surgical biopsy.

If you have a palpable breast mass and your breast physician or surgeon does not perform needle biopsies, then seek a second physician who is comfortable with these techniques. Given the choice for biopsies of palpable masses, either technique is adequate, but the core technique is preferable. The surgeon will choose the method he or she has had the most experience performing. In the next section we will see why the core technique is recommended for nonpalpable abnormalities. If, after the needle biopsy, the pathology report shows a malignancy, then lumpectomy, or surgical removal of the mass, is required—or less likely—a mastectomy, or removal of the breast.[2,3]

WHY MAMMOGRAMS ARE NOT RECOMMENDED FOR WOMEN UNDER FORTY

A young woman in her teens or twenties who finds a mass or thickening should not have a mammogram as the first diagnostic study. Since young breast tissue is sensitive to radiation and cancers are rare in women of that age, the first step should be referral to a breast surgeon for a thorough breast exam. At this stage of the evaluation, breast ultrasound may also be of value, although optional. If the breast surgeon believes the physical finding to be significant, step two should be needle biopsy. In most cases a surgical biopsy should not be the second step. If your breast surgeon does not perform needle biopsies (FNA or core) on palpable abnormalities, get another surgeon. Only when the biopsy shows malignancy should mammography and lumpectomy be performed.

﹏ The Mammogram Abnormality—Is It Real?

Many times a radiologist will recommend a biopsy of a mammogram abnormality that is not palpable. Most of the mammographic abnormalities requiring biopsy are too small to be palpable; therefore, the needle biopsy of a palpable mass described earlier cannot be used. Should you find yourself in this situation, you have several options. First, make sure the abnormality is "real." It should be shown to be a genuine finding, not just superimposition of normal breast structures causing an apparent abnormal density. Additional views of the abnormality will help distinguish this possibility. Again, make sure you have consulted with the radiologist who read your mammograms to discuss the findings. Ask the following questions: Are additional views needed to confirm suspicions? What is the quality of the mammogram study? How sure are you of your classification of the finding? When confronted with similar findings, what percentages of the abnormalities turn out to be malignant after biopsy? If you feel any doubt about any responses, make that second opinion appointment with another radiologist.

❧ *It's Real, You Can't Feel It—What Are Your Biopsy Options?*

The good news is that most of these abnormalities are benign, but a biopsy is needed to confirm this. After your need for a biopsy is established, there are important alternatives to consider. You may be sent to a surgeon for an open surgical biopsy. This technique has been the "gold standard" for decades but is rapidly being replaced in many parts of the United States and Europe with a newer nonsurgical technique performed by a radiologist. Since approximately 75 to 90 percent of these abnormalities that require biopsy are later proven to be benign, this nonsurgical technique is logical. In the case of a benign mammogram finding, the patient does not need to have the abnormality removed; she can just leave it alone. Once diagnosed as benign, these abnormalities will be continually monitored on subsequent screening mammograms. Keep in mind that if you have ever had a benign breast tumor, you will have a slightly increased risk for later development of breast cancer in either breast. The condition that causes the risk is that breasts with benign tumors contain cells that are more prone to divide and multiply. Despite what you may have heard, benign tumors do not become malignant tumors. A breast cancer begins its life as a single cell or a tiny group of malignant cells that continue to grow and divide until a tumor is produced. These malignant tumors are not created from benign tumors.

WHAT IS STEREOTACTIC NEEDLE BIOPSY AND WHY SHOULD YOU CHOOSE IT?

This newer, nonsurgical type of breast biopsy is called stereotactic needle biopsy. As with needle biopsies performed by general surgeons, it can be performed using FNA or core gun techniques. The FNA is the older method, but, as previously mentioned, the more advantageous core procedure is rapidly becoming the acknowledged standard. It has been proven successful in more than 10,000 women. Unlike core biopsies performed by surgeons on palpable masses, stereotactic needle biopsy uses a unique type of mammographic equipment designed only for breast biopsies. The woman lies facedown on a padded table, with the breast in question extending through an opening. Below the table is a special mammogram unit that is capable of taking stereo mammographic views of the breast. This procedure requires multiple stereo views, hence the term *stereotactic*. Using a special computer, the radiologist views the two stereo images of the breasts to determine the exact three-dimensional coordinates of the abnormality's location. A core needle biopsy is then performed by a biopsy gun mounted in a calibrated holder. Unlike most surgical breast biopsies, this nonsurgical biopsy does not even require sedation. Local anesthesia is used, similar to that used in dentistry and other forms of needle biopsy of the breast. This technique, which has a very high rate of diagnostic accuracy (equal to that of surgical biopsy), can locate and biopsy abnormalities much smaller than a pea deep inside the breast. This procedure can be done even when implants are present.[4] The stereotactic core technique takes approximately forty-five minutes to an hour, and the patient is able to return to work that day, if she desires. She will have a small dressing over the puncture site, which can be removed in a day or so. There is no painful recuperation period. The puncture site in the skin heals completely, leaving no trace after a month. And after healing over the first month, the mammogram shows no evidence of internal scarring.

COMPLICATIONS AND ACCURACY

Stereotactic biopsy is a relatively new method of accurately determining the exact nature of very small, nonpalpable breast tumors. The development of the special equipment, allowing precision stereo views, allows either needle biopsy technique to enjoy a high rate of accuracy. At Scripps Clinic in La Jolla, California, more than nine hundred stereotactic core biopsies have been performed with excellent results and no complications. Side effects are minor, almost nonexistent.

Some critics state that theoretically, cancer cells could be spread into normal breast tissue as the needle is withdrawn from a cancerous tumor. Conceivably, this is true; however, women in whom malignancies are found using nonsurgical biopsies would eventually undergo lumpectomy, followed by radiation therapy (XRT). XRT would kill any scattered cancer cells that had been inadvertently spread throughout the normal tissue. Those few women who choose mastectomy, which is not followed by XRT, would have these cells eliminated with surgical removal of the breast.

HOW IS ULTRASOUND USED FOR NEEDLE BIOPSIES?

Some facilities use ultrasound guidance to perform the core biopsy of a nonpalpable abnormality, instead of guidance by the stereotactic mammogram unit.[5] The accuracy of the ultrasound technique is comparable to that of the stereotactic core biopsies. If the abnormality can be well seen with ultrasound, then ultrasound imaging—not stereotactic technique—is used to guide the gun core biopsy. However, if the abnormality cannot be well viewed by ultrasound, the stereotactic mammogram unit is used. An advantage of ultrasound is that it takes less time. In some centers, up to half of all core biopsies are performed using ultrasound guidance.

HOW MUCH DOES BIOPSY COST?

Although the cost of the stereotactic biopsy varies from one part of the country to another, its cost is approximately one-third of the total cost of a surgical biopsy. Of course, your breast surgeon may not give you the option of a stereotactic core biopsy. Regardless of what biopsy method is recommended, remember that a breast surgeon cannot perform a needle biopsy of a nonpalpable mammogram abnormality in his office because he or she needs to clearly feel the structure before using such a procedure.

YOU NEED A BIOPSY BUT DON'T HAVE A PROPER FACILITY IN YOUR AREA

If there are no centers in your county using stereotactic needle biopsy, and if you have a nonpalpable mammographic abnormality for which biopsy is recommended, ask your physician for the nearest locations outside your area. It would be worthwhile to travel to a major center that has significant experience in this state-of-the-art technique.

HOW DO GENERAL SURGEONS FEEL ABOUT THIS PROCEDURE?

Currently, there are few valid reasons for a surgeon to perform a diagnostic surgical biopsy for a small nonpalpable mammographic abnormality when the nonsurgical biopsy is available. Many breast surgeons, trained in the older surgical biopsy technique, do not have much experience (or confidence) in sending patients to radiologists for nonsurgical biopsies, and therefore tend to be prejudiced against the newer procedure. Another possible reason for a bias against the nonsurgical technique is economic. Surgeons who refer numerous breast biopsy procedures to radiologists may be doing women a favor, but they are doing little for their revenues. Obviously, a patient's well-being should come before a physician's financial concerns. You have a basic right to have all of your options explained to you without bias.

THE IMPACT OF NONSURGICAL BIOPSY ON THE COST TO SOCIETY

Even if we disregard, for the moment, the many important advantages for women of nonsurgical gun core biopsies of the breast, the impact of this technique on lowering our nation's medical expenses would be immense. As more and more women observe recommendations for screening mammograms, more women will have suspicious findings—which require biopsies—diagnosed. As you may recall, in 1994 approximately 850,000 breast biopsies were performed, and this trend will only continue upward. It has been said that the major cost to our society for providing screening mammography is not the actual cost of performing and interpreting the mammograms, but the cost of the surgical breast biopsies generated by abnormal mammogram reports. While the total cost of surgical breast biopsy varies throughout the nation and even within cities, it probably averages about $1,500 to $3,000, whereas stereotactic core biopsy averages $750 to $1,200. If all 850,000 women had had surgical biopsies, this would have cost our health-care system $1.275 to $2.5 billion. If all these women had had the nonsurgical biopsies, the total cost would have been under $800 million, a savings of at least 53 percent.

✿ Summary

One of this book's purposes is to let women know their options so they will take a proactive role in practicing and maintaining their health. If biopsy is recommended, don't let the biopsy method be chosen for you. Be informed about the nonsurgical methods of biopsy and discuss them with your physician. Challenge him or her with the facts (including medical references) in this chapter. If your doctor insists on a surgical biopsy, get a second opinion.

Chapter 5

Breast Self-Examination

"Early detection is your best protection," we have heard again and again as an argument for performing breast self-examination (BSE) once a month for our entire adult lives. Silently we resist, not fully understanding why we don't consistently embrace this potentially lifesaving technique. Do we not like to touch ourselves? Are we afraid of what we might find? Is it possible we don't really know what we are looking for? Maybe we cannot fathom the possibility that we may be at risk for breast cancer. Or perhaps we don't really believe breast self-exam will do any good.

Unfortunately, BSE is a practice that by its very nature seeks disease. If the purpose of BSE is to look for cancer, it is no wonder that less than 50 percent of all American women regularly practice BSE, although over 95 percent are aware of the recommendations to do so.[1]

We would like to suggest another way to think about this

critical issue. We propose considering BSE as a fundamentally important health practice, one that allows you to know your body better, to know yourself better, and ultimately, to enhance the sense that you have a measure of control in your health and life. Let's examine our attitudes and the issues surrounding BSE in the hope we may begin to generate a new perspective and stimulate a greater desire to give ourselves the consistent attention and care we deserve.

❧ Is Breast Self-Examination Necessary?

The recommendation for breast self-examination is based on the assumptions that it is a technique available to all women and that early detection leads to greater survival.[2,3] There are many good reasons to practice BSE, which we will discuss throughout the chapter, but first let's focus on why it is a necessary technique.

You may recall our earlier discussion on the breast cancer epidemic that we all face. The incidence of breast cancer has risen 250 percent in the last thirty years, and despite a twenty-year "war on cancer," the mortality rate has not changed in the last fifty years. As early as 1964, the World Health Organization concluded that 80 percent of cancers were due to human-produced carcinogens, and in 1979 the National Institutes of Health identified environmental factors as the major cause of most cancer. Despite this information a minute fraction of all cancer research has focused on prevention.[4]

The reality of the situation is that the United States remains diagnosis- and treatment-oriented. In the hundreds of scientific papers on BSE that we have reviewed, over and over we have encountered statements such as "Since there is no practical method of primary prevention of breast cancer immediately available at the present, screening resulting in the diagnosis and treatment of breast cancer at an early stage seems to be a rational approach to reducing mortality from this common tumour."[5] While we hope to convince you that there are many effective preventive measures available, the fact remains that the earlier you can detect a cancerous lump and the less nodal involvement there is, the greater your survival rate and the less severe your treatment options. Being aware of any breast changes on a monthly basis can assist you in early detection.

Furthering the case for BSE, recall that breast cancer is now the leading cause of death for all women between the ages of thirty-five and fifty-four, and the leading cause of cancer death for all African-American women. Furthermore, it is the leading site of cancer incidence and cancer mortality for women between the ages of fifteen and fifty-four.[6] Mammography, the most effective method of early detection, is not recommended for women under forty, is being debated for women forty to forty-nine, and is still largely unavailable to minority or lower socioeconomic status women. A high percentage of certain groups of women, especially the elderly and minorities, never receive referrals from their physicians for a mammogram.[7] Moreover, mammography does not detect 10 percent of all tumors and may miss even a greater percentage in younger women. In light of these conditions, BSE becomes a very important aspect of early detection.

Clinical breast exam (CBE), an important player in early detection, has its own limitations. Published guidelines recommend breast examination by a physician once a year. A tumor, particularly one that is more aggressive, not estrogen dependent, and often develops in premenopausal women, can become palpable in much less than a year. Relying on CBE alone can leave you largely unprotected.

Studies indicate that most physicians are not well trained in CBE and have limited experience with palpation of the breast.[8] One study found that physicians were much more successful in their detection techniques when they took adequate time for the procedure. Unfortunately, the actual average exam time is very short, only 1.8 minutes per breast in a normal screening procedure. In the same study, while physicians were able to detect 87 percent of the tumors one centimeter or larger, the percentage of detectable tumors under one centimeter dropped to 23.5 percent.[9,10] The point here is not to evaluate physician competence based on a couple of studies, but to recognize that a clinical exam is only one piece of the equation in maintaining your breast health, and that your own personal examinations are critical to fill in the previously mentioned detection gaps.

One of the most convincing arguments for the use of BSE is the fact that many women find their own tumors, usually accidentally rather than during purposeful breast self-examination. Statistics also show that 50 percent of all cancers found have already metastasized. This means we are not finding them early enough.[11]

This is a sobering string of facts, to be sure, yet we offer this information not to scare you, but to bring a certain reality into focus: we need to take control of our own breast health. Breast self-exam gives us one viable method.

⋅⋅ Does Breast Self-Examination Affect Survival?

Most medical researchers in this field will say, to date, there is no hard scientific evidence that BSE reduces mortality rates or increases survival time. Others, particularly those reviewing the medical literature in the last few years, will present a more positive picture. Much of the controversy centers around the study designs, in which certain types of studies are debunked because they are epidemiological or retrospective (i.e., studying populations or women who already have cancer). The prospective, randomized, controlled study design, considered to be in the top echelon of studies and the only one accepted by many scientists, does not lend itself well to a variety of issues. BSE, in the opinion of numerous medical researchers, is one of these issues. There are too many variables that are difficult to control in studies of this nature.[12,13]

In review of the BSE literature in which approximately five

hundred scientific articles have been published in the last fifteen years, favorable evidence is mounting for the practice of BSE, despite the controversy. However, this evidence has less to do with actual death rates and more to do with the stage at which a tumor is found. More studies indicate that women who are inclined to practice regular BSE, and who become more aware of their breasts, are finding tumors at an earlier stage and with less nodal involvement. A critical aspect of these findings is the level of competence a women demonstrates in her BSE practice.[14,15,16,17,18,19,20]

Much of the research on BSE has been unable to assess the quality of breast self-exams that are being performed in these studies. Those studies that do account for proficiency have found it to be severely lacking. One scientist states, "Because data obtained elsewhere show that most women performing BSE do not perform it competently, the significance of the positive evidence on BSE value is heightened."[21]

So in simple terms, what does all this mean? BSE is a noninvasive, low-risk, inexpensive screening procedure that may help you detect a cancerous lump before it spreads to the lymph system or other parts of your body, particularly if you do it proficiently and regularly. So, why don't we all do it?

☙ Problems with Breast Self-Examination

Researching and writing this chapter has forced Taffy to examine her own BSE technique. Before, she would have said that she was proficient and regular. However, the sobering truth is that she was not thorough, did not know exactly what she was looking for, and only performed BSE when she felt a pain or unusual sensation or when she was feeling particularly fearful about breast cancer. She admits that it has been a long, slow evolution and a process of fear desensitization to reach a place where she is able to carefully and seriously examine her breasts.

Equally sobering, Taffy found that as she talked with other

women and researched the literature, her experience is a normal one. Fear and anxiety about finding something that may lead to loss of a breast, illness, harsh treatments, and death are the most commonly cited barriers. Other women may not believe they are at risk or they are not confident of their abilities to perform the procedure. They think there is no real benefit, and they realize that BSE assures no diminished chance of contracting the disease. They feel uncertain of their ability to cope with the possibility of finding a lump, or perhaps it just seems too complicated. Some women believe that regular mammograms and clinical breast exams are sufficient.[22,23,24,25]

A most commonly cited problem for the elderly, who are at highest risk and who practice BSE the least, is the difficulty in remembering to do so. They also report feeling embarrassed to touch themselves, not liking to look at their bodies in the mirror, and having less interest in their long-term health.[26,27,28]

One medical doctor who wrote an editorial in a cancer medical journal concludes that low compliance in the practice of BSE is based upon "simple dislike." She writes:

> . . . a much more persuasive explanation is that women may not like doing breast self-examination because it generates tensions that heighten the mind-body dichotomy. . . . The problem is that the fingers, breasts, and mind all belong to one individual. The act of distancing one's mind from one's physical being can be an unpleasant and depersonalizing experience. It requires objectification of a body part that is associated with the most important of sensuous human experiences: lovemaking and suckling. With breast self-examination, feeling seeks disease instead of producing pleasure. The act of examination requires not only the repugnant splitting of mind from body, but also repetition of a behavior that by its very purpose implies an inwardly directed hostility, suspicion, and distrust. It is as though the woman is saying "These breasts of mine cannot be trusted; I must monitor them constantly to discover if they have betrayed me by becoming cancerous."[29]

We suggest that you examine your own thoughts and feelings about BSE. As you read about these common barriers, see if you can identify with any of the feelings and difficulties mentioned. We recommend that you discuss your thoughts and feelings with someone you trust. It certainly can take much of the stigma out of these often undisclosed feelings and heighten your sense of safety and control. If you find that you cannot get past your negative feelings about BSE and it is really something you don't want to do, accept that as your reality. Just make sure you schedule breast exams with a health professional on a regular schedule and follow American Cancer Society standards for mammography.

Breast self-examination is really a way to honor yourself and your life. Rather than promoting a mind-body split, your goal should be to make your breasts a very important part of your whole being. Performing BSE regularly and carefully can be a good way for you to learn to love and appreciate your breasts in all the roles they play in your life.

COMPETENCE AND COMPLIANCE

Study after study concludes that women who feel confident in their ability to competently perform breast self-examination are more likely to do so on a regular basis.[30,31,32,33,34,35] Yet proficiency seems to be a key problem. Is our exposure and training inadequate? There is no question most of us have encountered the pamphlets with pictures and thorough descriptions on how to do BSE. However, the breast is a complicated structure with ducts, glands, and fibrocystic conditions, and no two breasts are the same, including your own. Numerous studies indicate a pamphlet is not adequate, and direct training with a health professional is the most effective way to get immediate feedback and build your self-confidence.[36,37,38,39,40]

Many women have managed to get through their entire premenopausal life without one doctor or nurse suggesting a direct training. Sometimes not even one doctor asks about BSE. Furthermore, exposure to plastic self-examination models, with various sizes of tumors embedded in them, is extremely limited. The labor-intensive aspect of teaching women BSE techniques appears to be the primary problem in effectively promoting the procedure. It is said that the amount of time to accomplish this is not a very good return on a busy physician's investment.[41]

We suggest it is no longer appropriate for us to be passive in our exposure to good BSE training. It is time to demand the opportunity to know if we are performing our examination competently. Most clinics and medical centers offer BSE classes led by registered nurses using self-exam breast models. If these are unavailable, ask your doctor to show you her breast model. Ask for one with a nodular background. Place the model on your chest and familiarize yourself with what an abnormality feels like. You may have an aversive response, as many women do, feeling lumps that remind you of your worst fears. Try to stay with the feelings and let them pass through you. It will help next time you examine your own breasts.

❧ *The Baseline Self-Examination*

"Women should be as familiar with the feel and appearance of their breasts as they are with the lines on their faces," says Elin Greenberg, vice chairman for education at the Susan G. Komen Breast Cancer Foundation. Once we understand the necessity for BSE, getting to know our breasts should then be our primary objective. It is not our job to evaluate any lumps we may find, but to know when our breasts are undergoing changes and allow professionals to do the diagnosis.

Unless you have been trained in BSE and practice regularly, start with a "baseline" self-exam with a health professional, just as you do a baseline mammogram. This is the first exam in which you get to know your breast tissue, and then use this information as the basis of comparison in subsequent examinations. As you feel the various lumps of the breast, you can receive immediate reassurance about what is normal. Then diligently perform this technique at the same time again for the next few months so that you can remember what you learned, and truly become familiar with your breast tissue. This "baseline" exam can relieve any fears, especially if done in conjunction with a mammogram. From then on, you will know that you can be your own best monitor should you find a new lump or a thickening, or recognize any other changes in the skin or tissue. If you are premenopausal and you are following all breast health guidelines, do not panic at the onset of a change. Breasts go through constant changes throughout your lifetime, particularly during your menstrual cycles. Wait a cycle to see if the change is persistent. Then see your doctor.

In speaking to members of a support group of breast cancer survivors, we asked if there was any one thing they would urge women who had not yet encountered breast cancer to consider. Their unanimous and resentful response was not to allow a doctor to "watch" a suspicious lump for several months but to demand further investigation immediately. These women were adamant about seeking another opinion if a doctor dismisses the lump as unimportant. It appeared that many in this group had unnecessarily delayed diagnoses.

If you feel panicky about a lump or change in your breast or have a deep instinct something is wrong, trust yourself and make an appointment immediately. Do what is necessary to give yourself peace of mind and don't worry that anyone will think you are a hypochondriac or just another "hysterical woman." One of the registered disadvantages frequently mentioned in the scientific literature regarding BSE is a concern about "overuse" of physician time by women who may be fearful and frequently generate only "false positives" (a benign or normal lump).[42,43] Remember, we *pay* doctors for their services. They would not exist without our need for them. When we pay, we are in charge. If a doctor has less than a positive attitude toward your anxious feelings and is not totally supportive of your diligence regarding your health, speak your mind and find a new doctor. There are plenty of good physicians around who will be happy to team up with you in your efforts to stay well.

The following BSE instruction pamphlet is reprinted from

the latest American Cancer Society materials. These instructions are basic and similar to ones that you can find in any health-care provider's office. Reread them occasionally as a reminder and verification of your technique.

☙ *Breast Self-Examination: A New Approach*[44]

All women over 20 should practice monthly breast self-examination (BSE). Regular and complete BSE can help you find changes in your breasts that occur between clinical breast examinations (by a health professional) and mammograms.

Women should examine their breasts when they are least tender, usually seven days after the start of the menstrual period. Women who have entered menopause, are pregnant or breast feeding, and women who have silicone implants, should continue to examine their breasts once a month. Breast feeding mothers should examine their breasts when all milk has been expressed.

If a woman discovers a lump or detects any changes, she should seek medical attention. Nine out of ten women will not develop breast cancer and most breast changes are *not* cancerous.

Remember the seven P's for a complete BSE:

1 Positions
2 Perimeter
3 Palpation
4 Pressure
5 Pattern
6 Practice with Feedback
7 Plan of Action

• *1 Positions*

VISUAL INSPECTION: STANDING
In each position, look for changes in contour and shape of the breasts, color and texture of the skin and nipple, and evidence of discharge from the nipples.

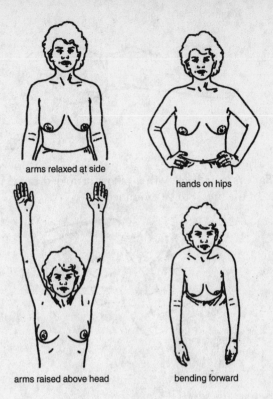

arms relaxed at side

hands on hips

arms raised above head

bending forward

PALPATION: SIDE-LYING & FLAT

Use your left hand to palpate the right breast, while holding your right arm at a right angle to the rib cage, with the elbow bent. Repeat the procedure on the other side. The side-lying position allows a woman, especially one with large breasts, to most effectively examine the outer half of the breast. A woman with small breasts may need only the flat position.

SIDE-LYING POSITION:

Lie on the opposite side of the breast to be examined. Rotate the shoulder (on the same side as the breast to be examined) back to the flat surface.

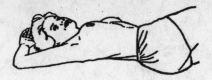

FLAT POSITION:
   Lie flat on your back with a pillow or folded towel under the shoulder of the breast to be examined.

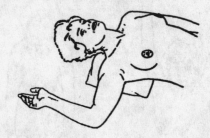

- *2 Perimeter*
   The examination area is bounded by a line which extends down from the middle of the armpit to just beneath the breast, continues across along the underside of the breast to the middle of the breast bone, then moves up to and along the collarbone and back to the middle of the armpit. Most breast cancers occur in the upper outer area of the breast (shaded area below).

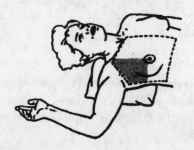

- **3 *Palpation with pads of the fingers***
  Use the pads of three or four fingers to examine every inch of your breast tissue. Move your fingers in circles about the size of a dime.

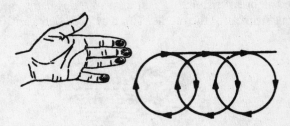

Do not lift your fingers from your breast between palpations. You can use powder or lotion to help your fingers glide from one spot to the next.

- **4 *Pressure***
  Use varying levels of pressure for *each palpation,* from light to deep, to examine the full thickness of your breast tissue. Using pressure will not injure the breast.

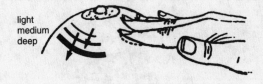

- **5 *Pattern of search***
  Use one of the following search patterns to examine all of your breast tissue. Palpate carefully beneath the nipple. Any incision should also be carefully examined from end to end. Women who have had any breast surgery should still examine the entire area and the incision.

VERTICAL STRIP:

Start in the armpit, proceed downward to the lower boundary. Move a finger's width toward the middle and continue palpating upward until you reach the collarbone. Repeat this until you have covered all breast tissue. Make at least six strips before the nipple and four strips after the nipple. You may need between 10 and 16 strips.

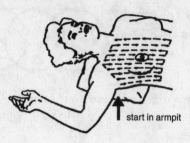

start in armpit

WEDGE:

Imagine your breast divided like the spokes of a wheel. Examine each separate segment, moving from the outside boundary toward the nipple. Slide fingers back to the boundary, move over a finger's width and repeat this procedure until you have covered all breast tissue. You may need between 10 and 16 segments.

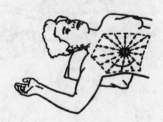

CIRCLE:

Imagine your breast as the face of a clock. Start at 12 o'clock and palpate along the boundary of each circle until you return to your starting point. Then move down a finger's width and continue palpating in ever smaller circles until you reach the nipple.

Depending on the size of your breast, you may need eight to ten circles.

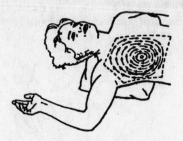

NIPPLE DISCHARGE:

Squeeze your nipples to check for discharge. Many women have a normal discharge.

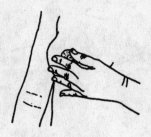

AXILLARY EXAMINATION:

Examine the breast tissue that extends into your armpit while your arm is relaxed at your side.

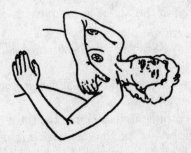

- **6 Practice with feedback**

  It is important that you perform BSE while your instructor watches to be sure you are doing it correctly. Practice your skills under supervision until you feel comfortable and confident.

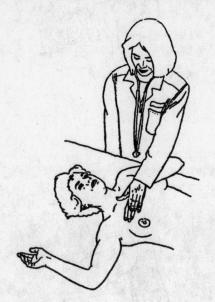

- **7 Plan of action**

  Every women should have a personal breast health plan of action:

  ✔ Discuss the American Cancer Society breast cancer detection guidelines with your health care professional.

  ✔ Schedule your clinical breast examination and mammogram as appropriate.

  ✔ Do monthly BSE. Ask your health professional for feedback on your BSE skills.

  ✔ Report any changes to your health care professional.

If this seems complicated and involved, the nipple squeeze step can be dropped. One medical researcher, who is concerned that this step is disagreeable to many women and adds to the complexity of the procedure, has suggested that the necessity of the nipple squeeze be reconsidered in BSE. She states there is no evidence other than personal opinion to justify this maneuver.[45] Dr. Susan Love, in *Dr. Susan Love's Breast Book*, says, "Don't squeeze your nipples to see if there's discharge; any discharge that comes only when you squeeze your nipple is fine anyway. Remember that at this stage you're not looking for anything in particular—you're getting to know what your breasts feel like so that, eventually, you'll know them well enough to feel when there's something unusual."[46] However, it is important to pay attention to any spontaneous discharge that may appear on your bra or clothes. This can be considered a change that warrants a visit to the doctor.

If you are not sure which search pattern to use, it may help to know a study was done assessing the various methods. It concluded that the vertical strip pattern generated considerably more thorough coverage of the total breast area.[47] Checking your breasts while standing is not particularly useful for women with medium or large breasts, so it is generally recommended that all women lie down for the exam.

As you become acquainted with your breast tissue, changes you may want your doctor to examine will most likely be obvious. Dr. Love says that a "really dangerous lump or other cancer symptom isn't subtle."[48] Others say a minor thickening can be a signal worth heeding. The primary signs to pay attention to are skin swelling, superficial veins, skin dimpling, an inverted nipple, and a single, firm, nonmobile lump that is most often painless and does not change with your cycle.

THE SENSOR PAD

Many of you may have become familiar with the controversy surrounding an early detection device for breast cancer, the Sensor Pad. On the market for ten years, it is currently being sold in many other countries, but has been denied approval by the FDA for use in the United States. It is a simple latexlike polyurethane pad, ten inches in diameter, filled with a small amount of silicon lubricant. Its function is to allow your hand to glide more easily over your breast to heighten the sense of touch. The pad eliminates friction so that a finger can explore the contours of an object as small as a grain of salt.

On face value, it seems bizarre that we might be denied a lifesaving device as simple as this one. Apparently, the FDA has expressed concern about the indirect risks of using this product. The agency claims that using it could lull women into complacency (if they use the pad, they might think they have the ability to detect any tumor), potentially allowing a cancerous lump to go undetected. The FDA indicated that, if approved, the pad could be sold only by prescription and could carry no reference to breast cancer. It appears that each step of the way, as the manufacturers of the Sensor Pad attempted to comply with FDA requests, the agency demanded more sophisticated trials of efficacy and safety, categorizing the product as a "medical device." The manufacturers, not agreeing that this pad is a medical device, began to market it to hospitals. This began what appears to be a hostile, unresolvable conflict between the company and the FDA.[49]

For purposes of this book, we contacted the manufacturer and unsuccessfully attempted to purchase a Sensor Pad. We were offered the alternative of ordering this device through a company in England for $25 (see Appendix B). "The thing that amazes me," says manufacturer Grant Wright, "is that the research spending [on breast cancer] keeps going up and I can't get this simple $7 product into the hands of women who want it."[50]

Another way to get to know your breasts is in a hot tub, spa, pool, or deep bathtub, where your breasts can float. This method can be alarming initially because you are likely to feel previously undetected lumps. Don't panic. This is only meant to increase your awareness, and you may find you are already familiar with this tissue in a different way from BSE conducted when lying down.

Take the time to get to know your breasts. Remember, this is your time to give to yourself. You might want to set the stage so your environment is comfortable and relaxing. Breathe deeply as you explore your breasts. If you are comfortable with your mate or loved one's participation, allow a ritual to form around this monthly examination. Do whatever is necessary *not* to let this become a distasteful, hurried, and fearful search for cancer.

🕯 Summary

We are in the midst of a cancer epidemic, and we are all at risk. It is generally agreed that early detection is associated with better prognosis. Remember that mammograms and clinical breast exams alone are not fully adequate for early detection, and most women find their own lumps. Fifty percent of all diagnosed breast cancers have already spread to other parts of the body, making treatment more difficult and outcomes less favorable. You can see how important it is that we take control of our own bodies and stay aware of the health of our breasts. When we feel as if we have control, we generally also experience greater self-esteem and less fear about our bodies and health. Generating a positive cycle, we are then more likely to reward ourselves with self-care and good health practices such as monthly breast self-examination.

Chapter 6

Estrogen: The Real Story

It may shock you to learn that estrogen is a breast carcinogen! This chapter will discuss the evidence for this declaration, and the associated risks for hormonal contraception and for hormone replacement therapy. We learned in Chapter 1 that the conditions leading to a cancer development are believed to be a "two hit" process: initiation and promotion. Carcinogens can act in either phase. It has been well established from animal and human epidemiological studies that estrogen acts as a promoter form of breast carcinogen. This is true whether the estrogen is from a woman's ovaries or from a hormone pill. As we discussed in Chapter 2, estrogen stimulates breast cells to grow, divide, and proliferate. Breast cancer is an exaggerated, uncontrolled proliferation of breast cells. So whether the woman's first "hit" was due to an inherited gene defect or to a gene defect that was caused by an environmental condition, estrogen can provide the crucial second "hit" required for cancer development. Estrogen stimulates already established breast cancers to grow, even ones that are only microscopic and too small to be detected by mammography. Some breast cancers develop the ability to enhance their sensitivity to estrogen, so they can grow even better in a woman's estrogen environment. Some breast cancers use this enhanced sensitivity to flourish even in conditions in which the estrogen levels are low, such as after menopause.[1]

OVULATORY CYCLES AND BREAST CANCER RISK

Many of the known risk factors for developing breast cancer are related to excess estrogen exposure. Other hormones may play a part in the risk, but most investigations point primarily to the role of estrogen. One risk factor for breast cancer is the number of ovulatory cycles a woman experiences during her lifetime. Ovulatory cycle number is directly related to estrogen exposure risk. Long ago it was found that there was an increased risk for breast cancer when a woman began menstruating early in life. Menarche before age twelve presents double the risk compared to menarche at age thirteen or older. Menopause late in life also presents a known risk. Either or both situations subject a woman to more ovulatory cycles and therefore a greater exposure to her own ovarian hormones, primarily estrogen. If exposure to these cycles is reduced, such as in premature or surgical menopause, there is a decreased risk for breast cancer for life. In the United States, the average woman will experience menarche at age twelve, have two children, and subsequently have 450 ovulatory cycles in her lifetime. Two hundred years ago she would have had menarche at age seventeen, eight children, and fewer than 150 ovulatory cycles.[2] Besides having more ovulatory cycles, girls who experience early menarche tend to have higher estrogen levels throughout the remainder of their lives. This situation exposes these individuals to a double threat: greater lifetime estrogen exposure and a higher level of estrogen exposure. While less clear for premenopausal women, there is established research to show that postmenopausal women with high estrogen levels have increased breast cancer risk.[3,4]

OBESITY AND ESTROGEN

Another established risk factor that is related to estrogen exposure is obesity. Obese women (20 percent over ideal weight) are at increased risk for breast cancer since they have higher levels of circulating estrogen because their bodies' fat cells have converted adrenal hormones into estrogen. This "converted" estrogen adds to the ovarian estrogen output, producing total levels higher than normal. Even in a postmenopausal state, obese women have higher estrogen levels than nonobese postmenopausal women because adrenal hormone levels do not fall off, as they do for ovarian hormones. Thus "converted" estrogen production continues.

Obesity can be broken down into several subgroups with even higher risks for breast cancer. When women gain excess weight in adulthood, especially during the postmenopausal years, there is extra risk. When the excess weight distribution is primarily abdominal in location (central obesity), this increases risk even more. These obese individuals have a demonstrated increased risk for postmenopausal breast cancer. Along with higher levels of estrogen, these women have higher levels of free fatty acids and insulin. And while the elevated estrogen level is responsible for the breast cancer risk, the elevated levels of the other substances may serve to further magnify that risk.[5]

One of the conditions associated with the early menarche risk just described is abdominal obesity. There is evidence that abdominal obesity in prepubescent girls can be correlated with early menarche, elevated insulin levels, and elevated estrogen levels. Again, these individuals have their breast tissue exposed to estrogen for a longer time and to higher levels of the hormone owing to central obesity. To lower this risk, it is very important for them to achieve ideal body weight through proper diet and exercise.[6]

WHY ARE THE FORMS OF ESTROGEN IMPORTANT?

Besides the breast cancer risk for elevated estrogen levels, there may be additional risk factors related to the *forms* of estrogen produced by women. Women produce three distinct forms of estrogen throughout their lives: estrone, estradiol, and estriol. It has been known for a long time that the first two forms are carcinogenic; the third form is a weaker estrogen and is noncarcinogenic. The relative amounts of these estrogens can be measured in the urine. It has been found that women who have breast cancer have *lower* percentages of the estriol, or noncarcinogenic, type.[7] Scientists know that in populations in which women are at low risk, there tends to be more noncarcinogenic estrogen produced than in populations of women with high risk for breast cancer. This difference is believed not to be genetically determined, but controlled by diet and lifestyle. Therefore, diet and lifestyle can influence the quality of estrogen production, not just the quantity.

In addition to what type of estrogen is originally manufactured by the women, one can look at how the body breaks down (metabolizes) estrogen. Estrogen (estradiol) is changed primarily into two forms: a "good form" (inactive or possibly anti-estrogenic form) and a "bad form" (producing estrogenic effects). The body levels of the good form are easier to change than the more stable bad form; however, there has been some debate over whether we should be trying to raise or lower the levels of the good form. Previous investigations have found that when good form levels are higher, there is more risk for estrogen-dependent cancers, such as breast and endometrial.[8,9] More significant studies have shown the opposite; there is less risk for these cancers when good-form estrogen is present.[10,11] We believe the latter studies to be more valid.

Why is this important for us to know? Because we are currently able to manipulate relative levels of the good and bad forms with changes in our diets or lifestyles. We can increase our levels of the good form by practicing aerobic exercise (keeping our bodies thin) and consuming vegetables from the cruciferous family (which includes cabbage, cauliflower, broccoli, brussels sprouts).[12] Lower levels of the good form are produced by obesity, high-fat diets, hypothyroidism, and certain anti-ulcer medications.[13] Intuitively, and with the available data, we feel that we should be attempting to increase levels of the good form. This increase will follow the intentional dietary and lifestyle changes described in this book, changes we already know to be beneficial in helping women avoid breast cancer.

ESTROGEN AND BREAST FLUID

Elevated estrogen blood levels in women may be the tip of an iceberg because some types of breast tissue have the ability to concentrate estrogen in breast fluid. Some investigators have measured breast fluid estrogen levels at forty-five times higher than the circulating blood levels.[14] This finding indicates that the breasts have the ability to remove estrogen from the blood and concentrate it in mammary ducts, thus exposing the ductal cells to very high levels of estrogen. Women with benign breast disease can have elevated levels of one of the carcinogenic estrogens (estradiol) in their breast fluid, but lactating or parous women (those who have had a full-term pregnancy) have lower levels. This is significant when we remember that women with many forms of benign breast disease have an increased risk for breast cancer development. Lactation and parity (the condition of having had children) decrease this risk. Perhaps the internal hormonal environment of the breast ducts is even more important than we have believed. After all, it is from within the ducts that most cancers arise. Having elevated blood levels of estrogen would represent a higher risk since the mammary ducts are exposed to even higher estrogen levels in the breast fluid.[15,16] In the future, measuring hormonal levels in nonlactating women's breast fluid may be used for measuring risk factors.

❧ *Physical Activity*

PHYSICAL ACTIVITY AND ESTROGEN

Physical activity during any stage in a woman's life can reduce estrogen exposure. This represents one of the lifestyle modifications a woman can make to substantially reduce her lifetime risk of breast cancer. Physical activity in the prepubescent girl can help prevent early menarche through prevention of obesity and other factors. It has been known for some time that strenuous exercise, such as regular ballet dancing, running, or swimming, can produce a considerable delay in the onset of menses. Recently it has been found that even moderate physical activity in adolescence, while not causing amenorrhea (absence of menstrual cycles), can produce cycles that are anovulatory (in which ovulation does not occur). Activity two or more hours a week involving aerobic exercise classes, swimming, jogging, or tennis can produce this effect.[17] These anovulatory cycles reduce the lifetime ovulatory cycle number, thereby reducing breast cancer risk. Conversely, girls who experience early menarche also have earlier ovulatory cycles. So throughout their lives, these individuals will experience more cycles, and more of them will be ovulatory.[18] Adequate exercise can result in the prevention of obesity at all ages, leading to the lowering of elevated estrogen levels. Experimental animal studies have shown that as exercise intensity increases, the incidence of breast cancer decreases.[19] Human studies show that the average number of hours spent in physical exercise activities per week from menarche to age forty is directly related to protection from breast cancer risk.[20] Moreover, human studies show that as physical fitness increases, death from all causes, including cancer, decreases.[21] (Exercise will be covered in more detail in Chapter 14.)

Other lifestyle changes that can reduce serum estrogen, such as increasing dietary fiber and eating more vegetables (including cruciferous vegetables, etc.), will be discussed in detail in later chapters. Alcohol consumption, which has also been associated with breast cancer risk, is another cause of elevated estrogens.[22] Reducing or eliminating alcohol from the diet is another practical method to reduce serum estrogen.

⋙ Hormonal Contraceptives and Breast Cancer Risk

ORAL CONTRACEPTIVES

Modern birth control uses a combination of an orally active synthetic estrogen with an orally active synthetic progesterone (progestin). Synthetic hormones are used because nonsynthetic natural hormones, if ingested, will be broken down by the body's digestive system before they can enter the blood. Oral contraceptives are progestin-dominant; the progestin is added to reduce the risk of endometrial cancer from the synthetic estrogen. It is not known, however, whether the progestin reduces the pill's risk for *breast* cancer. Some experts believe that it is the progestins, as well as the estrogen in the oral contraceptives, that are contributing to the rapidly increasing breast cancer risk in the United States.

How do we evaluate a synthetic hormone as more like estrogen or progesterone? Let's look at what it does to breast cells. Experimentally, in breast cell cultures almost all currently available progestins have estrogenic effects and can stimulate cell division and proliferation of breast cancer cells that have estrogen receptors (ER+). This does not seem to bode well for the theory of prevention of breast cancer by progestins. Another way to examine the question is to look at what blocks the activity of the hormone. If progestins were equal to true progesterone, their effects would be blocked by *antiprogesterone* drugs. This is not the case. Their effects are blocked by *antiestrogen* drugs. This further indicates the true estrogenic nature of the synthetic progestins. Why is this important? Because in modern contraceptives the estrogen and the progestin are *both* exerting synergistic estrogenic effects.[23,24] Conversely, progesterone produced by a woman's body does not behave in the manner of progestins; it does not stimulate breast cancer cells and can be blocked by antiprogesterone drugs. (Progesterone will be more thoroughly discussed in Chapter 7.)

From clinical experience it is known that the use of oral contraceptives reduces the risk for pelvic inflammatory disease, endometrial cancer, and ovarian cancer. However, their use in women *over the age of thirty-five* increases the risk of cardiovascular disease, stroke, thromboembolism (the last is especially increased in smokers). Numerous clinical studies concerning the risk of breast cancer from oral contraceptive use have been carried out. Many have shown mixed results and therefore the final answers are not yet conclusive. However, there is some consensus among most experts regarding breast cancer risk. The data show that there is some *slight* increase in relative risk for breast cancer in women beginning oral contraceptives at an early age (shortly after menarche), using them before a first full-term pregnancy, taking them for a long duration, and using a high-progestin-potency variety. A recent French study did not show increased risk of breast cancer with the use of this class of progestins, but possibly some protection.[25] More studies are needed to fully understand the possible causal relationship of oral contraceptives on breast cancer.[26,27,28,29,30,31,32,33,34]

In the quest for safer contraceptives, future designs will probably involve drugs that suppress the pituitary hormone responsible for stimulating ovarian function. This will dramatically reduce a woman's number of ovulatory cycles and thereby reduce her estrogen levels. Replacement sex hormones could then be used at safer levels, well below both those in current contraceptives and those in normal ovulation.[35,36]

IMPLANTABLE CONTRACEPTIVES

One form of nonoral hormonal contraceptive is the type that is implanted beneath the user's skin. The currently available implantable contraceptive is Norplant. It consists of small Silastic (silicone-based polymer) capsules measuring 2.4 by 34 millimeters and filled with a progestin. Although containing no estrogen, the package insert nevertheless states that studies have shown some increased risk of breast cancer with oral contraceptives (long-term and/or high-dose) and that the risk should be considered similar with this product. Since long-term data on Norplant is not available, only time will tell what the true risk is. Known or suspected breast cancer is a contraindication for the use of this contraception.

INJECTABLE CONTRACEPTIVES

Another form of nonoral hormonal contraceptive is a long-active injection. In some parts of the world, injections of this synthetic hormone product are very effective and the contraceptive of choice. Although used worldwide since 1964, it has been licensed in the United States only since 1992 because of concerns about breast cancer risk. This product, called Depo-Provera, has been shown in two recent studies to possibly increase breast cancer risk in very young users, prior to first full-term birth, and in very recent users.[37,38]

❧ Hormone Replacement Therapy

NATURAL MENOPAUSE AND HORMONE REPLACEMENT

There are over 470 million women fifty years of age or older living in the world today. These women are beyond the age for natural menopause. Several generations ago the average woman did not live to the age of fifty. Thus, today more women are spending larger portions of their lives in the postmenopausal state. In the United States, the average postmenopausal life expectancy is twenty-eight years. This stage of life exposes women to the associated chronic diseases of reproductive cancers (breast, ovarian, endometrial, cervical), osteoporosis, and coronary heart disease. In fact, cardiovascular heart disease is the leading cause of death in this age group. Nonlethal, but nevertheless important, menopause is also associated with varying degrees of vasomotor symptoms (hot flashes), related interference with sleep, and resultant interference with alertness, mood, and enjoyment of life. There can also be genitourinary symptoms (stress incontinence and painful sexual intercourse).

BENEFITS AND RISKS

There are an estimated 1.5 million fractures caused by osteoporosis in the United States annually. We know that estrogen replacement reduces the risk for osteoporotic fractures by approximately 50 percent, while estrogen alone increases the risk for endometrial cancer by 200 to 300 percent. Estrogen can also reduce the risk of heart disease by 50 percent. However, in countries where heart disease in women is much less common, the risk of using estrogen therapy for heart disease is not appropriate because of the possible risks of long-term therapy on breast cancer development.[39] Physicians use hormone replacement therapy (HRT) believing that the number of deaths from breast cancer caused by the therapy will be overshadowed by the number of lives saved from heart disease. This scenario is known as a desirable risk-to-benefit ratio. If we can produce a situation in which the chances for heart disease and osteoporosis are markedly reduced, then there would be no rationale for prescribing HRT. The risk-to-benefit ratio would be too large. Deciding whether to undergo HRT for symptoms of menopause is not easy for either the woman or her physician. (Since HRT is such an important subject for so many women, it will be covered in detail in Chapter 7.)

BREAST CANCER PATIENTS AND HRT

Most physicians feel that any woman who has been successfully treated for breast cancer should not be treated with estrogen hormone replacement therapy because of its cancer-promoting effects.[40] This contraindication is printed on the HRT package inserts. Of course, a problem occurs in that successfully treated breast cancer can be associated with earlier menopause, which may in turn call for HRT. As more and more localized breast cancer is diagnosed through the use of screening mammography, "adjuvant chemotherapy" (chemotherapy prescribed in addition to standard lumpectomy and radiation therapy to increase their effects) is increasingly being used. Survival rates for earlier stages of breast cancer are improving. One of the side effects of chemotherapy, however, is earlier menopause.[41] Therefore, we will have a growing population of women who have had breast cancer treated and who now have to deal with early menopause. The dilemma is what menopause therapy, if any, will be safe for this increasing number of women. To help answer these questions, the Women's Health Initiative, a new fifteen-year, $625 million federal study examining the effects of HRT, among other things, was formed. (The Women's Health Initiative Study is discussed more fully in Chapter 10: Dietary Fat.)

✥ *The Importance of Estrogen Receptors*

Certain breast cancers are made of cells that have a chemical "socket," or receptor, for estrogen on their surfaces. The measurement of this receptor's presence is made during pathologic examination of biopsy tissue. About 50 to 70 percent of all breast cancers have estrogen receptors and are referred to as being positive for estrogen receptors (ER+). This leaves 30 to 50 percent without such receptors, which are defined as negative for estrogen receptors (ER–). ER+ breast cancers are stimulated by the presence of estrogen more than are ER– cancers. Cutting off the estrogen supply to ER+ tumors often stops or slows their growth rate. This is important because two-thirds of patients with ER+ tumors respond to hormonal therapy, compared to less than 10 percent with ER–. Therefore, being estrogen receptor positive is a good prognostic sign. In general, ER+ breast cancer is more common in older than younger women and in post- than premenopausal women. The reason for the older women having more estrogen receptor positive breast cancers is unknown, but it could be due to the fact that cancer cells need to grow in an environment with a lower level of estrogen. It is possible the estrogen receptors make the cancer cells more sensitive to these lower levels. Another explanation may be that there are lower levels of progesterone in these older women since progesterone inhibits ER development.

FACTORS AFFECTING ESTROGEN RECEPTORS

Studies of whether oral contraceptives, estrogen replacement therapy, and opposed hormone replacement therapy (estrogen replacement plus an added progestin) are risk factors for the development of ER– tumors are not conclusive. Some studies have shown higher percentages of estrogen receptor negative cancers in women who have used oral contraceptives or in those who have had many children. Women who are present or past smokers also seem to have a higher percentage of ER– breast cancers. Breast cancers in black women are more likely to be ER–, compared with those in white women.[42]

Some investigators have shown that high dietary fat, not obesity itself, is associated with more breast cancers. High dietary fat also leads to an overall poorer prognosis for all breast cancers, regardless of ER status.[43] We know that the amount of dietary fat is related to a woman's blood estrogen levels. When pre- and postmenopausal women switched from a high-fat to a low-fat diet, there were significant reductions in estrogen levels.[44,45] Some dietary fats are good for you. Increasing dietary consumption of one type of "good fat" (omega-3 fatty acids), found in certain fish, flaxseed oil, etc., lowers the production of estrogens and other tumor growth factors. Therefore, it is important not only to reduce total dietary fat, but also to increase the percentage of omega-3 "good fats" in your diet. (Dietary fat is covered in more depth in Chapter 10.)

✒ Summary

We see that the female hormone estrogen is a double-edged sword, having beneficial properties as well as cancer-promoting effects. Furthermore, longer exposure to the hormone increases the risk for breast cancer. It is important to maintain an ideal body weight to minimize estrogen levels: exercise and weight control are beneficial at all ages, even in prepubertal girls, for lowering the risk of breast cancer. Additionally, a healthy diet and lifestyle can increase the percentage of noncarcinogenic "good" estrogen, lowering risk. Women should be aware that long-term hormonal contraceptives are associated with some risk of breast cancer. Similarly, postmenopausal hormone replacement therapy is associated with breast cancer risk, and should be used only when other means of controlling hot flashes, lowering cardiovascular risk, and raising bone density are not effective. HRT should not be used in women who have had breast cancer. Estrogen receptor presence on breast cancer cells, a prognostic factor, is affected by age, menopausal status, race, hormone contraception, parity, and dietary factors. While estrogen plays a role in the development of breast cancer, you have the power to alter its influence on your individual risk.

Chapter 7

The Pros and Cons of Hormone Replacement Therapy

Hormone replacement therapy (HRT) is a medical treatment that has redefined a natural rite of passage or life transition into a condition or disorder that needs to be treated. In fact, to many women menopause feels much like an illness, with severe symptoms that require relief. Women in the industrialized Western world are under enormous pressure to act and appear youthful since this society does not revere the wise older woman. Unfortunately, women in and approaching menopause have few, if any, models for embracing this transition as a natural part of life, a way of coming into a new kind of power. Furthermore, most modern women have developed little tolerance for tumultuous hormonal conditions, and they think something is wrong with them when they feel the changes associated with menopause. Hence, hormone replacement therapy seems like a godsend to many women, while others are deeply concerned about its potentially life-threatening risks.

Today more women than ever are spending a larger portion of their lives in the postmenopausal state. You may recall that in the United States, the average postmenopausal life expectancy is twenty-eight years. As a result, millions of women have to confront the issue of hormone replacement therapy. In this chapter we will address the issue of whether or not HRT increases a woman's risk of developing breast cancer. We will discuss how these hormonal therapies work, and examine the benefits and risks associated with their use. Our intent is to provide women with some important new options that offer fewer risks and greater protection against breast cancer.

❧ *Menopause*

Menopause, which usually occurs sometime between the ages of forty-five and fifty-five, is the permanent cessation of a woman's menstrual activity. Perimenopause, sometimes called the "change of life," refers to a transitional period of five to seven years before and several years after menopause. During this time a woman's menstrual cycles become less regular and ovulation does not consistently occur with each cycle. The term *climacteric* also refers to this period in a woman's life. Menstruation may stop suddenly, but most women experience a gradually decreased flow each month, and/or longer intervals between periods, until complete cessation.

Menopause is caused by a normal decline in ovarian function. Eventually, the decreased secretion of estrogen is no longer sufficient to produce menstrual cycles. A woman's fat cells, which normally convert small amounts of adrenal compounds into estrogen, now become the body's sole source of this hormone. The estrogen continues to support the structure and function of the hormone-dependent sex tissues (breasts, vagina, vulva, oviducts, and urethra) for several years. Eventually, the production of adrenal estrogen precursors declines, and these tissues undergo varying degrees of atrophy.

SIGNS OF MENOPAUSE

Most women begin to experience a number of changes as they enter the perimenopausal period of their lives. Hot flashes (referred to as Power Surges by some women of the nineties) are probably the most commonly associated signs of approaching menopause. These uncomfortable and unpredictable waves of intense body heat usually produce noticeable red flushing and profuse sweating on the head, neck, and chest. Some women wake up during the night totally drenched in sweat, necessitating a change of nightclothes and bedsheets.

The heat from hot flashes is the result of hormonal changes affecting the hypothalamus, which is the heat regulatory center in our brain. At the same time, a dilation of the blood vessels on the surface of the skin causes a sudden increase in blood flow which produces the characteristic flushing or redness.[1]

Hot flashes can last anywhere from a few seconds to several minutes, and when they occur in social or business situations they can be very embarrassing. Some women experience only one or two episodes a week, while others are plagued with several hot flashes per hour and many per day. For most women, hot flashes gradually decrease and eventually stop within one to two years, but they can go on for as long as five to ten years.

Menopause also causes changes in the vagina and the external genitalia. These tissues become thinner and less elastic. During this period the labia major becomes smaller, and the amount of pubic hair decreases.[2] A reduction in the normal secretions in these tissues leads to vaginal dryness, which predisposes the vagina to more frequent bouts of inflammation and infection. Vaginal dryness often results in another major frustration associated with menopause: varying degrees of pain and discomfort during sexual intercourse.

Sometimes an inflammation develops owing to the drying and thinning of the tissues in the urinary tract. This can cause painful or frequent urination and occasional urinary incontinence, which is often experienced following a hard cough or a sneeze.

Many women also experience emotional and psychological changes during this period of their lives. These effects range from mild to severe and can include occasional irritability, fatigue, insomnia, a temporary decrease in libido, anxiety, and depression.

There are two other conditions with potentially life-threatening implications that usually develop during the perimenopausal period. A woman's hormonal changes during these years substantially increase her risk to cardiovascular disease, including high blood pressure, atherosclerosis, and heart attacks.[3] The other condition that develops rapidly during this time in a woman's life is osteoporosis.[4]

At this point, let's summarize the symptoms associated with menopause. They include hot flashes, dryness and thinning of tissues that can cause problems with both intercourse and urination, psychological changes such as anxiety and depression, and an increased risk to osteoporosis and heart disease. Is there anything that will help? The answer is an emphatic YES!

✺ The Benefits of Hormone Replacement Therapy

It was initially discovered that the effects of menopause, produced by declining levels of estrogen, could be treated by giving women small daily doses of replacement estrogen. Hot flashes and vaginal dryness were quickly and easily eliminated. Most studies also show that estrogen replacement substantially reduces the risks of cardiovascular disease and the frequency of osteoporotic fractures. Estrogen replacement therapy (ERT) worked almost like magic for approximately two decades. However, the magic disappeared when long-term follow-up studies started to reveal that women taking supplemental estrogen were experiencing substantially higher rates of endometrial (uterine) cancer.[5]

In response to this problem, a new protocol called hormone replacement therapy was developed. HRT utilizes both estrogen and a synthetic form of progesterone in a manner that more closely approximates a woman's normal hormonal cycle. This quickly became the accepted protocol for women with an intact uterus.[6] Women who have had a hysterectomy can still utilize ERT because they cannot develop uterine cancer.

Using therapeutic estrogen alone resulted in what is called unopposed estrogen. In a woman's cycle, estrogen normally causes a proliferation of tissue in the uterus and breast each month. When the monthly supply of progesterone is secreted, the estrogenic tissue growth effects stop, the excess uterine tissue is sloughed off in menstruation, and everything returns to normal until the next cycle begins. The ERT protocol was supplying estrogen on a constant basis, but there was no progesterone to balance its effects. Therefore, women were constantly under the influence of estrogen's tissue growth effects, and an increase in uterine cancer was the result. The addition of a synthetic progesterone to this protocol successfully solved the problem. Consequently, HRT has been the therapy of choice in recent years.

To summarize, we can say that hormone replacement therapy works wonders at alleviating the symptoms of menopause, slowing the bone loss associated with postmenopausal osteoporosis, and decreasing the risk of cardiovascular disease. However, a nagging question remains unanswered. Does giving additional estrogen to a woman to treat the symptoms of menopause increase her risk of developing breast cancer?

✣ The Risks of Hormone Replacement Therapy

As mentioned, the question of whether or not the various therapies for menopause cause an increased risk for breast cancer is fraught with contradiction and controversy. An examination of the research provides some insights into the nature and complexity of the problem.

Over the past five decades, more than sixty studies and a

number of meta-analyses have been published on this topic.[7] Meta-analysis, a relatively new study design that combines data from multiple studies, enables researchers to spot trends, increase statistical reliability, and generalize results with greater accuracy.

One analysis of sixteen studies reported a slightly increased risk of breast cancer after five years of estrogen replacement therapy, and a 30 percent increased risk of developing breast cancer after fifteen years of estrogen use.[8] The results of two other meta-analyses showed no significant increase in breast cancer risk with estrogen replacement therapy.[9,10] A fourth meta-analysis reported that short-term use of estrogen (less then fifteen years) caused no increased risk, whereas long-term use could cause up to a 25 percent increase in risk.[11] A fifth meta-analysis, evaluating thirty-one different studies, reported that women with more than ten years of estrogen use had a 23 percent increased risk for developing breast cancer.[12] Obviously, even the conclusions from these meta-analysis studies do not provide women with clear-cut answers regarding the risk of breast cancer with hormone replacement therapy.

A look at the many variables involved with breast cancer studies helps explain why this substantial volume of research has not come up with definitive answers. Prior to the 1980s estrogen alone (ERT) was primarily prescribed for the treatment of menopausal symptoms. A low dose of estrogen was generally given for a relatively short period, usually a few years. Therefore, it was necessary to study short-term use of estrogen therapy and the risk of breast cancer.

In the 1970s doctors began putting women on long-term estrogen replacement therapy to reduce their risks of developing heart disease and osteoporosis. This trend made it necessary to conduct studies on the long-term use of estrogen therapy and breast cancer.

Long-term, unopposed estrogen therapy was then discovered to cause up to an eightfold increase in the incidence of uterine cancer.[13] This finding resulted in the addition of synthetic progesterone to the therapy. It then became necessary to study the relationship between combination hormone replacement therapy and breast cancer.

To date, only a few trials of long-term HRT have been conducted. An initial study published in 1983 reported that the addition of a synthetic progesterone resulted in a decreased risk of breast cancer.[14] However, several years later a Swedish study reported just the opposite findings. These researchers found that women taking estrogen plus a synthetic progesterone had a 4.4 times greater incidence of breast cancer.[15] As you can see, a review of the literature still leaves us without any conclusive answers.

ESTROGEN SKIN PATCHES

A new dosage form of estrogen has recently become available—a skin patch (trade name Estraderm) containing the natural estrogenic hormone estradiol. The hormone is easily absorbed transdermally (through the skin). Remember that of the three types of estrogen, estradiol is the most carcinogenic form. Therefore, with regard to breast cancer, this form of hormone replacement should not be considered any different from the pill therapy.

Although there is some controversy, a majority of the studies agree with the following summary statements about the traditional medical therapies for menopause and their relative risk to breast cancer. Taking some form of estrogen successfully treats the symptoms of menopause, but there is probably a slightly increased risk for breast cancer, a risk that continues to increase with the length of therapy. Women with an intact uterus who need treatment should use the combination HRT therapy in order to avoid an increased risk of uterine cancer. Also, most physicians believe that women who have already been diagnosed with any kind of cancer, or who are at high risk to breast cancer, should not take any form of hormone replacement therapy.

However, this is not the end of the story. We have some exciting new menopause treatment options to report.

a Alternative Hormonal Therapies

Two hormones, natural progesterone and estriol, are important alternatives to the drugs that are usually prescribed to treat the symptoms and conditions associated with menopause. The amount of research on both substances is limited, but the results of the studies that have been published are very promising. Each hormone has been shown to be more effective than the traditional drugs used in hormone replacement therapy. Instead of increasing risks, they each provide *greater protection* against the development of breast cancer.

NATURAL PROGESTERONE

Natural progesterone refers to the actual chemical that is produced in a woman's ovaries. In nature, a compound called diosgenin, which closely resembles progesterone, occurs naturally in over 5,000 plants; its content in Mexican yams and soybeans is quite high. For commercial use, diosgenin is usually extracted from these sources and converted by a simple chemical process into progesterone. This form of progesterone is molecularly identical to the hormone produced by the female ovary.

Natural progesterone products are commercially available without a prescription as a 3 percent topical cream or in an oil base to be used as sublingual (under-the-tongue) drops. Additionally, higher-strength creams can be obtained by prescription from some specialty pharmacies. These products have been used successfully to treat many of the PMS-related problems experienced by premenopausal women, and is very effective when used to treat the symptoms of menopause. To top it off, natural progesterone has been shown to both prevent and reverse osteoporosis.

Progesterone is one of the two main female sex hormones (the other, of course, is estrogen) produced by the ovaries in premenopausal women. Made by the corpus luteum just after ovulation, it is secreted in the second half of the menstrual cycle and is primarily responsible for the early development of the embryo and fetus.

Progesterone also increases a woman's libido. During the second half of the cycle when an egg is released, progesterone levels are highest. An increase in sex drive during this time is nature's way of promoting procreation.

Another interesting fact is that progesterone functions as a mild antidepressant. During pregnancy tremendous quantities of progesterone (a hundred to two hundred times above normal) are produced by the placenta.[16] This may be responsible for the proverbial "glow" observed in many pregnant women.

If conception does not occur, progesterone levels drop off and menstruation ensues. Progesterone also plays an important role in regulating a wide variety of other biological activities and is the main precursor for the development of estrogens, adrenal hormones, and testosterone.

⊱ *Progesterone and Breast Cancer*

A number of studies have examined the relationship between progesterone and breast cancer in women. Nine different studies have reported that women with breast cancer excrete lower levels of progesterone in their urine.[17]

In another study, endometrial biopsies were examined. These researchers reported that women with Stages I and II breast cancer had deficient production of progesterone.[18]

Three prospective trials have examined the incidence of breast cancer in women with clinical evidence of progesterone deficiency.[19,20,21] All three studies showed a higher incidence of breast cancer in progesterone-deficient women. One of these studies examined 1,083 women and found that premenopausal women who were progesterone-deficient had a 5.4 times greater incidence of breast cancer.[22]

It is important to note that these studies are consistent in reporting decreased progesterone levels in women with breast cancer. In fact, this is one of the few areas of breast cancer research which has shown some consistency. These findings suggest that a deficiency of progesterone may be an important key in our understanding of the breast cancer epidemic.

One possible explanation offered is that many women start having anovulatory cycles a number of years before menopause. This means that the ovaries secrete estrogen, but there are no ova follicles left to mature, hence, no progesterone gets produced. This means that in perimenopausal women, anovulatory cycles produce the high-estrogen/progesterone-deficient condition of estrogen dominance that was reported in the previously mentioned studies. Thus, natural progesterone may be an important substance for the prevention of breast cancer.

☙ *Natural versus Synthetic Progesterone*

The importance of progesterone cannot be overemphasized. It is one of the most important master-control hormones in the human body. Since naturally occurring substances cannot be patented, pharmaceutical companies had to make slight alterations in the structure of natural progesterone in order to formulate a unique drug they could patent. This class of drugs is called progestins. However, slight changes in nature's design can make big changes in how a drug is metabolized and in its biological effects in the body. In fact, there are vast differences between natural progesterone and the slightly altered synthetic progestins that drug companies have created to use in birth control pills and the drugs used to treat the symptoms of menopause. Provera is the trade name of the progestin most commonly given to menopausal women.

In order to highlight and emphasize the difference between natural progesterone and the synthetic analogs, we will compare the side effects of natural progesterone with those of Provera. The progestins are available only by prescription, and they have a substantial number of possible side effects. The following list summarizes the adverse reactions for Provera.[23]

Pregnancy: Use during pregnancy may cause birth defects.

Breast: Breast tenderness and abnormal milk flow have been rarely reported.

Skin: Sensitivity reactions consisting of urticaria and pruritus (types of allergic itching), edema, and generalized rash have occurred in an occasional patient. Acne, alopecia (hair loss), and hirsutism (excessive hair growth in unusual places) have been reported in a few cases.

Thromboembolic Phenomena: Thromboembolic phenomena (blood clotting), including thrombophlebitis (clot and inflammation of a vein, usually in leg) and pulmonary embolism (clot in artery of the lung) have been reported.

General: The following adverse reactions have been observed in women taking progestins including Provera:

breakthrough bleeding
fever
spotting
change in menstrual flow
amenorrhea
edema
nausea
insomnia
prolonged drowsiness

cholestatic jaundice (yellow skin from bile blockage)
allergic reactions (anaphylaxis)
allergic rash with and without itching
mental depression
fever
changes in cervical erosion and cervical secretions

Compare with this the fact that natural progesterone is nontoxic, is virtually without side effects, and is available without a prescription. It is quite easy to see the vast difference between the two. Now let's examine the relationship between estrogen and progesterone.

PROGESTERONE AND ESTROGEN

There are many examples of two substances, such as calcium and magnesium or sodium and potassium, working together to regulate some function in the body. In these cases, the amount of one substance is usually not as important as its ratio to the other, so together they can achieve the proper balance in their activity and function. This is also true for progesterone and estrogen.

In the first half of the female cycle, estrogen levels are high. During the second half of the cycle, progesterone is released and actually stops estrogen's activity, counterbalancing its effects. It is well known that estrogen promotes tissue growth in the breast and uterus, and is the main breast cancer–promoting substance in women. Progesterone opposes these activities, and when the two are in proper balance everything works according to nature's design. The following list compares the counterbalancing physiological effects of estrogen and progesterone:

Estrogen's Effects	Progesterone's Effects
Tissue growth in the breast	Helps prevent breast cancer
Tissue growth in the uterus	Helps prevent uterine cancer
Slows down osteoporosis	Prevents and reverses osteoporosis
Decreases libido	Restores libido
Increases body fat	Helps utilize fat for energy
Breast stimulation	Helps prevent "fibrocystic" change
Salt and fluid retention	Natural diuretic
Depression and headaches	Natural antidepressant
Interferes with thyroid hormone	Improves thyroid hormone function
Increases blood clotting	Normalizes blood clotting

Impairs blood sugar control	Normalizes blood sugar levels
Promotes growth of endometrium	Maintains endometrium
Reduces zinc and retains copper	Normalizes zinc and copper levels
Reduces oxygen levels in cells	Restores proper cell oxygen level
Reduces vascular tone	Necessary for survival of embryo
Lowers cholesterol; Increases HDL, lowers LDL cholesterol	Precedes production of adrenal hormones, estrogen hormones, testosterone

This list may make it seem that estrogen is bad and progesterone is good. This is definitely not the case. Estrogen produces a wide variety of important benefits and functions. In addition to its role in the development of the female breasts and genitals at puberty, estrogen influences the cardiovascular system, blood chemistry, and skeletal structure.

The problem arises when the estrogen/progesterone ratio gets out of balance. The dangers of this imbalance were tragically discovered after many of the women taking supplemental estrogen to treat menopausal symptoms began developing uterine cancer. As previously mentioned, it was the unopposed estrogen (estrogen without progesterone) that caused an increase in the incidence of uterine cancer.

There are several other sources of estrogen exposure that may contribute to an imbalance of the estrogen/progesterone ratio, thus increasing the risk of breast cancer. In 1954 the U.S. Department of Agriculture approved the use of estrogen-related drugs as growth stimulants in cattle, poultry, and hogs. Notice in the previous list that one of estrogen's effects is to increase body fat. Mixing these drugs into their feed enables the animals to attain their market weight faster and on less feed, producing fat-streaked or "marbleized" meat.[24] Although this practice has been discontinued in pigs and poultry, it is still in widespread use in the cattle industry.

The current technique is to implant a time-release pellet of estradiol under the skin of cattle. If you recall, estradiol is the most carcinogenic form of estrogen. It is estimated that treated beef cattle reach their market weight of about 1,000 pounds approximately thirty-five days sooner than untreated animals, saving about 500 pounds of feed per animal. This process is still widely used in the 1990s. It is great for business, but it may not be great for your health. Meat eaters are continually ingesting trace amounts of estrogens. Although the Code of Federal Regulations lists the levels of estradiol that are allowable in heifers, steers, calves, and lambs that are reportedly safe, some health professionals question this.[25]

There are two other sources of estrogen exposure of which to be aware. The pesticides and herbicides used in agriculture act like estrogens. When they are ingested, they remain in the body for a long time, exerting estrogenic effects. This topic is covered in detail in Chapter 13. Alcohol also increases estrogen levels in a woman's body. Read more about this topic in Chapter 16. It has not been proven that these sources of low-level estrogen exposure cause an increase in breast cancer. However, we feel that these areas should be thoroughly researched, and at the very least women should be warned about as many external sources of estrogen as possible.

❧ Estriol

In Chapter 6 we discussed three different naturally occurring forms of estrogen, and expressed our primary concern about estrogen therapy and its risk for breast cancer. Among the three estrogens, estradiol is the most stimulating to the breast. Estrone is slightly weaker, and estriol is much weaker. For example, estradiol is about a thousand times more potent than estriol.[26] In fact, estriol has actually been shown to be cancer protective, whereas estradiol and estrone have both been shown to promote cancer.

Estriol has been shown to be effective in alleviating the hot flashes and vaginal dryness associated with menopause without side effects.[27] One of the most remarkable aspects of utilizing estriol is that unlike the other estrogens, it does not cause uterine proliferation and shedding. This means that most women taking estriol will not experience uterine bleeding. Thus, estriol solves the problem of breakthrough bleeding, which is one of the most frequent and bothersome side effects experienced by women taking other forms of estrogen.

In Germany, a five-year multicenter study of menopausal women taking a daily dose of estriol reported effective elimination of unpleasant symptoms. There was no uterine bleeding and no side effects. The following statement from that study is worth noting: estriol "is considered by patients and physicians to be a remarkable advantage for women in this period of life."[28]

Estradiol and estrone are the forms of estrogen most frequently used in the United States. While estriol is commonly used in Europe, it has encountered only limited acceptance here. On the other hand, a growing number of health-oriented doctors are beginning to learn about and prescribe estriol for menopausal hot flashes and vaginal dryness. Because it is a weaker form of estrogen, higher doses of estriol are necessary, but the results are usually effective, and it provides a slight protection against—rather than an increased risk for—breast cancer.

Although estriol is not available in regular drugstores, several specialty mail-order pharmacies make it available in a variety of strengths and dosages. Doctors can order it for their patients, and women can call to request information about its use. The pharmacies that carry these products will be referenced in Appendix B, Other Resources.

In addition to relieving the symptoms of menopause, hormone replacement therapy (ERT or HRT) is frequently prescribed because of estrogen's effectiveness in preventing both cardiovascular disease and osteoporosis. Recognition of these benefits has resulted in a high increase in the number of estrogen prescriptions dispensed in the United States, from 14 million per year in 1980 to over 35 million in 1993.[29]

Hormone Replacement Therapy and Heart Disease

Estrogen's effect on cardiovascular disease was discovered in 1981 when a study revealed that women who had both ovaries removed (resulting in a loss of estrogen) during a hysterectomy had a 7.2 times greater risk of having a future heart attack.[30] Since then a number of studies have shown that women taking estrogen replacement therapy have a substantial protection against atherosclerosis and heart disease.[31,32] Subsequent research has revealed that estrogen's cardiovascular-protective effects are due to its ability to improve blood cholesterol by raising HDL (the "good" cholesterol), lowering LDL (the "bad" cholesterol), and lowering total cholesterol.[33] These changes definitely decrease a woman's risk of cardiovascular disease.

The cardiovascular effects of combination hormone replacement therapy still seem unresolved. One study reported that adding a progestin (Provera) to estrogen (HRT) canceled the beneficial effects on cholesterol that estrogen alone produces.[34] A second study reported that some forms of synthetic progesterone reversed estrogen's beneficial effects, but that Provera did not.[35]

We acknowledge that heart attacks and other forms of cardiovascular disease are major killers, and promising therapies should be well researched and evaluated. However, we think that it is important for women to know that the long-term effects of estrogen therapy (ERT or HRT) are still not well known, and that there are definitely some increased risks associated with its use. In fact, it appears that doctors have enrolled millions of women in what may be considered to be one big on-going experiment.

The health aspects of the breast cancer prevention program presented in this book (which includes a health-oriented low-fat diet, appropriate nutritional supplements, and regular exercise) are also the things that help to prevent heart disease. For women who don't want to make these diet and lifestyle changes, estrogen replacement may be an acceptable therapy to reduce cardiovascular risks. However, that choice obviously does not embrace the breast cancer prevention program. Now let's examine the use of hormone replacement therapy in the treatment of osteoporosis.

❧ Hormone Replacement Therapy and Osteoporosis

Each year women experience approximately 1.2 million osteoporotic fractures at an estimated cost of over $6 billion.[36] Since the 1970s estrogen (ERT) or estrogen plus a progestin (HRT) has been given to millions of women to help prevent osteoporosis. Although estrogen is successful at slowing down the advancement of osteoporosis, no research has ever shown that it can stop or reverse its progression.

The results of recent research reported in the *New England Journal of Medicine* show that taking estrogen for just five or ten years after menopause does not effectively prevent women from having hip fractures in their later years because once estrogen is stopped, bone loss proceeds at its usual pace.[37] Thus, by the time a woman reaches her mid-seventies, when susceptibility to hip fractures is greatest, there is little difference in bone density between women who have used hormone replacement and those who have not. So for maximum protection from osteoporotic fractures, women have to continue taking estrogen for the rest of their lives. However, as was previously mentioned, some studies report that taking hormone replacement for longer periods of time significantly increases one's risk to breast cancer.

❧ Natural Progesterone and Osteoporosis

In 1990, John R. Lee, M.D., published the results of a landmark study on the use of natural progesterone in the treatment of osteoporosis.[38] The participants included one hundred postmenopausal women ranging in age from thirty-eight to eighty-three. At the beginning of the study the average age was 65.2 years old, and the average number of years since menopause was sixteen. A majority of the women had already experienced a loss in height, some as much as five inches. All of the women were followed clinically for over three years, and sixty-three of the patients were able to have their bone density monitored by a relatively new technology called dual photon absorptiometry.

The women were instructed to rub a small dose of cream containing 3 percent natural progesterone into their skin at bedtime for twelve to fourteen days each month. Most of the women were also taking a low dose of estrogen. They were encouraged to eat a healthy diet, take some recommended nutritional supplements, and exercise twenty to thirty minutes three times per week.

The results of this study were quite astounding. Within three months most patients were expressing an improved sense of well-being. During the three-year study patient height was stabilized, aches and pains diminished, mobility and energy levels increased, and normal libido returned. As an added bonus, there were no side effects.

The most dramatic finding was that bone densitometry studies actually showed an increase in bone density. Dr. Lee reported that it was common to see a 10 percent increase in bone density in the first six to twelve months, followed by an annual increase of 3 to 5 percent until bone density stabilized at the levels of healthy thirty-five-year-olds. Several patients showed a remarkable 20 to 25 percent increase in bone density during the first year. Another very significant result was that the occurrence of osteoporotic fractures dropped to zero.

Now, if natural progesterone is so great, why haven't you heard about it and why hasn't your doctor prescribed it for you? The answer to this question will take us into some very sensitive and controversial issues dealing with the politics and economics of our health-care system.

Since naturally occurring substances cannot be patented, pharmaceutical companies are not motivated to research and develop a product like natural progesterone. Unfortunately, the system as it currently works puts economic considerations ahead of health concerns. Therefore, we need to change our values to change the system. Somehow we need to pressure our political representatives to transform how the FDA and the NCI function. The government needs to create incentives so drug companies will be willing to research products like natural progesterone. Also, a much higher percentage of research dollars needs to be appropriated for therapies that offer prevention rather than for development of more drugs for after-the-fact treatment.

✿ Ongoing Research

Recent studies suggest that when estradiol is metabolized in the liver, some of its metabolites may actually be more carcinogenic than estradiol itself.[39] More research is needed to understand how the various forms of estrogen are metabolized and how women can maximize their protection against the toxicity of estrogen metabolites.

Another important area of research that is required is the measurement of the urinary excretion of estrogens. In such studies the level of estriol is compared to the combined level of estrone and estradiol. Researchers refer to this as comparing the level of noncarcinogenic estrogens to the level of procarcinogenic estrogens. Healthy women have high estriol excretion, whereas women with breast cancer have low estriol and high estradiol plus estrone excretion.[40] In the future, a test measuring urinary estrogen levels may provide an important indicator of a woman's risk for breast cancer.

❧ *Summary*

Whether or not to begin hormone replacement therapy is a difficult decision for many women to make. We feel that women should be aware of the risks associated with this type of therapy and should also be informed about their options. Natural progesterone and estriol are two important options that are usually not presented to most women. We hope that the information in this chapter will help you make the healthiest and best decisions for yourself.

Diet: Eat Right for Life

Can what you eat either promote or protect you from breast cancer? Literally hundreds, if not thousands, of studies have examined the relationship between various aspects of our diets and breast cancer. Although this topic is one that stirs up great controversy, we feel that some important answers are beginning to emerge. Results from worldwide research suggest that dietary fat, fiber, and sugar each have some influence on the risk of developing breast cancer. In addition to these dietary components, this chapter will discuss the new anticancer compounds called phytochemicals found in many fruits and vegetables and the benefits of a vegetarian diet compared to the standard American diet (SAD).

♨ Government Alarm

In 1976 the U.S. Senate Select Committee on Nutrition and Human Needs was organized to study eating habits and dietary trends in America and the health effects of the modern American diet. In January 1977 the results of this landmark study, titled *Dietary Goals for the United States*, were made public.

The report made the following alarming observation: "During this century, the composition of the average diet in the United States has changed radically. Complex carbohydrates—fruit, vegetables, and grain products—which were the mainstay of the diet, now play a minority role. At the same time, fat and sugar consumption have risen to the point where these two dietary elements alone now comprise at least 60 percent of the total calorie intake."[1]

The study's concluding statement said, "Most major health problems today are diet related. Almost all of the health problems underlying the leading causes of death in the United States could be modified by improvements in the diet. The eating patterns of this century represent a public health concern as critical as any now before us."

Even though we as a nation still have horrendous eating habits, this study was responsible for stimulating a great deal of scientific research into the relationship between diet and disease. It is now generally recognized that diet does play a role in the causation of certain cancers, especially breast cancer, and substantial progress has been made in identifying some of the major dietary cancer risk factors.

The standard American diet is killing people. Women, if you accept the challenge to take charge of your health and prevent breast cancer, one of the most important and effective things you can do is change your diet.

A substantial body of research now suggests that high-fat, low-fiber diets, like those consumed in the United States, increase cancer risk, while plant-based diets rich in fruits, vegetables, legumes, and whole grains are protective. In fact, the fat content of the average American diet is approximately 38 to 42 percent.[2]

✸ *Dietary Fat*

Targeting dietary fat as a risk factor for breast cancer makes scientific sense. In the past decade, scientists have gained a new understanding of the intimate relationship between body fat and female hormones. Although fat may feel like dead weight on your tummies and thighs, it is chemically quite active. You might recall from previous chapters that fat cells make estrogen, which promotes breast cancer.

Most epidemiological studies on breast cancer have shown that high fat–consuming societies have higher rates of carcinogenic malignancy.[3] However, in 1992 the authors of the much-publicized Nurses' Health Study caused great controversy when they reported finding no such link.[4] On evaluation, the Nurses' study has been criticized because the lowest fat diets were only in the range of 29 to 30 percent fat, whereas diets in Asia, where breast cancer is much lower, contain only 15 to 20 percent fat.

In his book *Save Yourself from Breast Cancer*, Robert Kradjian, M.D., makes the following comment about the Nurses' Health Study: "This report has done incalculable damage to responsible efforts to reduce the incidence of breast cancer in American women."[5] Dr. Kradjian also addresses a point that we continue to stress. Data from the worldwide epidemiological literature clearly and consistently show that dietary fat must be 20 percent or less (the "20 percent solution") in order for the individual to gain meaningful protection against breast cancer.

The relationship between dietary fat and breast cancer is so important that we have devoted Chapter 10 to it.

✸ *Fiber Fights Cancer*

Fiber is the partially indigestible carbohydrate material (formally called roughage) that occurs abundantly in fruits, vegetables, legumes, and whole grains. It consists of substances such as cellulose, lignin, gum, and pectin that provide structure and strength to plant cells. Even though fiber is mostly indigestible, it is a vital component in a healthy diet, primarily because it provides bulk and increases the water content in the stool.

Fiber provides important protection against breast cancer because it also has a mechanism that works to decrease the amount of estrogen in a woman's body. Estrogens circulating in the blood pass through the liver, where they are bound into biologically inactive compounds. These inactive estrogen complexes are then passed via the bile into the intestines for excretion. However, intestinal bacteria free up much of this estrogen, making it available for reabsorption.[6]

Recent studies suggest that the amount of fiber in the diet affects the activity of intestinal bacteria, which in turn affects the amount of reabsorbed estrogens. In meat-eating women, the bacteria are more capable of freeing up the previously bound estrogen, increasing both reabsorption and breast cancer risk. On the other hand, intestinal bacteria in vegetarians free up less estrogen, and these women excrete more estrogen in the feces.[7]

In addition to these effects on intestinal bacteria, excretion of fecal estrogens can be enhanced by binding to certain types of fiber in the intestinal tract. The water-insoluble fibers that occur in high concentrations in vegetarian diets have a high capacity for binding both estradiol and estrone.[8]

By increasing the bulk and water content in the gastrointestinal tract, fiber also speeds up the transit time of the stool through the intestines. Faster transit through the intestines decreases the amount of time that estrogens and other carcinogens remain in the bowel, thereby reducing the chance they will be reabsorbed.

❧ Constipation

Millions of women have digestive problems and regularly use laxatives. Is it possible that women's digestive problems could be contributing to breast cancer? This issue was directly addressed in an article in *The Lancet* by Drs. Petrakis and King.[9] They note: "In the past, many physicians believed that bacterial fermentation in the large bowel led to autointoxication through the formation and absorption of toxic waste products. Furthermore, it was thought that this process was causal in many diseases which were likely to result from consumption of a Western diet which contains large amounts of meat and refined carbohydrates."

During the first two decades of this century, a number of distinguished surgeons were writing about the relationship between constipation and breast problems, including cancer, in medical journals. For example, in 1912, British surgeon Dr. W. Arbuthnot Lane published an article in the *British Medical Journal* listing the main symptoms of chronic constipation.[10] Here are his comments on breast symptoms: "The changes in the breast which are always present in a varying degree when autointoxication has existed for any length of time are very characteristic. Indeed, they may be regarded as a measure of the amount of poisoning to which the tissues of the body have been exposed."

He continues: "The change begins as a hardening in the upper and outer zone of the left breast, and later in the same area on the right side. As time goes on this hardening becomes a more marked feature and extends to the rest of the breast, the change in the upper and outer segment being still in excess of that in the rest of the breast."

He ends by saying: "Later cystic and inflammatory changes arise, followed after an interval of time by intracystic growths or by cancer. In almost every case of cancer of the breast a previous history of chronic constipation can be demonstrated."

Another interesting paper on this topic, entitled "Benign Mammary Tumors and Intestinal Toxemia," was presented by Dr. William Bainbridge at the thirty-third annual meeting of the American Association of Obstetricians, Gynecologists, and Abdominal Surgeons in 1920.[11] Dr. Bainbridge reported on a series of twenty-five patients with abnormal breast changes apparently caused by autointoxication. He stated: "When these cases are seen in their early stages the breast condition is often overlooked; when they have developed into a more easily recognized state, frequently a diagnosis of malignant disease is made." Dr. Bainbridge also noted that these cases of chronic intestinal toxemia produce a condensation or lobular hardening of the upper, outer quadrants of the breasts and that terms such as *toxic breasts* and *lumpy breasts* are descriptive of this condition.

In his summary, Dr. Bainbridge stated that intestinal toxemia produces definite abnormal changes in the breast tissue. He also noted that various forms of treatment which result in curing the intestinal constipation often result in the complete return of the lumpy or toxic breasts to normal. His closing statement is especially important: "In this connection, an important question must be noted: Would an early recognition of a toxic breast and timely and efficient treatment of the underlying intestinal causes, tend to lessen the danger of malignant degeneration? If this is so, then we have here an important contributory factor in the etiology of cancer of the breast."

The present-day research by Drs. Petrakis and King supports these earlier clinical observations, suggesting that there is an association between severe constipation and breast disease. In their study, they found that healthy women with a history of chronic constipation had a higher incidence of abnormal cells in the breast tissue.[12]

These previous reports are very suggestive and may help to explain the link between a poor-quality, low-fiber diet, digestive problems, and an increased risk for breast cancer.

Hence, we may be starting to understand how such a diet is a major contributor to the epidemic of breast cancer. The low-fiber diet causes constipation. This results in an increased reabsorption of estrogens, which stimulates breast tissue abnormalities.

A number of studies have demonstrated the fiber intake of different dietary patterns. One study showed that vegetarians, on average, consumed 28 grams of fiber daily, whereas people consuming the meat-based standard American diet averaged only 12 grams of fiber daily.[13]

Another study reported significant reductions in estrogen concentrations in the blood of premenopausal women when their usual diet was supplemented with an amount of wheat bran that approximately doubled their daily fiber intake.[14]

It is generally accepted that a high-fiber diet decreases the risk of colon cancer, cardiovascular disease, and diabetes. Now there is direct evidence that the amount of fiber in the diet also influences breast cancer risk in both pre- and postmenopausal women.

ᴥ *Phytochemicals Fight Cancer*

Phytochemicals are the nutritional breakthrough of the 1990s. On April 25, 1994, the cover of *Newsweek* magazine read, "Better Than Vitamins, Can 'Phytochemicals' Prevent Cancer?" Phytochemicals are substances that occur only in plant foods, and although not classified as nutrients, many of them have substantial anticancer benefits, and in general, they profoundly affect our health.

One of these compounds, indole-3-carbinol (I3C), which occurs only in cruciferous vegetables, specifically protects against breast cancer. A study at the Foundation for Preventive Oncology in New York gave twelve subjects 350 to 500 mg of indole-3-carbinol (the equivalent of 10 to 12 ounces of raw cabbage or brussels sprouts) daily for one week. They found that the indole-3-carbinol metabolized estrogen into a harmless metabolite rather than the active form linked to cancer.[15] Subsequently, the researchers duplicated the effect of this cruciferous vegetable extract on a larger group of women and obtained the same estrogen-lowering results.

Your mother's encouragement to eat your broccoli was not unfounded. A phytochemical called sulforaphane found in broccoli and other cruciferous vegetables has also been proven to have important anticancer properties. Sulforaphane was found to increase the synthesis of an important group of enzymes that are capable of detoxifying cancer-causing compounds.[16]

Drs. Zhang and Talalay at Johns Hopkins achieved over a 50 percent reduction in the occurrence of mammary tumors in animals treated with sulforaphane. Evidently, sulforaphane was responsible for the neutralization of carcinogens before they could trigger tumor growth. The authors of this study stated: "The induction of detoxication enzymes by sulforaphane may be a significant component of the anticarcinogenic action of broccoli."[17]

Noncruciferous vegetables can also be helpful. Tomatoes contain a substance called lycopene which may prove to be more powerful than beta-carotene in preventing some forms of cancer. Two additional phytochemicals in tomatoes, p-coumaric acid and chlorogenic acid, have been shown to protect against certain types of stomach cancer.

Soybeans are another rich source of dietary anticarcinogens. Scientists have identified five phytochemicals in soybeans that provide protection against cancer. One scientist researching the value of soy phytochemicals feels that one serving of soy foods per day may be the most effective dietary means of preventing breast cancer. The National Cancer Institute is so excited about the importance of phytochemicals that it has launched a multimillion-dollar project to identify, isolate, and study them. Chapter 12 contains a complete discussion of soy foods and their breast cancer prevention characteristics.

But, why wait? It will take years before enough studies have been done for scientists and organizations like the NCI, the FDA, and the American Medical Association to make recommendations. You can start today to include more fresh fruits and vegetables in your diet. Cruciferous vegetables, including broccoli, cabbage, cauliflower, and brussels sprouts, are extremely rich sources of these newly discovered anticancer phytochemicals. We suggest you include some in your diet every day. Rotate among salads, vegetable soups, stews, and stir-fries.

❧ Sugar

The authors of another study suggest that there may be a connection between sugar consumption and the risk for breast cancer.[18] Data for this study were obtained by examining both mortality and detailed food consumption statistics from twenty-one countries belonging to the Organization for Economic Cooperation and Development.

A strong association was found between sugar consumption and breast cancer in postmenopausal women. Even though associations are not causations, they are more likely to be taken seriously if a plausible mechanism exists. The connecting link between sugar and breast cancer is insulin. The effect of insulin on normal breast tissue is similar to estrogen and prolactin. All three of these hormones are necessary for the growth and proliferation of breast tissue.

The fact that women with adult onset diabetes have a higher incidence of breast cancer supports the sugar/breast cancer hypothesis.[19]

❧ The Benefits of Vegetarian Diets

We now have a scientific explanation for why vegetarian diets help to protect against breast and some other forms of cancer. Vegetarian diets, which are lower in fat and sugar and higher in fiber, tend to lower a woman's level of circulating estrogen. Conversely, the high-fat, high-sugar, low-fiber standard American diet increases estrogen levels, thereby increasing women's risk for breast cancer.

In the September 1992 issue of *Nutrition and Cancer*, researchers from the University of California at Berkeley published an analysis of the results from 128 previously published studies related to the cancer-preventive effects of fruit and vegetable consumption. They noted that "the evidence of an association between fruit and vegetable consumption and cancer prevention is exceptionally strong and consistent." In their conclusion, they stated that few if any risk factors besides smoking confer the kind of risks posed by *low* vegetable and fruit consumption.[20]

The analysis of 128 studies makes a strong case for the cancer-protective effect of vegetarian diets. In light of this inverse relationship (low fruit and vegetable intake equals a much higher cancer risk), American eating habits are a disaster. Documentation from a one-day sampling of 12,000 Americans in the second National Health and Nutrition Examination Survey (NHANES II) revealed that 41 percent ate no fruit on the day of the sampling, and only 25 percent reported eating a fruit or vegetable rich in either vitamin C or beta-carotene.[21]

In summary, vegetarian diets provide a number of health benefits. By switching to more of a vegetarian diet, you will increase your intake of anticancer nutrients and the important anticancer phytochemicals. A health-oriented vegetarian diet also increases your quantity of fiber and decreases your intake of fat and sugar, all of which will decrease your risk for breast cancer.

↔ How to Avoid Toxins

Another very important factor in considering switching to a vegetarian diet has to do with the amount of toxic chemicals ingested. In fact, the primary source of pesticides and other toxic chemicals for most Americans is the consumption of high-fat foods including commercial meat, eggs, and dairy products. These toxins are fat soluble, hence they accumulate in the fatty tissues of these animals and are passed into our food supply.

In a paper titled "Organochlorine Contamination of Breast Milk," the authors state that over 95 percent of all the toxic chemicals ingested in the American diet come from meat, fish, eggs, and dairy products.[22]

In *How to Survive in America the Poisoned*, pesticide authority Lewis Regenstein writes: "Meat contains approximately 14 times more pesticides than do plant foods; dairy products $5^1/_2$ times more. Thus by eating foods of animal origin, one ingests greatly concentrated amounts of hazardous chemicals."[23]

The link between environmental toxins and breast cancer will be explored more deeply in Chapter 13. However, from the information cited, you can see that one of the most important aspects of a vegetarian diet is that it is both low fat and low pesticide.

One of the classic questions about vegetarian diets is whether or not you get enough protein. This concern is unjustified and can be laid to rest. In the 1970s, Frances Moore Lappé's best-selling book *Diet for a Small Planet* introduced the world to the concept of protein combining. This taught people how the strengths and weaknesses of the amino acid contents in two plant foods could complement each other. In the introduction to the tenth-year anniversary edition of her book, the author clearly states that adherence to protein combining is not necessary.[24] In fact, we now know that if people eat several servings of grains, beans, and vegetables throughout the day, it is virtually impossible to be protein deficient.

The only nutritional concern related to a vegetarian diet has to do with vitamin B_{12}. Strict vegetarians should either take a vitamin B_{12} supplement or get an occasional B_{12} intermuscular injection.

❧ *Organic versus Commercial Foods*

Another important dietary issue to consider is organic versus commercial foods. We unhesitatingly recommend organic when possible, for two very compelling reasons.

The first reason relates to the quantity of nutrients in foods. According to the findings of a recent study published in the *Journal of Applied Nutrition*, organic foods have about double the nutrient value of the same type of commercial foods.[25]

The second benefit is that organically grown foods are raised without the use of pesticides and insecticides. Hence, not only can organic food increase your protection from breast cancer through better nutrition, but it will also protect you against some environmental risks.

Organic farming is slowly increasing year by year; however, in many areas the demand does not support distribution. Magazines like *Vegetarian Times* and *Natural Health* often list companies that ship organic produce, grains, and a variety of other products anywhere in the United States. Going organic may require a little extra time and money. We hope you will find that this extra effort increases your enjoyment of natural foods, as well as providing long-term health benefits.

✹ *The Breast Cancer Prevention Diet*

What to eat, what not to eat, what causes cancer, what doesn't cause cancer—it can be a truly confusing area with advice coming from so many different sources. It is hard to know who and what to believe. Although assimilating a cancer-protective diet into your life may require time and education, a few basic parameters can serve as a guide and help you get started. The majority of your diet should come from plant-based foods, which include fresh vegetables, fresh fruit, whole grains, breads, and pastas made from whole grain, whole grain cereals, beans, and legumes. Add variety by exploring grains such as quinoa, millet, barley, buckwheat (as in soba noodles), and wild rice. There is also a wide range of beans and legumes and an infinite number of ways to prepare them. Keep fruit juices to a minimum (high sugar content), and enjoy fresh vegetable juices frequently.

Should you wish to have some flesh food in your diet, fish is preferable. In the process of eliminating animal foods from your diet, make sure that what you buy is lean and raised free of hormones and antibiotics.

Avoid milk products as much as possible, using nonfat and low-fat options when available. Remember, in addition to increasing *your* fat cells, the fat content in these foods carries the highest concentration of pesticide and hormone residuals. Organic cheese and butter are available in some areas, and low-fat cheese can be found nationwide. Your egg usage should also be minimal, and again you should make a special point to buy eggs from hormone-free chickens.

Avoid all white flour products, which include most pastas, prepared mixes, crackers, cookies, and commercial breads. These foods are bereft of nutrients and play havoc with your digestive system, particularly with regard to elimination. It is also important to minimize or delete use of sugar, alcohol, and caffeine.

The type of fat you use is one of the more important dietary considerations. The best oils to use are expeller pressed, unfiltered, and monounsaturated, such as olive, canola, or peanut oil. If you can find them in dark bottles, all the better. It is best to keep them refrigerated. This reduces the possibility of exposure to light and oxygen, which make oils dangerous to your health. Minimize use and intake of polyunsaturated vegetable oils such as safflower, sunflower, and corn oils, as they are more likely to become rancid than the monounsaturates and are implicated in cancer incidence. It is best never to cook with flaxseed oil; however, it can be blended with another oil for salad dressings if made in small portions, covered, and used within days.

Totally avoid all products containing partially hydrogenated fats and oils, especially margarine and shortening. This will be tricky if you do not have good health food stores around because all commercial cookies, crackers, cakes, and chips contain partially hydrogenated oil in order to extend shelf life. When there is a choice to be made between butter and margarine, butter is best, but use as little as possible.

This is not a healing diet. For that, we would suggest a plan far more radical than this, such as completely cutting out all animal proteins, especially milk products, as well as sugar, alcohol, and caffeine. Our goal is to help you avoid the diseases, particularly breast cancer, associated with daily and excessive intake of high-fat, high-sugar, animal-based diets. Therefore, it is a good idea to make changes in your diet at a rate that feels comfortable to you. Sometimes a radical change can stimulate feelings of deprivation, which are often followed by overeating or bingeing on sweet and fatty foods. Assuming you have your own best interests at heart, you can gradually begin to enjoy the flavors of fresh natural food, and you'll be amazed how the standard American diet, in time, has less and less appeal. As you educate yourself and experiment with a natural foods diet, you will become the expert on the diet best suited for your particular needs and desires. We have listed numerous books and publications in Appendix C to assist you in this journey.

✦ *Summary*

An ever-increasing body of research indicates that a vegetarian-based diet is substantially healthier than the standard American diet, which is based on animal proteins. Balanced, whole-food vegetarian diets (organic when possible) will increase your intake of nutrients, anticancer phytochemicals, and fiber, as well as decrease intakes of fat, sugar, and environmental toxins. Eat well and stay healthy . . . for life!

Antioxidants: The First Line of Defense

Antioxidant nutrients are effective anticancer agents because they can disarm, or neutralize, cancer-causing substances called free radicals. This chapter will explain antioxidants and free radicals, and discuss how to utilize antioxidant nutrients as the cornerstone of a breast cancer prevention program.

In 1956, Denham Harman, M.D., Ph.D., published a hypothesis he called the Free Radical Theory of Aging.[1] His theory enabled us to make a quantum leap in our understanding of how and why we age.

In order to understand free radicals, we need to discuss a little chemistry. Throughout the entire universe everything is held together by pairs of electrons called chemical bonds. These electrons are spinning in opposite directions at incredibly high rates of speed (nearly the speed of light, or 186,000 miles/second).

When an electron is displaced or somehow dislodged, we have a free radical. By definition, a free radical is a molecule, or a molecular fragment, with a free or unpaired electron. At the cellular level, a free radical, spinning wildly without its mate, rampages through your system and quickly rips an electron from something else in order to regain its stability. However, in the process of stealing an electron for its own stability, the free radical damages or destroys something else. This free radical damage is literally the cause of the aging process. In order to understand the true nature of free radical reactions, visualize the following scene.

ᴥ *Mousetraps and Ping-Pong Balls*

Picture an entire football field neatly filled with row after row of mousetraps. Each mousetrap is cocked in its ready-to-spring position, and a Ping-Pong ball rests on the springing arm of each trap.

As you stand contemplating this scene, you pull one extra Ping-Pong ball from your pocket. This ball represents a single free radical. You throw it out onto the field and watch it set off a chain reaction. Within seconds there are literally hundreds of thousands of Ping-Pong balls flying around. This is the true nature of free radical reactions. They are self-generating, self-perpetuating chain reactions that are capable of inflicting tremendous amounts of damage at the cellular level.

Some of the major sources of free radical exposure and/or generation include cigarette smoke, trace amounts of pesticides and insecticides in our food and water supplies, lipid peroxidation (oxygen attacking fats in the body), any kind of stress (physical or emotional), and suboptimal levels of oxygen in the cells and tissues of the body, as well as our body's natural metabolism.

It has been well documented that free radicals are capable of causing cancer. Therefore, one of the important ways that people can prevent cancer is to minimize their exposure to free radicals and/or free radical–generating substances. However, we all know that in today's world it is impossible to live a totally pure, stress-free life. So what is a person to do?

Fortunately, nature has provided us with a group of substances that can counteract the destructive effects of free radicals. These "good guys" are called the antioxidant nutrients.

❧ Antioxidant Nutrients

The four main antioxidant nutrients are vitamin C, vitamin E, beta-carotene, and the trace mineral selenium. Although other nutrients possess antioxidant activity, these four are the most important ones. They are also the four main anticancer nutrients and play a major role in keeping the immune system strong.

The main job of antioxidant nutrients is to do battle with and neutralize free radicals. Thus, antioxidant nutrients function like an alert police force, always on guard, ready to protect you. When an antioxidant neutralizes a free radical, it actually accepts or takes on an extra electron. This changes the electrical charge of the antioxidant, which renders it useless. The antioxidant sacrifices itself, but in the process saves the life of a cell that would have been damaged or destroyed by the free radical.

Therefore, antioxidant nutrients are continually being depleted in the process of protecting you. Optimal intake of antioxidant nutritional supplements is your front line of defense. Whenever you are deficient in an antioxidant nutrient, you are vulnerable to free radical chain-reaction destruction, which results in the aging process.

❧ What Is Optimal?

How do you determine optimal antioxidant intake? That is a very difficult question to answer. Prospective human studies have not been done because they would take many years and would be far too expensive. However, what can be said with assurance is that intake of antioxidant nutrients should be substantially higher than the Recommended Daily Allowance (RDA) levels.

To date more than ninety studies have shown a link between higher intakes of vitamins and a lower risk for cancer. Studies show that women who develop breast cancer have lower blood levels of the antioxidant nutrients than matched healthy controls.[2] Also, a large Chinese study showed that dietary antioxidants provide a protective effect which helps in the prevention of breast cancer.[3]

Because these antioxidant nutrients are so important, we will take a look at each one individually.

✒ *Vitamin C*

In September 1990 the National Cancer Institute cosponsored a landmark symposium in which about forty papers were delivered on the relationship between vitamin C and cancer. One of the most important aspects of this conference was the basic fact that the NCI, after years of ignoring vitamin C, is now acknowledging its potential in the prevention and treatment of cancer.

Two-time Nobel Prize winner Dr. Linus Pauling gave the opening speech at the conference. He told the audience that his initial interest in the value of large doses of vitamin C was mainly due to his discovery of the amazing fact that most animals manufacture the human equivalent of about 10,000 milligrams (mg) of vitamin C per day.[4]

Dr. Balz Frei began his presentation by pointing out that lipid peroxidation and free radical reactions can cause cancer. He then discussed his research studies in which he exposed human blood plasma to various types of known cancer-causing chemicals, including cigarette smoke. Dr. Frei reported that as long as sufficient vitamin C was present in the blood, no cancer-causing chemical reactions like lipid peroxidation occurred. However, as soon as vitamin C was depleted, lipid peroxidation activity began again.[5]

Dr. Gladys Block from the National Cancer Institute ended the conference with a paper that attracted worldwide attention. She presented an impressive summary of all the human epidemiological studies on vitamin C's ability to prevent cancer. Out of forty-six studies, thirty-three showed that vitamin C had a statistically significant preventive effect against cancer at various sites, with high intakes providing about two times the protective effect of low intakes.[6]

In another important paper, researchers examined twelve case-controlled studies in a major meta-analysis of dietary factors and breast cancer. In the conclusion, the authors state: "Vitamin C intake had the most consistent and statistically significant inverse association with breast cancer risk."[7] This means the more vitamin C a woman ingests, the less chance she has of developing breast cancer, and conversely, the less vitamin C one ingests, the more chance there is of developing breast cancer.

A recent study that documented vitamin C's life extension capabilities is also worth mentioning. Researchers at UCLA evaluated 11,348 adults and found that men with the highest intake of vitamin C live approximately six years longer than men with the lowest consumption of vitamin C, while women with the highest vitamin C intakes live approximately one year longer.[8]

In summary, a substantial body of research now shows that higher intakes of vitamin C confer a significant protective effect in the prevention of various cancers, including breast cancer. A number of health professionals suggest eating a healthy diet and taking about 1,000 mg of vitamin C per meal as a nutritional supplement.

** *Vitamin E*

Vitamin E is our most abundant and efficient fat-soluble antioxidant nutrient. It resides primarily in the fatty layer of cellular membranes, where it protects against potentially cancer-causing, lipid peroxidation free radical reactions.

Recently, scientists have begun to understand the importance of studying nutrient interactions in the body. For example, when vitamin E scavenges a free radical, the electrical charge is changed and the vitamin E is essentially dead. It is now known that vitamin C can "repair" or regenerate vitamin E back to its active antioxidant form again.[9,10]

In one study, excess dietary vitamin E effectively reduced chemically induced breast cancer in rats.[11] In another study, rats fed diets with either no vitamin E or one-half the minimum recommended level had a significantly greater incidence of mammary tumors compared to those whose diets contained either adequate or excessive amounts of vitamin E.[12] Vitamin E alone was not effective in reducing chemically induced mammary tumors in rats fed a high-fat diet,[13] but in a similar study vitamin E, although ineffective by itself, did enhance selenium's effectiveness in reducing chemically induced mammary tumors in rats fed high-fat diets.[14]

Another study looked at various antioxidants in relation to the future risk of breast cancer. The results showed that low levels of plasma vitamin E were strongly associated with a higher risk of developing breast cancer.[15]

In a study evaluating the risk of female cancers, it was found that women with lower serum levels of vitamin E had an increased cancer risk. The authors of this study state that low serum vitamin E levels can be used to predict the development of some cancers in women. However, this association was reported to be stronger for cancers occurring in epithelial cells but is less reliable in predicting epithelial cell cancers in hormone-related sites such as the uterus, ovaries, and the breast.[16] Epithelial cells are the cells that line the internal surface of glands and organs.

The results of some studies failed to support these findings; therefore, to date, the effectiveness of vitamin E in preventing breast cancer remains somewhat controversial and inconclusive.

Vitamin E plays many roles in our biological systems. Therefore, we should not let the breast cancer issue be the only reason to consider taking vitamin E. For example, numerous studies have reported vitamin E's ability to boost the immune system.

Researchers looking at the major risk factors for cardiovascular disease recently published a study that sent shock waves throughout the medical and scientific communities around the world. They found out that the number-one risk factor for cardiovascular disease is not high blood pressure or elevated blood cholesterol levels, but rather the amount of circulating serum vitamin E in the blood. Evaluations of more than 130,000 people with no history of heart disease found that taking 100 IU of vitamin E daily for at least two years lowered the risk of heart disease by 46 percent in women and 26 percent in men.[17]

Although the studies we have just discussed have not related directly to breast cancer, they do show how important vitamin E is in promoting and maintaining good health. A dosage of between four hundred IU to eight hundred IU of natural vitamin E daily is considered appropriate for a prevention program.

❧ Beta-carotene and Vitamin A

Beta-carotene and vitamin A are chemically related. Beta-carotene occurs only in fruits and vegetables, whereas all the vitamin A in our diets comes from animal sources. Both have gained recognition as important nutrients in the prevention and treatment of cancer.

Structurally, beta-carotene is two molecules of vitamin A linked together head-to-head. Whenever the body needs more vitamin A, enzymes split a molecule of beta-carotene in half, yielding two molecules of vitamin A.

Approximately 90 percent of all cancers originate in epithelial cells. These are the cells that make up your skin, the lining of all your glands and organs, and other thin tissues throughout the body. This includes the linings of the globules and ducts within the breast tissue. An accumulating body of research now shows that both beta-carotene and vitamin A help to prevent mutations in epithelial cells, which can lead to cancer, as well as strengthen the immune system.[18]

Although earlier studies tended to focus on vitamin A, recent evidence indicates that beta-carotene is the more important anticancer agent. This conclusion stems from the relatively recent discovery that beta-carotene (but not vitamin A) is a powerful antioxidant capable of neutralizing a very dangerous type of free radical called singlet oxygen.[19,20]

Many studies have been published showing decreased rates of cancer at various sites in individuals with higher intakes of beta-carotene;[21] however, in this book we want to focus primarily on the relationship between beta-carotene and breast cancer.

❧ Breast Cancer

Several studies have shown that either high dietary and/or serum level of beta-carotene is associated with a decreased risk of breast cancer. An Italian study reported a strong inverse relationship between intakes of beta-carotene–rich foods and breast cancer risk.[22] A study of women in Athens, Greece, showed that higher intakes of both vitamin A and beta-carotene contributed to a reduced risk of breast cancer.[23] Results from an Australian study found no correlation for vitamin A, but supported the previous study's findings by reporting that higher intakes of beta-carotene provided statistically significant decreased risk for breast cancer.[24]

Beta-carotene's power as an anticancer nutrient seems to be due to its antioxidant activity, not to its function as the precursor to vitamin A. Beta-carotene's proven ability to quench free radicals in the epithelial membranes of the breast tissues makes it one of the most important nutrients in the prevention of breast cancer.

A dosage of 25,000 IU per meal (75,000 IU per day) as a nutritional supplement should be adequate for a preventive program. However, it is also advisable to eat a diet rich in fresh green leafy vegetables to get regular intakes of the other mixed carotenoids from nature.

Before leaving the beta-carotene topic, we would like to comment on the highly publicized Finnish study published in April 1994, in which beta-carotene failed to provide any protection against lung cancer.[25] This study was poorly designed. Beta-carotene would not be expected to reverse lung cancers that had probably already been growing for a number of years in long-term heavy smokers. Also, the dosages of beta-carotene that were given were far too small and the length of the study too short to expect earth-shattering results.

Health professionals from around the world were disappointed that a respected publication like the *New England Journal of Medicine* would allow such a poorly designed study to be published. It was also unfortunate that the media chose to sensationalize this story in such a way as to question the effectiveness of all nutritional supplements, as evidenced by the April 25, 1994, cover story in *Newsweek* magazine entitled "Are Supplements Still Worth Taking?" One piece of bad science cannot overturn years of research reporting the benefits of beta-carotene; it remains one of our most important antioxidant, anticancer nutrients.

✷ *Selenium*

Recent research has drawn attention to the multiple ways selenium functions as an inhibitor of carcinogenesis. It is one of the strongest, most versatile anticancer substances known to man. This remarkable anticarcinogenic nutrient has several different mechanisms of action. It boosts the immune system, prevents free radical damage, eliminates toxic heavy metals, and inhibits or modulates the rapid proliferation of cells which is so often seen in breast cancer.

It was only in 1959 that selenium was discovered to be an important essential nutrient. Therefore, we have only had about three decades to begin learning about selenium deficiencies and their effects on our health and longevity.

Selenium first became recognized for its potential in the prevention of breast cancer in the 1970s. In studies with mice prone to developing breast cancer, selenium-supplemented diets produced a remarkable 72 percent reduction in the incidence of mammary tumors.[26]

Another study of particular interest demonstrated that selenium's anticarcinogenic activity is exerted in both the initiation and the promotion phases of carcinogenesis.[27] This suggests that selenium is not only effective in prevention, but can also be used as a chemotherapeutic agent in the treatment of cancer.

GLUTATHIONE PEROXIDASE

Selenium is perhaps best known in its relationship to the enzyme glutathione peroxidase, a major antioxidant detoxification enzyme that protects us from potentially cancer-causing free radicals. Every molecule of this important enzyme contains four atoms of selenium. There are many people who are deficient in their selenium intake and therefore suffer the decreased functional capacity of this important anticancer detoxification mechanism.

HEAVY METAL DETOXIFICATION

Selenium actively detoxifies heavy metals such as mercury, lead, arsenic, cadmium, nickel, and tin. These toxic elements are proven environmental and occupational carcinogens. During the process of detoxifying these substances, selenium gets depleted. It has been suggested that a significant health hazard now exists in industrialized countries because many people get combined exposures to these toxins which significantly exceed the amount of dietary selenium available for detoxification.[28] Thus, a higher intake of selenium will improve heavy metal detoxification and ensure that extra selenium is available for all the other important anticancer and immune system functions it provides.

ANTIPROLIFERATIVE PROPERTIES

Proliferate means "to divide rapidly," which is what happens to cells in breast cancer and other solid-tumor cancers. It has been proposed that selenium exerts some of its anticarcinogenic effects by modulating the rate of cellular division.[29] Slowing the rates of certain phases of cellular division could prevent the expression of cancer genes and create conditions favorable for DNA repair and carcinogen detoxification.

IMMUNE SYSTEM ENHANCEMENT

Another mechanism of anticarcinogenic activity is selenium's ability to stimulate the immune system. Enhancement of the immune system by selenium has been demonstrated in numerous experiments.[30] Selenium-mediated immune system enhancement may increase an individual's resistance to cancer. This makes selenium an important therapeutic agent for both the prevention and treatment of cancer.

EPIDEMIOLOGICAL STUDIES

Numerous epidemiological studies have shown that human cancer mortality is lower in areas where soil concentrations provide adequate dietary intake of selenium. One study divided states and cities in the United States into high, medium, and low selenium groups. The results showed an inverse association between selenium availability and deaths from cancer.[31]

A worldwide study correlated age-adjusted cancer mortalities with selenium intakes calculated from food consumption data by measuring blood selenium levels. In nations of the world and states of the United States, higher rates of cancers of the breast, colon, rectum, prostate, ovary, lung, and leukemia were found in areas with lower levels of selenium.[32]

In another study, blood samples were collected in 1973 from more than 10,000 men and women. Within the next five years, 111 of these individuals developed cancer. It was found that blood selenium levels had been significantly lower in those who subsequently developed cancer. Subjects with selenium levels in the lowest quintile, or 20 percent range, had twice the cancer risk of those in the highest quintile.[33] This study is of great significance because the blood samples were collected prior to the diagnosis of cancer, showing that the lower blood selenium levels were not caused by the cancer, but instead could possibly be related to the cause of the cancer.

BREAST CANCER STUDIES

Several epidemiological studies have specifically shown that women with higher blood levels of selenium have significantly lower rates of breast cancer.[34,35,36]

One study specifically looked at selenium levels in the blood of Japanese and American women with and without breast cancer and fibrocystic disease. This study also demonstrated that low blood selenium levels are associated with increased risk for breast cancer.[37] The results revealed that higher blood selenium levels in healthy Japanese women, compared to healthy American women, were due to differences in dietary intakes.

The average Japanese diet was shown to provide approximately twice the amount of selenium as the average American diet. It has been estimated that a lowering of the individual dietary selenium intake from 250 micrograms (mcg) per day to 125 mcg per day could cause approximately a four- to fivefold increase in the risk for breast cancer.[38] This difference in selenium intake is reflected by the breast cancer rate, which is five times higher in U.S. women than in Japanese women.

A recent study from Sweden showed that higher blood levels

of selenium provided a significantly greater preventive effect against the development of breast cancer in postmenopausal women.[39]

SELENIUM SUPPLEMENTATION

Many areas of the United States have soils that are deficient in selenium. Modern farming techniques continually deplete and do not replace selenium. Also, the increasing environmental problem of acid rain reduces a plant's ability to incorporate selenium.

It is also well known that the milling of grain and other food-processing techniques removes additional selenium from our food supply. Thus, it appears that most people in the United States do not get adequate dietary selenium and that daily nutritional supplementation with selenium can be of major importance in helping to prevent cancer. This is especially relevant for women and the prevention of breast cancer.

Dr. Gerhard Schrauzer is one of the world's most respected scientists studying selenium, and many of his studies have examined the relationship between selenium and breast cancer. According to Dr. Schrauzer, the evidence that selenium protects against cancer is strong enough to justify advising almost everyone to supplement their diets with 250 to 300 mcg of selenium daily. He has said that this would probably result in a substantial reduction in the incidence of breast cancer.

Another study reported that selenium supplements of up to 500 mcg daily can be considered safe for American adults, presuming that the diet itself will provide no more than 250 mcg of selenium daily.[40]

SIDE EFFECTS AND TOXICITY

Selenium is a trace element that can be toxic if excessive levels are taken. The National Research Council reports that toxicity occurs after long-term consumption of 2,400 to 3,000 mcg daily. The symptoms of toxicity include loss of hair, nails and teeth, skin inflammation, lassitude, paralysis, and eventual death. However, selenium toxicity in humans is very rare since the symptoms of excess occur long before the risk of death. The real danger with selenium lies in its deficiency, not its toxicity.

Research over the past two decades has shown that selenium is one of the most powerful nutritional anticancer agents yet discovered. It is also well established that higher intakes of selenium definitely reduce a woman's risk of contracting breast cancer.

⁊ Summary

Antioxidant nutritional supplements are an important part of a breast cancer prevention program. They are easy to incorporate into daily practice and are relatively inexpensive. Simple tests are currently being developed that reportedly will make antioxidant tests as easy as cholesterol testing. But why wait? Start taking antioxidant nutritional supplements now to gain added protection against breast cancer.

Chapter 10

Dietary Fat: The 20 Percent Solution

As a nation, we love fatty foods. Fat makes up about 40 percent of all our consumed calories. Eating this quantity of fat is detrimental to our health in many ways. It is important to remember that while "the fat you eat is the fat you wear" is true, fat represents much more of a problem than physical plumpness. Excess fat consumption creates significant health problems, including shortened life span, more chronic disease, cardiovascular heart disease, strokes, high blood pressure, adult onset (type II) diabetes, and several cancers, including breast cancer.

This chapter will explain what part dietary fat plays in the risk of developing breast cancer. We will describe the types of dietary fats and what part each plays in your health.

OUR MODERN DIET

In spite of a plethora of low-fat, fat-free foods on the grocery shelves, weight-loss counseling companies, weight-loss support groups, and articles from popular magazines and newspapers, we continue to eat large quantities of fat. We are getting fatter—as children and adults. Between 1960 and 1980 adults in the United States had a stable obesity rate of 25 percent. Currently, adult obesity stands at about 33 percent. Along with increasing dietary fat consumption, there is an increasing rate of breast cancer.

Primitive mankind ate wild game, fruits, and plants. This type of diet was very low in fat; probably fewer than 10 percent of its calories were derived from fats. This was the "normal" diet with which mankind developed. Modern humans developed ways to process plants and seeds for the extraction of oil to use in food preparation. Animal husbandry developed to breed and fatten up captive animals for consumption, producing meat with a much higher fat content. For reasons such as these, we began to rapidly increase dietary fat beyond a level for which our genetic makeup was adapted. Now we freely prepare home meals using cooking oils, shortening, butter, and margarine.

Over the past few decades we have become a nation in which both spouses are employed and more meals are eaten outside the home. We have less time for physical activity in our lives and to prepare home-cooked meals. Fast-food franchises are springing up everywhere, providing high-fat foods for adults and children of dual-income families who never seem to have enough time to eat properly. These eateries also provide a large portion of the diet of our adolescents. During adolescent years the developing breasts of girls may have an increased sensitivity to the deleterious effects of such a diet. Cheeseburgers, pizza, tacos, and fried side orders make up much of the adolescent diet. Adults eat these items, too, in addition to steaks, sour cream, butter, oil-saturated salads, and "sinfully" tempting high-fat desserts. We have become habituated to fat-filled food. Let's face it, fat tastes good. It gives food a certain richness, transports and intensifies flavors for our taste buds, fills us up, and keeps us feeling full longer.

❧ *All Calories Are Not Created Equal*

One of the most important lifestyle changes that can lower our risk for breast cancer is to reduce our dietary fat intake. Numerous animal and human studies have shown that the risk for cancers, including breast cancer, increases as dietary fat increases. This holds true whether the dietary fat is measured in daily fat-gram intake or as fat percentage of total calories (fat calories divided by total calories). Remember that each gram of fat contains 9 calories, while each gram of carbohydrate or protein contains 4 calories. Fat is, therefore, the most concentrated form of calories we consume. This means that even small portions of high-fat foods can contain high quantities of calories. In addition, the body's fat cells store excess calories as fat, since fat stores the most calories in the smallest space. If we consume too many calories in the form of fat, the body stores the excess in the fat cells.

When we eat too much carbohydrate or protein, our bodies must convert these excess calories to fat before storage in fat cells. This conversion uses energy (calories). It has been estimated that up to 27 percent of the excess carbohydrate or protein calories are burned up just in the conversion process. Therefore, if an extra 100 calories of carbohydrate are eaten, only 73 calories will be converted to fat and stored in your body. If you eat an extra 100 calories of fat, almost all 100 will be stored. Clearly, all calories are not created equal. In fact, it is very difficult to become obese by eating a low-fat, high-fiber, high–complex carbohydrate, vegetarian noncaloric restricted diet. Without caloric restriction, there is none of the constant hunger one experiences with a low-calorie diet. Without constant hunger pangs, people are able to stick with the healthy way of eating.

❧ *Categories of Dietary Fats*

SATURATED OR UNSATURATED

Most dietary fat can be divided into saturated and unsaturated forms. Unsaturated fats are then divided into monounsaturated and polyunsaturated forms. In China, where breast cancer risk is lower than in the United States, people consume almost twice the percentage of monounsaturated fats as Americans do. The Chinese also consume about one-half the total fat Americans consume. We can conclude that while the total fat in the diet must be lowered, the types of fats consumed are also important.

TRANS FAT

When iron combines with oxygen it forms rust, a material that is worthless and much changed from the original metal. Polyunsaturated fats, too, are prone to combine with oxygen, becoming rancid (oxidized), potentially harmful, distasteful, and much changed from the original fat. Because of this, these types of fats are not used in processed foods, as they would cause these foods to have short shelf lives. To counteract the problem, fat processors partially or completely hydrogenate the fats, making them capable of longer shelf lives. The hydrogenation is performed by superheating the polyunsaturated fats to 1000°F while bubbling hydrogen gas through the liquid. The hydrogen binds to the fat, making it less able to bind with oxygen and become rancid. Although this makes for a durable food product, it significantly alters the nature of the fat. The original polyunsaturated fat molecule has now become twisted and is no longer able to fit into the normal cell membranes. Consequently, the hydrogenated fat molecules are no longer able to protect and promote proper cell functions. These twisted molecules of hydrogenated fats are called trans fats. Trans fats now make up a significant percentage of the fats in processed foods. Unfortunately, these trans fats have the same deleterious effects as saturated fats, including raising serum LDL ("bad" cholesterol) and lowering serum HDL ("good" cholesterol).

⮥ Are Dietary Fats Linked to Breast Cancer?

In 1982 a group of experts convened by the National Academy of Sciences (NAS) concluded that the strongest evidence of an association between the incidence of certain cancers and dietary components points to dietary fat, particularly in the development of breast cancer. They were able to come to this conclusion after reviewing numerous scientific investigations, some dating back half a century.[1] Others were not yet convinced of the degree of the fat–breast cancer connection.[2,3] However, a more recently published study agrees with the original findings of the NAS.[4]

U.S. IMMIGRANTS AND BREAST CANCER

One way to study the problem is to look at similarly industrialized countries such as Japan where the prevalence of breast cancer is much lower than in the United States. It used to be thought that the Japanese had "good genes" and therefore didn't get breast cancer, but now we know better. When a Japanese immigrant to the United States has been in our country for a decade or so, her chance of developing breast cancer begins to increase. When she has a daughter who is born in this country, the daughter's breast cancer risk is the same as for any other U.S. woman. And in Japan itself, where the diet is becoming more Westernized, the breast cancer rate is starting to increase.

Epidemiological studies of developed countries other than Japan have confirmed the association: countries with high dietary fat intake post higher breast cancer rates than countries with low dietary fat consumption.[5,6,7] As with the Japanese, other immigrants to the United States, such as the Poles, Italians, and Chinese, soon experience the same increased risk of breast cancer after becoming Westernized and adopting our high-fat diet.[8,9,10,11,12]

Using this knowledge, we conclude that the risk for breast cancer is related to our Westernized diet. (A complete discussion of diet and risk for breast cancer was discussed in Chapter 8.) Because dietary fat is one of the significant risks for the development of breast cancer, we are devoting a complete chapter to this subject.

THE 20 PERCENT SOLUTION

An increasing number of scientists believe that a threshold may exist at which only dietary fat percentages below 20 percent have a beneficial impact upon breast cancer. In Japan, the traditional diet contained less than half the fat of the U.S. diet; 10 percent to 20 percent of total calories were derived from fat. Since 1975 the breast cancer rate in Japan has increased 58 percent. Correspondingly, over the same period dietary fat consumption in Japan has increased from 18 to 27 percent of total calories.

Many studies that fail to correlate dietary fat to breast cancer risk are faulty because they compare normal U.S. diets to experimental so-called low-fat diets in which the percentages of fat are significantly higher than the ideal 20 percent. The Nurses' Health Study, reported in 1987 and updated in 1992, is an example of such a faulty investigation. It concluded that reducing dietary fat had no effect in reducing breast cancer.[13] When results of such studies show no lowered risk for low-fat diets, one must question the validity of the conclusions. As it turns out, the two groups tested in the study took in 40 percent fat and less than 27 percent, respectively. Both of these quantities are too high for an effective test. Would it not be far better, when designing such a study, to set the low-fat dietary percentage to a level similar to that found in an existing large population group displaying low breast cancer risk?[14] Most U.S. investigators do not test the validity of the 20 percent fat diet because they feel that it is "extreme" and would be unpalatable for U.S. women. This is not true, as several studies have shown. Women can adhere to a palatable low-fat diet for extended periods without relapse.

DIETARY FATS AND BREAST CANCER

Breast cancer risk, especially in postmenopausal women, has been linked to percentage of calories from dietary fat. Studies have shown increased risk with the type of fat consumed, as well as the total grams of fat in the diet.[15,16] This holds true even with a population consuming lower fat and with lower breast cancer risk, such as the Chinese, in whose population 34.3 percent fat was associated with more risk than 13.8 percent fat.[17] It should be noted that daily consumption of a large number of fat grams is associated with a large daily consumption of calories. This is why some studies have shown increased cancer risk from overall higher caloric intakes as well.[18] Therefore, breast cancer risk is related to the combined elements of dietary fat percentage, total grams of fat, and total calories consumed.

HOW DOES HIGH DIETARY FAT INCREASE THE RISK OF BREAST CANCER?

Higher Estrogen Levels How do we believe dietary fat leads to breast cancer risk? Estrogen! As we learned in Chapter 6, estrogen is implicated as a promoter of hormone-dependent breast cancer. We have found that lowering dietary fat lowers estrogen levels in the blood. We also learned in that chapter that estrogen levels are elevated in girls who begin menstruation early. Finally, a high-fat diet is associated with early menarche, thereby contributing to an increased risk for breast cancer over a woman's lifetime.[19] One study of the effects of a low-fat diet showed that premenopausal women who reduced their dietary fat percentages from 35 to 21 percent lowered their estrogen levels by 33 percent in three months. Postmenopausal women needed six months to achieve a reduction.[20] Dropping dietary fat percentages to only 30 percent, as has been recommended by several national organizations (National Cancer Institute, American Cancer Society, and the National Academy of Sciences) to lower cancer risk, will probably have no positive effect, since serum estrogen levels might remain stable. One study of vegetarian women with dietary fat percentage of 30 percent had the same serum estrogen levels as a matched group of nonvegetarians with 40 percent fat in their diet.[21] Therefore, it is essential to reduce dietary fat to no more than 20 percent to reduce risk. Remember: *While obesity is a known risk factor for breast cancer, the risk factor of a high-fat diet is a separate matter and independent of body weight.*

Mammogram Changes Diets high in fat can be associated with increasing breast density on mammograms, making interpretation more difficult.[22] Less dense mammograms allow detection of smaller and earlier cancers. Besides reducing the risk for development of breast cancer, low dietary fat is associated with less advanced breast cancers which are detected earlier by mammography.

Colon Bacteria Changes High dietary fat changes the bacterial population and its actions in the colon. One investigator, who studied fecal bacteria in patients with colon cancer (also associated with high-fat diets), found that there were less aerobic (oxygen-dependent) bacteria and more anaerobic (oxygen-independent) bacteria present compared to normal controls. It was found that anaerobic bacteria are able to synthesize more estrogenlike hormones than the aerobic bacteria.[23] Again the finger points to estrogens as cancer-enhancing. Additionally, diets that are high in fat encourage the growth of bowel bacteria, which in turn reduce normal fecal estrogen excretion. The result is that more of the estrogen in the colon will be reabsorbed back into the circulation, leading to additional estrogen exposure.[24] Another detrimental effect of a high-fat diet could be its effects on protective antioxidants. It has been previously noted that increasing the antioxidant beta-carotene can decrease the risk of developing breast cancer. A recent study indicates that a high-fat diet may block this protective effect of beta-carotene intake.[25]

Animal Studies While not equating animals with humans, animal studies can shed light on disease mechanisms important to humans. There is clear evidence that high-fat diets promote breast cancers in animals.[26] When rats that were pretreated with a chemical breast carcinogen were fed a high-fat diet, they had a tenfold increase in breast cancers compared to rats on a low-fat calorie-restricted diet.[27] Even studies dating from forty to fifty years ago demonstrated that susceptible animals fed high-fat diets developed breast cancers earlier and in larger numbers compared to those on no-fat diets.[28,29]

From this data we learn that high dietary fats can raise blood estrogen levels in several ways, block preventive antioxidants, and promote cancer growth. Furthermore, a high-fat diet may be associated with more advanced breast cancers because body fat may inhibit early findings through mammography.

NOT ALL FAT IS BAD

Are certain types of fats more apt to be associated with breast cancer risk than others? There are conflicting data.[30,31,32] Numerous studies have associated breast cancer risk with higher intakes of polyunsaturated fats (corn, safflower, etc., known as omega-6 fats), including trans fats. Omega-6 fats have been implicated as promoters of cancer formation. Other investigators have shown a reduced risk for breast cancer with a certain form of polyunsaturated fats derived from fish and some plants (omega-3 fats).[33,34,35,36] Experimental studies have shown omega-3 fats to have an inhibitory effect upon breast cancer cells. The average U.S. diet has a dietary ratio of 20 to 1 for omega-6 and omega-3 fats, thought to be heavily tilted in the wrong direction. The authors believe that this ratio can be improved by increasing our intake of omega-3 fats so that the ratio becomes 6 to 1. This means eating marine, deep cold-water fish several times a week (such as salmon, mackerel, anchovies, sardines, herring, menhaden, bluefish) and/or taking supplemental omega-3 oils (fish oil or flaxseed oil). *[Warning: these omega-3 oils much be fresh. Rancidity occurs easily. Always look for expiration dates, and always refrigerate.]*

Some surveys have tied breast cancer risk to saturated fats in the diet. Some investigators believe that monounsaturated fats such as olive oil are not associated with higher risk, but lower risk. This was borne out in a recent study from Greece where it was found that olive oil consumption was associated with significantly reduced risk for breast cancer. Interestingly, margarine consumption (trans fats) was found to be linked to a *higher* risk.[37] Other investigators indict animal fats over those from plants. To be safe, we recommend reducing *all* dietary fats to a total of twenty percent or less,[38] while increasing omega-3 fats and olive oil in our diet. We should also attempt to minimize, if not eliminate, all trans fat from our diet, meaning all products that contain "partially hydrogenated" oils. We already know that saturated fats and trans fats promote atherosclerosis, so we have other reasons to keep them very low in our diets. A healthy low-dietary-fat diet program, in addition to reducing breast cancer risk, lowers the risk of cardiovascular heart disease, strokes, and cancers of the uterus, ovaries, colon, pancreas, prostate (for men), and skin.

As we learned in Chapter 6, obesity is linked to higher circulating estrogen levels owing to fat cell conversion of adrenal hormones into estrogens. Most obesity results from a high-calorie, high-fat diet. Changing to a healthy low-fat diet, even without conscious calorie restriction, lowers body-fat stores, thus reducing the body's exposure to estrogens. Adding exercise also enhances the benefits.

Women's Health Initiative Study

The Women's Health Initiative is a federal study conducted over fifteen years at the cost of $625 million and performed at forty-five centers. Sponsored by the National Institutes of Health (NIH) and involving 160,000 women aged fifty to seventy-nine, it is designed to assess the effect of modifying dietary fat/fiber and hormone replacement therapy on the development of coronary heart disease, stroke, and cancers of the breast, colon, and endometrium. It is also designed to evaluate calcium and vitamin D supplementation in relation to osteoporotic fractures.[39,40] While such studies are commendable, critics of this study state that its basic design makes it unlikely to ever be able to answer the central questions regarding low-fat diets and hormone replacement therapy.[41] These critics state that this trial was designed to placate the Women's Congressional Caucus, which discovered in 1989 that only 15 percent of the NIH budget went to women's health issues. Do not wait until the results of this study are in before making the change to a low-fat diet. There are enough animal, population, and case-control studies to show the benefit of such a dietary program.

❧ Dietary Fat and Breast Cancer Recurrence

BREAST CANCER PATIENTS AND DIETARY FAT

What are the recommendations for women who have already experienced breast cancer? We look to Japan again, as a population consuming less than 20 percent dietary fat, and we find that in postmenopausal women who have had prior breast cancer, the annual recurrence rate is 20 percent lower than in the United States, while the survival rate is 20 percent higher. This percentage is significant since it is equivalent to the benefit of being treated with an anti-estrogen drug or chemotherapy. A low-fat diet is also associated with less risk of metastasis. In animal studies the more fat the animals eat, the faster the breast cancer tumors grow and spread to other areas of the body.

Women who reduce dietary fat to 20 percent, without attempting to reduce overall calories, tend to lose some body fat. This also may play an important but independent part in lowering the risk of developing breast cancer and preventing its recurrence. For obese women, no matter how much their cancers have spread at the time of diagnosis, the prognosis is always worse. Even if women are not obese at the time of their breast cancer surgery, subsequent weight gain is equivalent to canceling out the beneficial effects of anti-estrogen drugs or chemotherapy. One study showed that women who were 25 percent over their ideal body weight had a 42 percent risk for breast cancer recurrence ten years after diagnosis, compared to 32 percent for nonobese women. Another investigation found that in women with breast cancer, the risk of dying from the disease at any one time increases 40 percent for every 1,000 grams of fat consumed monthly. Another one found the risk of dying increased by 50 percent for every 5 percent of additional dietary fat.[42] There is also a connection between high-fat diets and lymph node involvement after breast cancer.[43] Keep in mind that it is not necessary for us to understand the exact mechanisms of a low-fat diet in lowering breast cancer mortality risk—just that it is effective.[44,45]

Just how dietary fat worsens breast cancer prognosis is not known. Theories abound.[46] Perhaps the fat triggers genes that allow cancer cells to proliferate, making cancer cell membranes more pliable and enabling cancer to grow out of small blood vessels and into surrounding tissues. Another theory is that fats reduce the immune system's ability to kill cancer cells. It has been found that besides lowering serum estrogen, a low-fat diet seems to enhance the immune system, increasing the activity of a natural killer cell. It is possible that fats, especially polyunsaturated ones, become oxidized within the body, creating free radicals that damage both normal and already partially damaged cells, which lead to cancer development. We know that estrogen levels stimulate breast cancers that are positive for estrogen receptors (ER+), that such levels are elevated with high-fat diets, and that these tumors are more frequent in individuals on high-fat diets.[47] Another theory states that certain polyunsaturated fats (omega-6s) promote synthesis of unknown substances, which can stimulate cancer cell growth, proliferation, and/or invasion.[48] Conversely, the beneficial polyunsaturated fats (omega-3s) may help in suppression of breast cancer cells.[49]

THE NCI STUDIES BREAST CANCER PATIENTS AND DIETARY FAT

Currently, the NCI is performing a prospective study consisting of 2,000 women with breast cancer: Stage I (no lymph nodes involved) and Stage II (lymph nodes involved, but no other organs). All will be receiving standard therapy, but one-half will be put on a 30 percent fat diet, the other half on a 15 to 20 percent fat diet. These women will be followed for seven years. All forms of fat will be cut, not only specific types. A recent review suggests that dietary intervention in postmenopausal breast cancer patients should strive for 15 percent dietary fat intake, not 20 percent.[50]

DIETARY FAT GUIDELINES FOR BREAST CANCER PATIENTS

If you have had breast cancer, do not wait until the next century to make a decision to begin a low-fat diet. Right now, there is rational evidence supporting such adjuvant dietary change from epidemiologic observations, animal studies, cell-culture investigations, cellular biology, and human psychology. There are major differences in stage-by-stage survival of patients with breast cancer, when comparing countries with low-fat diets to those with high-fat diets, including correlation of biochemical and hormonal alterations. We have knowledge of the effects of dietary fat intake and factors related to survival of patients with breast cancer, such as effects of weight gain on breast-cancer survival. Animal studies show deleterious effects of high-fat diet on growth and metastasis of breast cancers. There are observed direct effects upon breast-cancer cell cultures with omega-6 fats. Currently, there is a reasonable understanding of the effects of high dietary fat on breast-cancer cell growth and spread in cell cultures. Finally, patient compliance to a low-fat diet has been demonstrated in women who have been treated for breast cancer.[51]

❧ *Summary*

Using the available evidence, we can state that a low-fat diet is beneficial to lowering the risk of developing breast cancer, as well as to preventing its recurrence and spread and increasing patient survival rates. It will not benefit you to wait for the results of the studies described or for future studies. We recommend you not "go on a diet." "Going on" suggests that sometime in the future you will be going off. Instead, why not make the decision to eat healthfully for the rest of your life? Some say that a true low-fat diet is too drastic for the American population. Is not the epidemic of breast cancer significant enough to warrant drastic treatment? A cancer-preventive diet does require a change of lifestyle, but recent studies have shown that it is a change that can be made and followed over the long term, using proper motivation and education.[52,53] The low dietary fat, *noncaloric-restricted, nonnutrient-restricted* lifestyle is not harmful to any adult or child over the age of four or five. It is especially beneficial to lower dietary fat intake in our children, to establish healthful dietary habits and beneficial hormonal patterns they can maintain for life. At the same time, while eating healthfully, we are enjoying other benefits, which include lowering our risks for many other chronic and life-threatening diseases.

Chapter 11

Taking Nutritional Supplements

America the beautiful is also America the sick. Our incidence of chronic degenerative disease is astronomical, and we spend more money on health care than any other nation in the world. It should be obvious that something is very wrong with this picture. In his book, *The University at the Crossroads*, medical historian H. E. Sigerist states, "The ideal of medicine is the prevention of disease, and the necessity for curative treatment is a tacit admission of its failure."[1]

This chapter deals with one of the most fundamental, controversial, and, potentially, important issues in human health: Should we take nutritional supplements, and if so, how much?

The U.S. Food and Drug Administration has traditionally been against nutritional supplements, as evidenced by the FDA pamphlet *Myths of Vitamins*, which states: "Foods can and do supply most Americans with adequate nutrients."[2]

However, the following information from the well-publicized

and respected National Health and Nutrition Examination Survey II (NHANES II) certainly seems to contradict the FDA's assurances that we get all of the nutrients we need from our food. These results showed that approximately 45 percent of Americans do not consume a daily serving of fruit and 22 percent do not eat a daily serving of vegetables. Furthermore, this study revealed that on any given day, 91 percent of the American population does not follow the recommended guidelines of eating two or more servings of fruits and three or more servings of vegetables.[3]

A substantial amount of information suggests that the standard American diet does not meet the nutritional needs of Americans. For example, a survey by the U.S. Department of Agriculture (USDA) revealed that the diet of most Americans is not providing the Recommended Daily Allowance (RDA) level of one or more of the following essential nutrients:[4]

USDA Survey

NUTRIENT	PERCENTAGE OF AMERICANS RECEIVING BELOW THE RDA
Vitamin B_6	80%
Magnesium	75%
Calcium	68%
Vitamin A	50%
Vitamin B_1	45%
Vitamin C	41%
Vitamin B_2	34%
Vitamin B_{12}	34%
Niacin (Vitamin B_3)	34%

&* Understanding Recommended Daily Allowance (RDA)

Most people misunderstand the meaning of the term *Recommended Daily Allowance*. The RDAs, formulated by the

Food and Nutrition Board of the National Academy of Sciences/ National Research Council, represent levels of nutrients thought to be adequate for most healthy people.

It is a little-known fact that the RDAs were not determined by scientific studies for optimal health. They are based on estimates of the level of nutrients already present in the standard American diet. Unfortunately, most people think the RDAs represent our government's scientifically determined levels of nutrients that will provide good health.

Nutrition as a science got started on the wrong foot. Initially, scientists discovered "things" in food that were apparently necessary for human health and well-being. Experiments were then designed to see what symptoms would appear if one of these substances (a vitamin or mineral) was totally removed from the diet. Then small amounts were added back into the diet to see how much of a particular nutrient was necessary to make the deficiency symptoms disappear. This was called the Minimum Daily Requirement (MDR). An extra amount was then added to provide a margin of error, and this was then called the Recommended Daily Allowance, or RDA.

The RDAs and most nutritional research have been based on minimalist thinking: looking at deficiencies and determining the minimal amount necessary to make the symptoms go away. The RDA can be compared to the minimum wage. Nobody envisions the minimum wage as their pinnacle of success or their goal. Neither should we allow the RDAs to be our nutritional goals of excellence.

Actually, the RDAs are only the estimated amounts that will prevent nutritional deficiency diseases in most healthy people. There are large groups of people who do not fit this nebulous RDA category of "most healthy people." These people, with specialized nutritional needs, can definitely benefit from taking nutritional supplements.

DIETERS

On any given day an estimated 40 to 50 million Americans (many of them women) are dieting. Low-calorie diets frequently fail to provide adequate nutrition. For example, a review of eleven popular diets revealed that none of them provided 100 percent of the RDA for the essential vitamins.[5]

BIRTH CONTROL PILLS

It is well established that birth control pills deplete a woman's body of vitamin B_6 and folic acid.[6]

OTC MEDICATIONS

Millions of people take over-the-counter products that interfere with an individual's nutritional status. For example, mineral oil and other laxatives prevent the absorption of the fat-soluble nutrients vitamins A, D, E, and K. Aspirin depletes vitamin C and folic acid. Antacids interfere with the digestion and absorption of many nutrients.

PRESCRIPTION DRUGS

Antibiotics interfere with calcium absorption. Medication for high blood pressure often depletes B vitamins and minerals like potassium, calcium, magnesium, and zinc. The popular cholesterol-lowering drug Mevacor depletes coenzyme Q10.

TEENAGERS

Surveys have shown that a disturbingly high percentage of adolescent girls do not meet the RDA level of important vitamins and minerals. Many of them skip meals regularly, eat junk food frequently, and are often dieting.

THE ELDERLY

Numerous factors affect the nutritional status of the elderly, including poor absorption, altered taste perception, low calorie intake, and drug/nutrient interactions. In addition, several secondary factors can affect nutrition in seniors, such as loneliness, depression, low income, limited mobility, and lack of transportation.

⊷ *Questioning the RDA*

A major philosophical and scientific debate currently surrounds the RDAs and whether or not they are appropriate nutritional standards for Americans. The debate centers around the words *adequate* versus *optimal*. The RDAs are apparently adequate to protect most Americans from nutritional deficiency diseases; however, we need to realize that good health is not just the absence of disease. In fact, there is a growing dissatisfaction as more and more people believe that the RDAs are not sufficient to promote optimal health and wellness.

⊷ *Our Nutritionally Declining Diet*

Another important reason to consider taking nutritional supplements has to do with the declining nutrient value in today's commercially available foods. Modern-day agriculture and food-processing practices often substantially deplete the nutrients from food before it reaches your table. For example, food is often force-ripened, picked early, sprayed or gassed with chemicals, refined, canned or frozen, stored, and shipped around the country.

A recent study published in the *Journal of Applied Nutrition* documented the nutritional decline in the American diet. Researchers compared the nutritional content of organically grown foods with the same food from commercial supermarkets. The results showed that organically grown foods contained about twice the level of nutrients as the commercially grown foods.[7]

❧ *Supernutrition*

A revolution is in the making. A paradigm shift and a system of new beliefs in the fields of nutrition and health are beginning to emerge. We need to abandon the RDAs and begin to target levels of nutrition that will promote optimal health and wellness for people. We need to start thinking in terms of supernutrition.

Billions of dollars have been spent on cancer research, yet the death rates from cancer keep increasing relentlessly. Unfortunately, only a small fraction of the cancer research money has been focused on prevention. The vast bulk of those billions was spent on methods of early detection and treatment.

Ross once heard the charismatic black minister Reverend Ike say, "The best way to solve the problem of the poor people . . . is to not be one of them!" A similar statement can be made about cancer. The best way to solve the problem of cancer . . . is to get healthy, stay healthy, and not get it. One of the most important aspects of a proactive cancer-prevention lifestyle is a daily program of high-potency nutritional supplementation.

BEYOND THE RDAs

Writing on nutritional needs and biochemical diversity, noted researcher Donald R. Davis, Ph.D., states: "A large body of experimental data leads to the unavoidable conclusion that striking variations in individual nutritional requirements of 2-, 5-, or 10-fold or more commonly exist in normal human populations."[8] Because of these variations in nutritional needs within "normal people," doesn't it seem wrong to target a single RDA value for nutrients as being appropriate for everyone?

As a species, mankind tends to view ourselves as biologically, physiologically, and genetically similar. Overall, this is true; we are very similar, but not identical. The importance of our differences was highlighted by the pioneering nutritional scientist Roger Williams, Ph.D., with the publication of his classic 1956 monograph, *Biochemical Individuality*.[9] The importance of his premise is still overlooked and underestimated. Many people have average needs for a majority of the essential nutrients; however, many of these people also have individual requirements for several essential nutrients which may be far above average. Unfortunately, medical science has been slow, if not unwilling, to grasp this concept.

The FDA continues to promote the RDAs as the amounts of vitamins and minerals that most people need to ingest daily. In two FDA pamphlets, *What About Vitamin C?*[10] and *Vitamin E—Miracle or Myth?*,[11] the FDA claims that there is no evidence to support the idea that nutritional supplements that exceed the RDAs have any real benefit.

On the other hand, an ever-increasing volume of research contradicts the FDA's viewpoint by showing that levels of nutrients above the RDA can and do provide substantial benefits to people. For example, in a recent ten-year study of over 11,000 Americans, men who ingested eight hundred milligrams of vitamin C daily (mostly from supplements) lived about six years longer than men who received only the RDA level (60 mg) of vitamin C daily. There was also a 30 percent reduction in deaths from all causes in men ingesting the eight hundred mg of vitamin C daily. Women subjects taking the higher doses of vitamin C lived only about one year longer. The difference between men and women may be due to the fact that women already outlive men by a number of years.

A study involving more than 130,000 people with no previous history of heart disease indicated that taking one hundred IU of natural vitamin E daily for two years lowered the incidence of heart attacks by 46 percent in women and 26 percent in men.[12] The RDA for vitamin E is only forty-five IU.

In another study, a group of elderly subjects with *no* nutritional deficiencies were put on a vitamin and mineral supplement program.[13] The extra nutritional supplements enabled these elderly subjects to decrease their incidence of infections and experience substantial improvements in a wide variety of immune system indicators.

These reports are just a sampling of literally hundreds of studies concluding that levels of nutrients above the RDA values provide substantial benefits.

✺ Are Nutritional Supplements Safe?

The question of safety comes up frequently when discussing the use of above-RDA levels of nutritional supplements. Members of the medical establishment frequently respond with a combination of ridicule, scorn, and scare tactics. However, the following statistics from the American Association of Poison Control Centers tell quite a different story.

✺ Fatalities from Prescription Drugs, Non-prescription Drugs, and Nutrients[14]

	Year								
	'83	'84	'85	'86	'87	'88	'89	'90	Total
Number of centers reporting	16	47	56	57	63	64	70	72	
Analgesics (pain killers)	22	53	87	82	93	118	126	134	715
Antidepressants (mood elevators)	19	57	90	100	105	135	140	159	805
Asthma Therapies	4	10	11	21	16	27	34	37	160
Cardiovascular Drugs[1]	5	18	21	50	52	65	70	79	360
Sedatives and Hypnotics[2]	11	51	62	61	48	77	78	72	460
Deaths from Amphetamines[3]	1	4	6	11	11	12	5	6	56
Deaths from all above drugs	62	193	227	325	325	434	453	487	2506
Deaths attributed to all nutrients	0	0	0	0	1†	0	0	1	2†

1. Includes blood pressure medications.   2. Includes sleeping pills and tranquilizers. 3. Includes stimulants. †The 1987 vitamin-related death report was later determined to be an error. Table adapted from Donald Loomis, *Townsend Letter for Doctors*, April 1992. Original data from the American Association of Poison Control Centers. Statistics first published in the *American Journal of Emergency Medicine*.

This study shows that over a period of eight years, there were 2,506 deaths from various kinds of drugs, while there was only one death from a nutritional supplement. Every day literally hundreds of thousands of Americans take nutritional supplements at levels well above the RDAs. This documentation should be enough to convince most people that the use of above-RDA levels of nutritional supplements is very safe. However, we also want to interject a note of caution. We are not advocating the indiscriminate use of massive doses of supplements. As with anything in life, a level of caution and good judgment are necessary. If you need help, seek the advice of a nutritionist or another qualified health professional.

There are wide variations in nutritional supplement programs, and we do not promote any particular product or name brand. The listing that we present is somewhat of a composite average to give you an idea of the content in a formulation with above-RDA ingredients.

One thing we want to stress is that the old concept of taking a once-daily type of vitamin pill is an out-of-date, inappropriate method of nutritional supplementation, based on the out-moded RDA level of nutrients. A daily regime incorporating higher levels of supplements will usually necessitate taking two or more pills *per meal.*

ᴥ *Essential Nutrients*

It is important to understand the concept of essential nutrients. When the word *essential* is used in this context, it has two meanings, both of which are very important. First, essential nutrients are those that the body *must have,* virtually every day, in order to function properly. Secondly, essential nutrients are nutrients that the body *cannot* make on its own. Therefore, the only way the body can get these essential nutrients is from outside sources, either in the food you eat or from nutritional supplements.

There are forty-five essential nutrients for humans: twenty

minerals, fifteen vitamins, eight essential amino acids, and two essential fatty acids. The body's nutritional needs are like a finely tuned human symphony where everything must act in synchronism and harmony. We could use another analogy and say, "The chain is only as strong as its weakest link." It is a well-documented fact that many Americans are not getting all of the essential nutrients in their daily diets. Many people, in an effort to solve this problem, take a few extra supplements like vitamin C, vitamin E, and calcium, without realizing how important it is to get all of the essential nutrients every day. One of the best and easiest ways to solve this problem is to regularly take a high-potency vitamin/mineral supplement at each meal.

☙ Guidelines for Nutritional Supplements

1. Take a vitamin-mineral supplement with a daily formulation containing approximately the following nutrients:

A (beta-carotene)	15,000 to 25,000 IU
Vitamin D	200 to 400 IU
Vitamin C	1,000 mg or more
Vitamin B_1	15 to 50 mg
Vitamin B_2	15 to 50 mg
Vitamin B_3 (niacinamide)	30 to 60 mg
Vitamin B_6	30 to 50 mg
Vitamin B_{12}	50 to 150 mcg
Pantothenic Acid	50 to 100 mg
Folic Acid	250 to 400 mcg
Biotin	200 to 400 mcg
Vitamin E (d-alpha)	100 to 400 IU
Calcium	1,000 mg or more
Magnesium	1,000 mg or more
Potassium	10 mg or more
Iron	5 to 15 mg
Zinc	5 to 30 mg

Manganese	3 to 6 mg
Choline	50 to 500 mg
Iodine	50 to 150 mg
Selenium	50 to 150 mcg
Chromium	100 to 200 mcg

NOTE: Keep in mind that these represent suggested ranges. The main purpose of the list is to show you the difference between this type of nutritional supplement and a once-daily type of supplement. Quality products can be purchased from most health food stores or from a variety of mail order companies.

2. Take an additional 1,000 mg of vitamin C or more each meal.
3. Take an additional 400 to 800 IU of natural Vitamin E per day.
4. Take an additional 25,000 IU of beta-carotene each meal.
5. Take an additional 100 micrograms of selenium at each meal.
6. Take 1 tablespoon of flaxseed oil a day (keep refrigerated).
7. Take 30 mg of Coenzyme Q10 each day.

❧ *Coenzyme Q10 (CoQ10)*

Recent research, which has grabbed the attention of the world's scientific community, suggests that the nutrient coenzyme Q10 may play an important role in the prevention and treatment of breast cancer in the future. The discovery of coenzyme Q10 is considered by some scientists to be one of the most important medical breakthroughs of this century. As a nutritional supplement, CoQ10 holds great promise in the treatment of a number of conditions, including cardiovascular disease and breast cancer.

CoQ10 is a nutrient that occurs naturally in the human body and is essential to the life and health of every individual. At the cellular level, it is a vital catalyst for the creation of energy and also functions as a powerful antioxidant.

The story of CoQ10 has been told in the book *The Miracle Nutrient Coenzyme Q10* by Emile G. Bliznakov, M.D., and Gerald L. Hunt.[15] Their book reveals that CoQ10 gained its "miracle" status because of its effectiveness in the treatment of the number-one killer, cardiovascular disease. CoQ10 lowers high blood pressure and strengthens the heart muscle. In fact, a leading researcher has suggested that congestive heart failure may be largely due to a CoQ10 deficiency. CoQ10 also provides a powerful boost to the immune system, aids in weight loss, and is remarkably effective in treating periodontal disease.

CoQ compounds occur in all plants and animals throughout nature. Thus far, ten CoQs have been discovered, but CoQ10 is the only one found in humans. There has been only a limited amount of research on the availability of CoQ10 through dietary means; therefore, the exact human requirements are yet to be determined.

Dr. Karl Folkers, the leading CoQ10 researcher in the world, discovered the method of synthesizing CoQ10 while working for the international pharmaceutical giant Merck, Sharpe and Dohme. Since natural substances cannot be patented, Merck was not interested in pursuing work with CoQ10, and the synthesis technology was sold to a Japanese company. Subsequently, Dr. Folkers left Merck and for the past twenty years has devoted his life exclusively to CoQ10 research.

❧ CoQ10 and Cancer

Beyond CoQ10's remarkable effectiveness in the treatment of cardiovascular disease, Dr. Folkers became excited about the possibility that it could be a breakthrough in the treatment of cancer. His initial interest in this possibility began twelve years ago, when a neighbor with terminal metastatic lung cancer began taking therapeutic doses of CoQ10 and experienced a complete remission.

CoQ10 and Breast Cancer

In March 1994, Dr. Folkers, in conjunction with Dr. Karl Lockwood from Denmark, published the results of a study in which thirty-two women with "high-risk" breast cancer were treated with a variety of nutritional supplements, as well as 90 mg of CoQ10 per day. At the time of publication, six of the women reportedly showed partial tumor regression. In one of these six women, the dosage of CoQ10 was increased to 390 mg per day. In one month her tumor had decreased in size to the point where it could no longer be felt. After a second month, mammography confirmed that the tumor was gone.[16]

Encouraged by this first high-dosage success, another woman with a verified tumor that remained in the breast after nonradical surgery was treated with 300 mg of CoQ10 daily. After three months this patient was reportedly in excellent clinical condition with complete elimination of the tumor.

In their paper Dr. Folkers and his coauthors state: "The bioenergetic activity of CoQ10, expressed as hematological or immunological activity, may be the dominant but not the sole molecular mechanism causing the regression of breast cancer."[17]

CoQ10 Nutritional Guidelines

CoQ10 is an important nutritional supplement to consider since it is vital to the energy production in every cell of the human body. Studies from Japan involving thousands of patients over many years have shown that CoQ10 is virtually non-toxic and devoid of any side effects, even when administered at high dosages for extended periods.

Some companies now include a small amount of CoQ10 in their multivitamin formulations. Additionally, CoQ10 can be purchased as a separate supplement in most health food stores. The usual recommended dosage is from 10 to 30 mg daily.

A dosage of from 15 to 30 mg of CoQ10 once daily is suggested for a breast cancer prevention program. Women with breast cancer and other seriously ill patients should consider taking higher dosages of CoQ10, but only under the supervision of a qualified health professional who can help track their progress.

❧ *Summary*

Nutritional supplements represent one of the best insurance policies available to you in your efforts to prevent breast cancer, and we urge every woman to get started on a good supplement program. And don't just do this for yourself. Healthy diets, healthy lifestyles, and nutritional supplement are important for husbands and children, too. You can be leaders in helping to change the health of this nation. Remember, an ounce of prevention really is worth a pound of cure. The ounce of prevention usually starts with family values that originate in the home.

To your good health . . . and don't forget to take your vitamins.

Chapter 12

The Soy Phenomenon

Soybeans and their products have proven to be important foods in the prevention of breast cancer. In cultures in which the diet is high in soybeans and other soy products, breast cancer rates are extremely low. For years, scientists have been looking for possible relationships between diet and the ever-increasing incidence of cancer. Recent research indicates that soybeans contain relatively large amounts of five different compounds that possess anticancer properties.

The dietary anticancer effects of soy foods began to attract attention when epidemiological studies revealed that breast cancer rates for women in the United States were five to eight times higher than for Asian women.[1] These studies revealed that the differences in breast cancer rates between Japanese and American women are not due to genetic factors, but rather to environmental factors.[2] One of the most obvious dissimilarities between the two countries is the diet.

The standard American diet, which is high in animal protein, dairy products, and processed foods, averages about 40 percent fat, whereas the traditional Japanese diet contains almost none of those foods and is only about 10 to 20 percent fat. As was discussed in Chapter 10, several studies have shown that nations with higher fat intake have higher rates of breast cancer.[3,4]

Other factors in the Japanese diet might also contribute to the fivefold variance in the incidence of breast cancer. For example, American protein comes primarily from meat and dairy products, whereas the main source of protein in the traditional Japanese diet comes from soy-containing foods such as *miso* (soybean paste), *natto* (fermented soybeans), *fukujinzuke* (soy sauce–pickled vegetables), and *misozuke* (miso-pickled vegetables). Numerous studies have shown that the consumption of these traditional Japanese foods results in a lower incidence of breast (and other) cancer.[5] This evidence suggests that the soybean-rich foods in the traditional Japanese diet might be the source of important substances that prevent the occurrence of breast cancer. Recent research has now isolated dozens of other phytochemicals in soybeans that have important anticancer properties.

In 1989 the National Cancer Institute funded a $20 million study to research the potential role of common foods, including soybeans, in preventing cancer. In 1990 the NCI added another $2.9 million to focus specifically on the anticancer properties of soybeans. The results of this research were made public at a two-day workshop in June 1990 entitled "The Role of Soy Products in Reducing Risk of Cancer."[6]

❧ *Phytoestrogens*

Phytoestrogens (*phyto* is derived from the Greek word for "plant") are plant-based estrogenlike substances. They usually have relatively weak estrogenic activity, yet they are able to occupy the estrogen receptor sites on the surface of cells, thus blocking the activity of normal estrogen and lowering a woman's risk for breast cancer.[7] Soybeans contain a number of phytoestrogens, which may explain why soy-based diets help prevent breast cancer.

In a case-controlled study in Singapore, researchers found that higher intake of soy protein was protective against breast cancer in premenopausal women. It was suggested that the phytoestrogens in soy products were responsible for this anti-cancer effect.[8]

Vegetarians, who as a group have a lower incidence of cancer, have been shown to excrete higher levels of phytoestrogens in their urine.[9] Urinary excretion of phytoestrogens is not only a measure of dietary intake, but also an indicator of the anticancer properties of the diet. Thus high urinary excretion of phytoestrogens may, in part, explain why vegetarian women have lower rates of breast cancer.

ISOFLAVONES

Isoflavones are a large class (over 4,400) of compounds that occur naturally in the plant kingdom. Many isoflavones possess weak estrogenic activity and thus are also classified as phytoestrogens. Some plant isoflavones are converted by human intestinal bacteria into a weaker isoflavone named equol. Equol has only about 0.2 percent of the biological activity of estradiol. In one study, subjects who were given 40 grams of soy daily had urinary excretion levels of equol from fifty to a thousandfold times higher than original baseline values, which ranged from undetectable to 80 mg/day.[10] The high excretion of equol indicates that those women have high circulating levels of this compound, which competes with estrogen and thus lowers the risk of breast cancer.

GENISTEIN

Genistein is an isoflavone with powerful anticancer activity. In addition to its estrogen-blocking effects, genistein has the extraordinary capacity to convert malignant cells back to cells that behave normally.[11] This compound, which is found in high concentrations only in soybeans, has grabbed the attention of cancer researchers around the world. In fact, in the last several years more than two hundred scientific papers have been published about genistein.

One study discovered that genistein blocks angiogenesis, which, in effect, starves tumors. Angiogenesis refers to the formation of new blood vessels. As tumors grow, they need to continually develop new blood vessel networks, which provide the tumor with nutrients for growth. When angiogenesis inhibitors, like genistein, inhibit a tumor's ability to build its network of blood vessels, the tumor begins to starve from lack of nutrients, and tumor regression or necrosis (death) results.

In addition to its anti-estrogenic activity, genistein has been shown to have an inhibitory effect on several classes of enzymes, including tyrosine protein kinases, DNA topoisomerases, and the S kinases. The activity of these enzymes is increased in cancer cells. Inhibiting the activity of these enzymes inhibits the ability of cancer cells to grow. Therefore, scientists are speculating that genistein and other isoflavones may play an important role in the prevention of a wide range of cancers.[12]

PROTEASE INHIBITORS

Proteases are enzymes that perform the necessary physiological activity of splitting, or breaking down, proteins into smaller segments that can be used by the body. However, they also represent a potential hazard since, if overactive or uncontrolled, they can destroy the protein components of cells and tissues. These enzymes have been shown to play a variety of roles in tumor promotion and carcinogenesis.[13]

Protease inhibitors occur naturally in many foods, and studies support the theory that their intake may reduce the incidence of cancer in humans. Soybeans contain relatively high concentrations of two protease inhibitors with known anticancer activity, namely the Bowman-Birk trypsin and chymotrypsin inhibitor (BBI) and the Kunitz trypsin inhibitor.

When raw soybeans, which contained high amounts of protease inhibitors, were fed to laboratory animals, there was a substantial reduction in experimentally induced breast cancer.[14] Additionally, it has been reported that the Bowman-Birk protease inhibitor, derived from soybeans, either inhibits or prevents the development of experimentally induced cancers of the colon, mouth, lung, liver, and esophagus. [15]

PHYTIC ACID

Phytic acid, also called inositol hexaphosphate, is a compound found in a variety of fiber-rich foods such as cereals, fruits, and vegetables. Soybeans are one of the richest sources of phytic acid. In the past, phytates have had a bad reputation nutritionally because they bind minerals like calcium and iron, preventing their absorption. But phytates also have good properties, including the ability to help prevent breast cancer.

One study examined phytic acid's ability to lower early risk markers for breast cancer. The study showed that higher levels of phytic acid in the diet clearly decreased the rate of cellular division in samples of breast tissue.[16]

In terms of breast anatomy, the highest proliferative cellular activity and the more significant changes in the mammary gland were seen in the terminal end bud, rather than in the alveolar bud and terminal duct structures. This is significant because the terminal end bud is the structural component that is the most sensitive to mammary carcinogens and is more frequently the site of tumor development.

The same study reported that animals treated with phytic acid experienced a decrease in the amount of destructive changes within the nucleus of breast tissue cells. This study concluded that the addition of phytic acid definitely reduced the risk for mammary cancer.

PHYTOSTEROLS AND SAPONINS

Phytosterols and saponins are two other classes of compounds with known health benefits and anticancer activity. Their concentration in soybeans happens also to be particularly high. Although these compounds have not been shown to specifically protect against breast cancer, the fact that they have known anticancer activity makes them worth mentioning.[17] In addition to increasing immune function[18] and lowering cholesterol,[19] they have been shown to inhibit colon cancer and decrease the growth of several different lines of cancer cells.[20] If you become aware of the overall benefits of decreasing dietary animal protein and increasing the use of soy foods, you can use the knowledge for your own benefit.

❧ *Soybeans in the United States*

According to agricultural statistics, nearly half of the world's soybean crop is grown in the United States. Soybeans represent the second most important cash crop (next to corn) in the United States (about $200 million/year); however, the majority of it is used as animal feed.

Nevertheless, over the past decade, each year has seen a substantial increase in the consumption of traditional soy food products such as tofu, tempeh, miso, and soy milk. There has also been a steady increase in the development, acceptance, and use of second-generation soy food products such as soy hot dogs, tempeh burgers, soy sausage, soy cheese, and soy milk, which frequently simulate conventional meat and dairy products.

Surveys indicate the U.S. per capita intake of soy foods has increased by approximately 40 percent in the past decade.[21] Soy products are playing an ever-increasing role in commercial foods, employed as emulsifying, gelling, texturizing, fat-binding, and dough-forming agents. However, for most people in the United States, the daily nutrient intake of soy food products is still relatively minimal.

❧ Nutritional Value of Soy Foods

Whole soybeans have a very strong nutritional profile. In addition to the anticancer substances already mentioned, soybeans contain vitamins A, C, D, E, and K, several of the B-vitamins, the minerals calcium, iron, zinc, phosphorus, and magnesium, and essential fatty acids. Most importantly, soybeans are an excellent source of amino acids such as arginine, cystine, glutamine, lysine, methionine, phenylalanine, and tyrosine.[22] More than 90 percent of the soy food consumed by humans in the United States is in the form of soy-protein food products. Unfortunately, as is true with most foods, when soybeans undergo food processing, a significant amount of the nutritional value is either lost or destroyed.

There are over 10,000 varieties of the common soybean, Glycine max L., with significant variation in nutritional content.[23] Studies have shown that the isoflavone content in soybeans (and thus the anticancer activity) varies greatly depending on the nutritional content of the soil, degree of ripeness at the time of picking, temperature, amount of sunlight, and moisture during the growing season. Therefore, nutritionally speaking, all soybeans are not equal.

❧ Haelan 851

Haelan 851 is the trade name for an amazing soybean product that was initially developed in China to treat critically ill cancer patients. Organically grown soybeans, handpicked at the peek of ripeness, are treated with a special patented fermentation process that results in a soy-protein beverage, which contains a tremendous concentration of all of the soybean's nutrients and anticancer phytochemical compounds. Special care is given to enhance and concentrate the ingredients, to improve digestion and assimilation, and to ensure that the nutrients are not destroyed during processing. Approximately twenty-five pounds of organic soybeans are needed to make a single eight-ounce bottle of Haelan.

Ross had the opportunity to use Haelan with cancer patients in a hospital environment. He saw dozens of critically ill cancer patients dramatically reverse the course of their disease in just five to seven days when they began drinking eight ounces of Haelan daily. The dense concentration of ingredients seems to provide an enormous boost to a patient's energy, appetite, and immune system quite quickly. Based on these early observations and clinical responses, Ross began suggesting that all his cancer patients consider taking the Haelan 851 soybean product. As patients improve, the daily dosage is gradually decreased. However, many patients choose to remain on a small maintenance dose of one or two ounces daily for an extended period of time. For more information on Haelan, contact Haelan Products, Inc., as referenced in Appendix B.

We are taking the time to focus on Haelan because it highlights the power and importance of the anticancer phytochemicals contained in fresh, well-grown foods. Mankind evolved for millions of years eating live, fresh foods that contain a wide variety of these phytochemicals. However, our modern-day factory-farming and food-processing industries eliminate or destroy most of these important plant compounds before they get to us. Haelan, with its huge concentration of these compounds, has shown how powerful these phytochemicals can be in the treatment of cancer. We believe the same principle holds true for the prevention of cancer. A healthy diet of live, fresh, phytochemically rich foods is an important part of a healthy lifestyle.

❧ Switching to Soy

Unless you have been a vegetarian for a long time, adding soy foods to your diet can be a challenging lifestyle change to make. While soy products are readily available in most good health food stores, many supermarkets have yet to incorporate them on their shelves. Tofu is truly a wonderful food; it can be used in many ways and takes on the flavors of any sauce or spice you cook with it. The trick is to learn what to do with it. The best way to accomplish this is to simply buy a tofu or vegetarian cookbook.

Tempeh is another accessible soy product, often used in place of meat owing to its firm and chewy texture. And miso, a soybean paste, is a wonderful addition to the natural foods kitchen. It can be used in many dishes as a flavor enhancer, and it is particularly good in vegetable soups and stews. Miso is well respected for its healthful properties. Switching from cow's milk to soy milk can require time to change your taste, but many people find soy beverages preferable and easily interchangeable. Other products made from soybeans include frozen desserts, salad dressings, mayonnaise, puddings, and pies.

Soybeans themselves are seldom used, and that is unfortunate. They are great in soups, salads, and stews. They are firm, tasty, and hold their texture. If you want to try them, be sure to soak and cook them a little longer than most cookbooks advise, and change the soaking water several times to avoid the flatulence they can cause.

Along with a new culinary adventure, switching from the standard American diet, which is high in meat and dairy products, to one based on more organically grown soy food products will help prevent breast cancer in a number of ways. You will lower the fat intake in your diet, decrease the intake of ingested pesticides and herbicides, decrease the ingestion of hormones and antibiotics, and increase the intake of phytoestrogens and other important anticancer nutrients.

❧ Summary

Soybeans are currently one of the hottest items in cancer research. This is because they contain significant amounts of at least five different phytochemicals which possess anticancer

activity. Also, cultures eating high levels of soy foods traditionally have low rates of breast cancer. Therefore, we think that
soybeans are one of the most important foods to include in a
breast cancer prevention diet. We recommend having soy-
containing meals several times per week on a regular basis.

Chapter 13

The Danger of Pesticides

"Breast cancer cover up: despite mounting evidence, scientists have avoided investigating the environmental links to breast cancer. . . ." This was the cover story in the May/June 1994 issue of *Mother Jones* magazine.

Pesticides, herbicides (weed killers), and other environmental chemicals are finally starting to gain recognition as possible contributors to our breast cancer epidemic. This issue made national headlines in April 1993, when Dr. Mary Wolff, M.D., and her colleagues at New York's Mount Sinai School of Medicine published the results of a study showing a strong association between elevated blood levels of DDE (a metabolite of the pesticide DDT) and breast cancer. The researchers evaluated blood samples from 14,290 women and found that those with higher levels of DDE had up to a four times greater risk of developing breast cancer.[1]

❧ Early Research

In 1962, Rachel Carson issued an urgent warning to the world in her prophetic book *Silent Spring*.[2] She reported that fish, birds, and other wildlife were being killed off by pesticides at an astonishing rate. In fact, in several areas a number of species of wildlife were nearing extinction after the chemicals had been in use for only a few years. She also warned us that these substances were most likely toxic to humans, but unfortunately, her warnings were not enough to change government regulatory policy or stem the tide of industrial and agricultural pollution.

An early pesticide–breast cancer warning was announced in 1976 when Dr. M. Wassermann of the Department of Occupational Health in Israel published a study that was supported in part by the World Health Organization. Dr. Wassermann's research revealed that DDT and other pesticides were found in very high concentrations in the tumors of women with breast cancer.[3]

There is a question that is begging to be asked. If the scientific community knew in the mid-1970s that DDT was highly concentrated in breast tumors, why has the issue of environmental toxins and breast cancer been ignored for almost twenty years?

❧ Organochlorines

Although thousands of hazardous chemicals have been introduced into our environment, a class of compounds called the organochlorines is probably the most dangerous. Massive quantities of these chemicals began to be produced after World War II, and today over 11,000 organochlorines are reportedly used in pesticides, plastics, industrial solvents, and refrigerants. Our primary exposure to these compounds comes from their frequent use in agriculture, as well as from their residential use as pesticides and weed killers on lawns and gardens throughout America.

Generally we know these substances by their abbreviations rather than their chemical names. Some of the major ones include dichloro-diphenyl-trichloroethane (DDT), dichloro-diphenyl-trichloroethylene (DDE), polychlorinated biphenyls (PCBs), polybrominated biphenyls (PBBs), hexachlorobenzene (HCB), dieldrin, and chlordane.

The possibility that ingesting traces of organochlorines is related to breast cancer comes from several observations. Many of these compounds are known to suppress the immune system and cause cancer in animals. More recently it has been discovered that many of the organochlorines, including DDT and PCBs, also exert estrogenlike activity that is known to stimulate breast cancer.

Organochlorines are very stable and resist being broken down and detoxified. It is this stability that enables them to remain in the environment—and the body—for very long periods. These compounds are also fat soluble; hence they concentrate in the fatty tissues of fish, birds, and commercial livestock. After eating these foods, we store the toxins in our fatty tissues. Corn or grain may have only two or three ppm (parts per million) of one of these pesticides, but a cow ingests many million kernels of corn and grains of oats in its lifetime. When you drink the milk or eat the meat, you are ingesting the lifetime fat-accumulated pesticides from that animal.

The Pesticide Monitoring Journal, published by the Environmental Protection Agency, monitors scientific studies and research regarding pesticide use. In response to what numerous studies have shown, the journal published the following statement: "Foods of animal origin are the major source of pesticide residues in the diet."[4] The following chart illustrates the source of several common pesticides in the U.S. diet.[5]

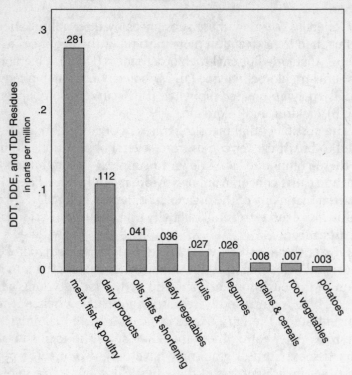

Pesticide Residues in the U.S. Diet

1964–68 Levels of DDT, DDE, and TDE
Data derived from: Corneilussen, P.E.,
"Pesticide Residues in Total Diet," *Pesticides Monitoring Journal*,
2:140–152, 1969

This chart clearly shows that the majority of pesticides come from meat and dairy products. However, it is also important to be aware of the following information. An article in the magazine *Vegetarian Times* suggests that "the government's latest figures on pesticide residues in fresh produce may spoil your appetite. According to a recent report from the U.S. Department of Agriculture's Pesticide Data Program (PDP), 61% of 6,000 fruit and vegetable samples tested had measurable residues from at least one pesticide, and many had residues from two or more different chemicals. That's not a real surprise, but here's the bad news: the samples were prepared as the consumer would eat them—washed, peeled, and cored."[6]

Pesticide tolerances are set and data are generally collected on food as the farmer harvests it in the field. An official from the EPA's Office of Pesticide Programs has been quoted as saying that this data and these "field tolerances" are "not ideal for deciding whether food is safe or not."[7] And yet these are the only tolerances to which we have access.

Richard Jackson, M.D., coauthor of a 1993 National Academy of Sciences study, *Pesticides in the Diets of Infants and Children,* is quoted as saying that current pesticide tolerances are like "setting the speed limit at 7,000 miles per hour and congratulating yourself that no one exceeds it. The tolerances are so high that clearly, there's very little food out there that breaks the law."[8] What we really need is a consumer uprising that forces a complete overhaul of the pesticide-regulation laws.

Fortunately, some environmental toxins have been discontinued. The use of DDT was banned in the United States in 1972, and PCBs were banned in 1977 after they were found to cause cancer in animals. However, just because they have been banned doesn't mean the problem has gone away. It is estimated that these compounds stay in the environment for decades, maybe even for centuries.

How big is the problem? Literally billions of pounds and billions of gallons of these toxins have been used. They are now in our soil and water, and they continue to make their way into our food chain.

❧ Pesticides in Breast Tumors

Several other recent studies have drawn attention to the pesticide–breast cancer hypothesis. Dr. Frank Falck and his colleagues did a pesticide chemical analysis of breast tumors from forty women (twenty with breast cancer and twenty with benign tumors). Their results showed that concentrations of

PCBs, DDE, and DDT were from 50 to 60 percent higher in women who had breast cancer than in women who did not.[9]

Another report chronicles the aftermath of an industrial accident in Germany that resulted in a large number of women being exposed to high levels of the toxic pesticide dioxin. These women are experiencing a higher incidence of breast cancer and twice the rate of cancer deaths as the German population as a whole.[10]

For years now it has been known that women who live in New York's Nassau and Suffolk Counties have one of the highest rates of breast cancer in the United States. The proposed explanation for this tragedy is that during the 1950s Long Island was heavily sprayed with DDT. A heart-wrenching documentary of this tragedy was aired on the popular TV program "Prime Time Live" on December 9, 1993.

Female professional golfers also have elevated rates of breast cancer. Many of these women, who have been playing golf since childhood, believe they have been poisoned by the pesticides and herbicides that are routinely sprayed on golf courses.

A survey by the U.S. Environmental Protection Agency has disclosed that counties where hazardous waste sites are located are 6.5 times more likely to have elevated rates of breast cancer.

ᴥ The Israeli Breast Cancer Story

Another study that strongly suggests a link between pesticides and breast cancer comes from Israel.[11] During the 1960s and 1970s breast cancer rates in Israel were among the highest and fastest-rising in the world. During this period milk and dairy products in Israel were contaminated with extremely high levels of three carcinogenic pesticides: DDT, alpha-BHC (benzene hexachloride), and gamma-BHC, also known as lindane. At the same time the breast milk in lactating Israeli women was found to contain extremely high levels of these pesticides.

In the spring of 1978 the women of Israel exploded in a dramatic public outcry of frustration and anger which ultimately caused their Supreme Court to ban use of those pesticides. The ban resulted in a substantial and almost immediate drop in the contamination of milk and dairy products in Israel. By 1980, a study of Israeli women in Jerusalem reported a 90 percent decline in the lindane content of breast milk, a 43 percent decrease in DDT levels, and an estimated 98 percent reduction in alpha-BHC.

More importantly, Israeli women also experienced a dramatic reduction in breast cancer. Previously, Israel had shown a twenty-five-year continual rise in breast cancer deaths. During the decade from 1976 to 1986, after the pesticide ban, Israel's breast cancer mortality rate actually fell 8 percent, while the rates in other countries continued to rise. During this decade younger Israeli women, aged twenty-five to thirty-four, experienced a spectacular 34 percent decrease in the incidence of breast cancer. The researchers also pointed out that when the 1976 rates and previous yearly increases were taken into consideration, the overall decline in breast cancer in the decade following the pesticide ban is probably closer to 20 percent. The dramatic drop in the incidence of breast cancer in Israeli women in the decade after the ban of these pesticides is powerfully suggestive of the link between pesticides and breast cancer.

On the other hand, a level of confusion exists because some studies on environmental toxins and cancer have reported negative findings. For example, a study in Denmark concluded that "the accumulation of PCB and DDT measured in breast tissue do not relate to the occurrence of mammary cancer."[12]

Scientists also continue to track the medical reports from Love Canal in Niagara Falls, New York. This area was used for over twenty years as a toxic waste dump site before being developed into a residential neighborhood in the 1950s. Although higher incidences of low birth weight and growth retardation have been reported, there has not yet been an increase in cancer mortality, as might be expected.

❧ *The Greenpeace Report*

In October 1993 the environmental group Greenpeace issued a sixty-seven-page report entitled *Chlorine, Human Health, and the Environment: The Breast Cancer Warning.*[13] The report states: "Organochlorines have been linked to large-scale hormonal disruptions, population declines, infertility and other reproductive problems, birth defects, impaired development, neurological and behavioral alterations, immune suppression and some types of cancer among people and wildlife."

Twenty scientists from a wide range of disciplines publicly endorsed the report, saying that it "provides an excellent public presentation of the growing body of evidence that links low-level organochlorine contamination of the environment to the risk of breast cancer in women."

Even with the publication of such reports, one of the saddest aspects of the pesticide story is that most people are not aware of the magnitude of the problem and the degree of cumulative exposure that comes from common, everyday commercial food choices. For example, at least nineteen pesticides with estrogenic activity are currently used on U.S. crops. This list includes atrazine (a weed killer that is the top-selling herbicide in the United States) and endosulfan (2 million pounds of which is applied each year to crops such as California grapes, lettuce, and tomatoes). The Environmental Working Group, a Washington-based nonprofit environmental policy organization, estimates that over 220 million pounds of pesticides with estrogenic activity are applied to sixty-eight different crops in the United States each year. The report by Greenpeace provides a much-needed public service by working to both educate and alert people about these dangers.

In their report Greenpeace also points out that safer alternatives to these pesticides already exist, and they issue an urgent call to all governments to phase out and discontinue the use of organochlorines.

An effort to educate medical doctors about the pesticide-breast cancer problem comes from David Perlmutter, M.D., whose letter to the editor was published in the *Journal of the American Medical Association*. After summarizing studies showing a relationship between organochlorine pesticides and breast cancer, he ends his letter with the following alarming report:

> The US government, hoping to stimulate the American economy, stands poised to approve the General Agreement on Tariffs and Trade (GATT). To stimulate worldwide agricultural trade, the GATT rules could allow substantially higher levels of pesticide residues on US import produce. Levels of DDT 5,000% higher than current US standards will be permitted on imported peaches and bananas with similar deregulation affecting grapes, strawberries, broccoli, and carrots.
>
> While recognizing the importance of national economics, this agreement, which affects safety standards of imported produce, demonstrates that the health of American women is not a primary concern.[14]

Consumer beware! In October 1994, President Clinton signed the GATT agreement. This means that starting in 1995, the relaxed standards will allow pesticide residues on imported produce that are enormously higher than what is allowed in the United States. Politicians will continue to put economic values ahead of health values . . . until we force them to change.

❧ Toxic Drinking Water

Hundreds of millions of pounds of five major herbicides—atrazine, cyanazine, simazine, alachlor, and metolachlor—are applied to agricultural crops in the United States every year. These toxic chemicals, which are known to cause birth defects, genetic mutations, and at least nine different types of cancer, have now thoroughly contaminated many of our lakes, rivers, and underground water supplies.

The Environmental Working Group recently published a disturbing report titled *Tap Water Blues: Herbicides in Drinking*

Water[15] which states that none of these herbicides are removed by the conventional drinking water treatment technologies that are used by more than 90 percent of the communities in the United States. Another problem is that the federal drinking water standards for these toxins are much weaker than they are for foods, making much higher levels of contamination legal in water supplies. For example, the drinking water standard for atrazine is nineteen times weaker than the EPA's food standard, and for cyanazine, which is the most toxic of all the herbicides, the drinking water standard is twenty-nine times weaker than the food standard. The health hazards represented by these discrepancies are a cause for concern.

❧ A Course of Action

What can you do to protect yourself and your daughters from pesticides and the other environmental risks for breast cancer? The answers lie in the interconnecting themes and topics that run through the various chapters of this book. Buy organic produce and reduce or eliminate meat and dairy products to minimize pesticide intake. Invest in a combination reverse osmosis/carbon filter water treatment system for your home. Taking extra antioxidant nutrients is also very important because they will help protect you against any future exposure, and against the pesticides you already have stored in your body.

For those of you who really want to detoxify yourselves, we suggest you seek out a certified clinical nutritionist or a health-oriented physician who can help you with a full detoxification program. These programs can include such elements as juicing, a detoxification diet, sauna sweats, colon cleansing, coffee enemas, and chelation therapy.

There is also a political course of action we hope many of you will take. Just what does that mean? To begin with, you can get mad as hell, and we hope you do! Write letters and/or make calls to your elected officials at the city, county, state, and federal levels of government. If possible, contact them personally and let them know that this is an important issue that you care deeply about. Threaten them with your activism and your vote. That is a language that politicians understand.

Contact Greenpeace and ask them how you can help locally and nationally. The organization's address and phone number are listed in Appendix B. One way or another, tens of millions of women in the United States, and hundreds of millions of women worldwide, need to collectively make their needs heard.

It is going to be a tough fight. Our suggestions on how to fight the breast cancer epidemic will challenge some of the biggest monolithic, multinational male-dominated industries in the world. For example, a low-fat, health-oriented, pesticide-free diet challenges the chemical and pesticide, agricultural, food processing, meat and dairy, and fast-food restaurant industries.

Can it be done? Yes it can! Big business and industry have enormous financial resources. They are making billions of dollars from the status quo; they have and will continue to resist change. On the other hand, women of America . . . you have millions of votes. You can force change to happen. If millions of women get committed and united, their voices and their votes can change the world.

You have a right to have a food and water supply that is safe and pesticide free. You also have a right to have a much greater percentage of your tax dollars channeled into programs that publicize, promote, and educate women about how to prevent breast cancer. Seize the opportunity. The time is now. Make yourself heard. Don't just get angry. Get active!

❧ Summary

This chapter has shown that there is mounting evidence indicating a possible association between environmental exposure to pesticides and the development of breast cancer. Although this link has not been conclusively proven, we think it is wise to understand the problem and do your best to minimize your exposure to these deadly toxins. One of the most important steps is to decrease your intake of meat and dairy products since these foods store and concentrate these chemicals. Other considerations include buying organically grown (unsprayed) food whenever possible and making sure that your source of drinking water is uncontaminated. We feel that a pesticide-free food and water supply are essential parts of the breast cancer prevention diet.

Chapter 14

Exercise: Feel Good and Live Longer

Regular exercise is an important, modifiable lifestyle activity that can substantially reduce a woman's lifetime risk of breast cancer. It is now known that exercise produces a more favorable pattern of menstrual cycles and also alters the production of female hormones.

A study published in the September 21, 1994, issue of the *Journal of the National Cancer Institute* reported that moderate regular exercise resulted in a substantial reduction of a premenopausal woman's risk of developing breast cancer.[1] The results showed that women who exercised from one to three hours per week could decrease their risk by about 30 percent compared to inactive women, and women who exercised four or more hours per week decreased their risk by more than 50 percent.

This study also reported that exercise for teenagers and young adults provided the greatest benefit. However, a very strong protective effect was also seen in women who started exercising as older adults. The results also showed that the protective effect of exercise against breast cancer was greater in women who exercised throughout their entire lives. This finding emphasizes the importance of creating a lifestyle that includes some form of regular physical exercise.

The authors of the study concluded: "Our data strongly suggest that continued participation in a physical exercise regimen can markedly reduce the risk of breast cancer in premenopausal women and emphasize the importance of beginning an exercise regimen early in life and maintaining it during adulthood."

◈ *Supportive Studies*

Dr. Rose Frisch at the Harvard School of Public Health examined the occurrence of breast cancer among female college athletes compared to nonathletes. Data were gathered from 5,398 women (2,622 former college athletes and 2,776 nonathletes) who were alumnae of eight different colleges from 1925 to 1981. Nonathletes had an 86 percent greater occurrence of breast cancer than athletes. The results were even more pronounced among women from both groups who had at least one full-term pregnancy. In this case, nonathletes had twice the risk of contracting breast cancer as the athletes. In their conclusion, the authors stated that "long-term athletic training establishes a lifestyle which somehow lowers the risk of breast cancer and cancers of the reproductive system." The study also found that the protective effects of exercise often overcame the existence of known risk factors such as age at menarche, hormone use, and age.[2]

A study evaluating the amount of physical activity in the workplace produced similar results. Women in occupations demanding higher levels of physical activity had a significantly lower incidence of breast cancer than women in jobs requiring less physical activity.[3]

In Finland, researchers evaluated the risk of breast cancer among female physical education and language teachers. As expected, language teachers were much less active than physical education teachers. And the results showed that language teachers had a 60 percent greater risk of developing breast cancer.[4]

❧ Moderate Physical Activity

There is also hope for the woman who is not an athlete and who doesn't plan on becoming one. When started in adolescence, even moderate levels of physical activity will produce the beneficial changes in menstrual cycle patterns and female hormones which significantly lower the risk of breast cancer later in life. According to the authors of this study, "Such moderate physical activity represents sustained participation of two or more hours per week in activities like aerobic exercise classes, swimming, jogging, or tennis."[5] Although this information only addresses adolescents, the following sections will demonstrate that exercise at any age provides women with protection against the development of breast cancer.

❧ Mechanism of Action

Based on a continually mounting volume of experimental and epidemiologic evidence, scientists agree that estrogen is a critical factor in the cause of breast cancer.[6] Therefore, anything that can modify the age of beginning menstruation, the frequency of ovulation, or the length of menstrual cycles could substantially reduce a woman's lifetime risk of developing breast cancer.[7] Exercise is one of those wonderful "magic bullets" that can make a significant difference.

In a study of breast cancer in very young women, researchers recorded not only the age at onset of menstruation, but also the age when "regular" menstrual cycles were established. Establishment of regular menstrual cycles within one year of the first menses—as opposed to more than five years—more than doubled the risk of breast cancer. Girls with early menarche (at age twelve or younger) and rapid onset of regular cycles have nearly a two times greater risk for breast cancer as girls with delayed menarche (at age thirteen or older) and longer time before regular cycles.[8] It has also been shown that girls who begin to menstruate early also establish ovulatory cycles more quickly than girls who have a later onset of menstruation.[9]

Numerous studies have shown that young girls who participate in some form of regular exercise substantially delay the onset of menstruation and the beginning of regular cycles. In one such study, a group of young ballet dancers were found to experience menarche at the age of 15.4 years. In the same study, music students experienced first menses at age 12.6 years and another group of girls who served as normal controls experienced their first menses at 12.5 years.[10] It is generally accepted that early menarche increases a woman's risk to breast cancer because it results in a greater lifetime exposure to estrogen.[11] This study indicates that nonexercising girls have a higher risk of developing breast cancer because they began to menstruate almost three years earlier than girls who exercise regularly during adolescence.

Another study found that high school girls who exercised two or more hours per week were more likely to have anovulatory menstrual cycles than girls who participated in minimal or no physical activity.[12] Other studies have supported this finding that exercising women[13,14] are more likely to have anovulatory cycles, thereby decreasing estrogen exposure and lowering breast cancer risk.

A third benefit from exercise is that it produces a beneficial shift within the menstrual cycle pattern. Cancer risk is greatest when cells are dividing. Biopsy[15] and autopsy[16] studies show that the rate of cellular division in breast epithelial cells is low during the follicular phase (second half) of the cycle and high during the luteal phase (first half). Thus, the amount of time spent in the luteal phase of the menstrual cycle is a significant determinant of a woman's risk to breast cancer. Research has shown that exercise shortens the length of the luteal phase of the cycle, resulting in a decreased risk to breast cancer.[17]

In summary, exercise-induced alterations in the female menstrual cycle help to reduce a woman's risk to breast cancer in three ways: in young girls, exercise delays both the onset of menarche and the beginning of regular cycles; in menstruating women, exercise causes a shortening of the luteal phase of the cycle; and lastly, women who exercise strenuously are more likely to have anovulatory cycles. Each of these alterations decreases a woman's overall exposure to estrogen.

✒ Exercising Women

Data on the health benefits of exercise continue to accumulate, showing that physical activity provides protective benefits ranging far beyond the prevention of breast cancer.

The good news is that more and more women are exercising regularly, as evidenced by the dramatic increase in the number of women competing in strenuous athletic events over the past two decades. For example, female participation in the New York Marathon increased from one runner in 1970 to 6,151 in 1993.[18]

Despite the important benefits of exercise, surveys of high school students and adults show that overall, few young people, and specifically few young women, exercise regularly. For example, the 1990 Youth Risk Behavior Survey showed that less than 40 percent of junior and senior high school girls were enrolled in physical education classes,[19] and only 20 percent of these girls participated in vigorous exercise three or more times per week.[20]

People who exercise regularly generally have a leaner physique and are closer to their ideal body mass. Body fat manufactures estrogen—about one-third of a premenopausal woman's supply—and virtually all of it after menopause.

Body fat also seems to influence or regulate how estrogen is metabolized. Women with a leaner body mass convert estrogen into a weaker, less carcinogenic, short-acting form, while heavier women produce more of the stronger, long-acting procarcinogenic type.

❧ Oxygen and Exercise

Understanding how oxygen functions at the cellular level explains another way that exercise helps to prevent breast and other types of cancers. Nobel Prize winner Dr. Otto Warburg discovered that cancer cells have a metabolic process that differs from that of healthy cells. Healthy cells are aerobic; they utilize oxygen in the production of energy. On the other hand, cancer metabolism is anaerobic, which means the cellular activity of cancer cells does not depend on oxygen. Dr. Warburg was able to demonstrate that certain cells exhibit cancerlike activity when there is a deficiency of oxygen, and when oxygen is reinfused back into the system the cells revert to normal behavior.[21]

Thus, optimal oxygen in the cells and tissues favors healthy, oxidative metabolism. Cancer metabolism, being anaerobic, favors a cellular environment with low levels of oxygen. Exercise stimulates the circulation of blood, which carries oxygen to the cells and tissues. This explains why exercise is one of the most important aspects of a health program.

❧ Strength Building

Researchers at the U.S. Department of Agriculture's Human Nutrition Research Center on Aging (HNRCA) at Tufts University have written a book that Ross feels is one of the most important books on exercise and health that has ever been written. The book is titled *Biomarkers: The 10 Keys to Prolonging Vitality*.[22] The authors of this book point out that weight lifting and other strength-building workouts are one of the most important, and yet, most frequently overlooked forms of exercise. This is especially true for women since strength-building is frequently thought to be more of a male/macho type of activity. Although these programs are universally beneficial, the comments in this section will be directed toward women.

Weight lifting and other strength-building exercises can make substantial biological changes for women in the following areas: decrease body fat, improve metabolic rate, increase muscle mass, strength, and aerobic capacity, and improve cholesterol, blood sugar, blood pressure, and bone density.

Improving aerobic capacity and cholesterol levels protects women from cardiovascular disease. Increasing bone density protects against osteoporosis. These are two of the greatest cripplers and killers of women.

Increasing muscle mass, strength, and improving metabolism helps women deal with a problem that a vast majority of them confront regularly, that of body fat and how it relates to their body image. This problem suggests the following connections to breast cancer. Excess body fat is a known risk factor for the disease (Chapter 10). Fats from animal products are more likely to contain pesticides, and fat cells store pesticides in our bodies—factors that have been linked to incidence of breast cancer (Chapter 13). For many women, being overweight seems like a helpless, hopeless predicament that produces a poor self-image and depression. In turn, depression can contribute to depressed immune function, which undermines the body's ability to fight off illness (Chapter 23).

Dieting and the many programs for weight control seldom produce long-term success. This is because they don't address or solve the underlying problem which is a combination of A.) too much fat; *and* B.) too little muscle. Body fat is metabolically inactive whereas muscle tissue's caloric needs are quite high. Simply put, building muscle helps to burn fat. Or, to put it another way, it is somewhere between difficult and impossible to successfully lose weight and keep it off by just going on a diet. Even if you are successful at losing some weight, keeping it off remains a battle. Most people gradually revert back to their old eating habits and put the weight back on again.

The real secret to success is changing the muscle-to-fat ratio in your body. This is called changing your body composition. You may feel you have too much fat, but the real problem is that you don't have enough muscle. If you really want to lose some weight and feel better about yourself, start lifting weights . . . build some muscle.

The authors of *Biomarkers* give the following explanation. "People with a high ratio of muscle to fat on their frame have a higher metabolism and a higher caloric need, and they don't have to worry as much about how much they're eating or about gaining weight. Conversely, because fewer calories are needed to maintain inactive fat tissue, obese people have a lower metabolism and a harder time losing weight no matter how little they eat."

Most people don't realize how extremely important muscle is in determining the overall vitality and well-being of your whole body. In fact, a strong, well-toned musculature provides a variety of wonderful contributions to your physical, mental, and emotional health. The benefits of muscle and strength building are so profound that we encourage all women to begin incorporating some form of this type of exercise into your workout program . . . just for the health of it.

Yoga

Yoga is one of the oldest organized fitness programs in the history of civilization. It is often misunderstood and thought of as an esoteric Eastern religion, when in fact it is a practical, systematic exercise program that has evolved over thousands of years and continues to provide an effective means of developing physical, mental, and spiritual well-being. The term *yoga* comes from the Sanskrit word meaning *yoke* or *union*, the bringing together of the mind, body, and spirit.[23] The first book to systematize yoga was the *Yoga Sutras* of Patanjali, which dates back to 200 B.C.[24] The aspects of yoga most practiced in the modern western world are hatha yoga (physical postures) and pranayama (breathing exercises).

Hatha yoga is a wonderful exercise for many reasons. One can begin this practice at any level of fitness or health, or at any age. Benefits are realized in a short period of time. Yoga is full-body conditioning, and when practiced regularly, one can develop agility, balance, strength, endurance, and great vitality. The postures (*asanas*) exercise and stimulate every muscle, nerve, and gland in the body.[25] Due to the slow, deliberate movements of the muscles, the lymphatic system, one of the body's primary structure's for detoxification, is activated. (See discussion on the lymphatics in Chapter 22.) Furthermore, the movements also bring more oxygen to the tissues.

Other types of exercises might also offer similar physiological benefits, however, what is special about yoga is that it is a "mindful" exercise. This term means that the physical exercise is performed with an inwardly directed cognitive component.[26] Benefits of mindful fitness are reduced stress, relaxation, enhanced mood, and greater vitality, perhaps resulting in greater immunity.

Referring you to Chapter 23, in which the impact of stress and depression on the immune system and general health is discussed, mindful exercise can be a crucial component in the prevention of breast cancer. In fact, many healing centers, such as the well-publicized Commonweal Cancer Help Program, Jon Kabat-Zinn's stress-reduction clinic, and Dean Ornish's program for healthy hearts, all utilize mindful exercise as a central part of their programs.

Unfortunately, Western medical science has produced few studies that support the benefits known by the practitioners of yoga. One study which compared the mood-altering benefits of swimming and yoga found the benefits of yoga to be equal for women and greater for men. Their conclusion was that aerobic exercise may not be necessary for mood enhancement. The authors of this study suggest that the deep, rhythmical, diaphragmatic breathing, which is a common element in stress-reduction techniques, may be responsible for the mood alteration. They theorize that other aspects of hatha yoga that may affect mood include stretching and relaxing large muscle groups in the body, an internal awareness, finding time for oneself, and a focus on the present moment thereby controlling the constant mind chatter.[27] Other unpublished studies report improvements in function and immunity in the respiratory system.[28]

Ross and Taffy have been practicing yoga for over twenty years. In fact, Taffy believes that if she had to choose only one type of exercise, it would be yoga. This choice is based on the fact that it can be aerobic, is strength-building, creates flexibility, helps detoxify the body, assists in the connection of all aspects of the self, and promotes an overall sense of well-being.

Most important, yoga is an excellent way to get to know your body. If you want to build and sustain health, it is critical that you gain greater awareness of the sensations of your body, where you hurt, what feels good, and how your bodily systems are functioning. A sustained practice of yoga can offer this. Initially, it is a good idea to take a class with a certified yoga teacher to learn the fundamentals and get feedback on your practice. It can then become a daily practice in the privacy of your home or with the use of the many videos available.

❧ Summary

Regular exercise is an area in which you can exert great control in the prevention of breast cancer. Ideally, three forms of exercise should be incorporated into your weekly schedule— strength-building and flexibility (yoga) workouts that target your muscles; and aerobic exercise that works your cardiovascular system.

Exercise appears to be more beneficial if started early and maintained throughout life, but no matter at what age you begin, you will reap immediate benefits. It is important to choose a form of exercise that you like. Rather than being a dreaded discipline, exercise can become an enjoyable part of your life.

Chapter 15

Smoking and Breast Cancer

Smoking, which has long been known to contribute to many health problems, is now being implicated in both the cause and promotion of breast cancer. In addition to explaining how toxins from cigarette smoke can affect the breasts, this chapter will discuss the seriousness of exposure to unfiltered sidestream smoke and the greater susceptibility of the developing adolescent breast to damage from smoke.

In the early 1980s it was initially proposed that smoking cigarettes might actually protect against the development of breast cancer. In fact, a possible connection between breast cancer and smoking was never even considered until 1982, when researchers discovered that women smokers actually had reduced urinary estrogen levels during the luteal phase of their menstrual cycles.[1] This antiestrogenic effect actually implied that smoking might lower the risk for breast cancer.

However, in 1986 a new hypothesis was proposed which suggested that cigarette smoke might exert carcinogenic effects on the breast that could override the possible benefits from reduced estrogen levels.[2] This hypothesis was based on two points: research had shown that cancer-causing agents from cigarette smoke concentrate in breast tissue fluids;[3] and that smoking causes an increased incidence of cancers in the cervix, pancreas, and bladder.[4] Since the smoke has no direct contact with these parts of the body, it became plausible to suspect that the toxins in smoke might also affect the breasts.

In the past decade over fifty different studies on smoking and breast cancer have yielded conflicting and inconclusive results. For the most part, these studies do not provide enough evidence to suggest that cigarette smoking substantially increases the risk of developing breast cancer. However, many studies have shown that smoking produces damaging effects on the immune system. For example, regular smokers are known to have lowered natural killer cell activity.[5]

Smoking also depletes the body's levels of antioxidants such as vitamin C, vitamin E, and beta-carotene.[6,7] As was discussed in Chapter 9, lowered levels of these key antioxidant nutrients increased the likelihood of free radical damage, which increases the risk of cancer.

A new understanding of the relative seriousness of exposure to sidestream smoke, the unfiltered smoke that is given off at the burning tip of a cigarette, may explain why previous research has provided so few answers regarding smoking and breast cancer risk.

✌ Passive Smoking

Passive smoking and involuntary smoking are terms that describe the involuntary exposure of nonsmokers to the tobacco combustion products, or sidestream smoke, generated by smokers. Sidestream smoke consists of the smoke that is not inhaled by the smoker, plus the portion of inhaled smoke that is exhaled.

Two studies have reported an increased incidence of breast

cancer in nonsmoking women who are married to smokers. One of these studies showed that nonsmoking women whose spouses smoked had twice the risk of developing breast cancer as nonsmoking women with nonsmoking husbands.[8] The risk was even higher for premenopausal women.

In a long-term study of 33,000 nonsmoking Japanese wives, it was found that women married to men who smoked one or more packs daily had a relative breast cancer risk four times greater than women married to nonsmokers.[9]

❧ A New Theory

Recently, A. Wesley Horton, Ph.D., of the Oregon Health Sciences University, has had two papers published on the topic of indoor tobacco smoke pollution. His papers provide some new insights into the possible link between exposure to cigarette smoke and the development of breast cancer.

To begin with, Dr. Horton notes that "a general lack of awareness of the difference in concentration of initiating and promoting factors in sidestream and mainstream smoke may well be an important factor in the current sad state of affairs in breast cancer epidemiology."[10] He points out that some very important information comes to light when the composition of cigarette smoke is examined more closely.

According to the 1986 Surgeon General's Report, indoor tobacco smoke is composed primarily of sidestream smoke, with less than 20 percent coming from the mainstream that has been inhaled and then exhaled by the smoker.[11] At the burning tip of the cigarette, red hot temperatures produce the sidestream smoke by evaporation and thermal decomposition of the tobacco, the paper, and the many curing agents, additives, and a wide range of pesticide residues also present in the tobacco. These combustion products are either completely vaporized or released as a suspension of microscopic particles in the smoke. The gas phase of smoke contains approximately twenty toxic and carcinogenic gases, and over 1,200 chemicals have been identified in the particulate phase of smoke, many of them known carcinogens and tumor promoters.[12]

This sidestream smoke is extremely dangerous because the toxic and carcinogenic chemicals that are released from the burning tip of a cigarette enter the atmosphere totally unfiltered. For example, in poorly ventilated enclosed areas, such as bars, automobiles, and conference rooms, allowing one pack of cigarettes to burn has produced levels of certain carcinogens that are ten times higher than in inhaled smoke itself.[13] The 1986 Surgeon General's Report, entitled *The Health Consequences of Involuntary Smoking*, states that sidestream smoke, when compared to mainstream smoke, contains from 20 to 150 times more (by weight) of carcinogens such as benzo(a)pyrene, nitrosamines, and aromatic amines than mainstream smoke.[14]

We know that smokers get a double load, breathing in both mainstream and sidestream smoke. However, what has long been overlooked is the exposure nonsmoking women have had to sidestream smoke. According to Dr. Horton, an important and often neglected variable in the study of breast cancer may well be how much exposure women have had to indoor tobacco smoke, generated by themselves, family members, or coworkers, particularly in the fifteen to thirty years before diagnosis.[15]

Both active and passive exposure to cigarette smoke result in increased estrogen levels. Noted researcher Dr. Henry Lemon states: "Many epidemiologists now believe that the majority of breast cancers are initiated within five years of menarche, as shown by the striking protective function of childbirth or competitive athletic exercise within this time frame on postmenopausal cancer risk."[16] This highlights the potential seriousness of exposure to cigarette smoke in adolescent girls.

A failure to consider and accurately adjust for exposure to indoor tobacco smoke may explain why so many studies on smoking and breast cancer have had conflicting and confusing results. Thousands of other cancer studies may also be somewhat flawed because exposure to sidestream smoke was not evaluated in both test and control subjects.

❧ Adolescent Exposure

The female breast is most susceptible to damage during the time of puberty, menarche, and for several years thereafter. During this period of rapid sexual development the initiating event for the future development of breast cancer may be a relatively short period of exposure to insults like radiation and/or chemical carcinogens, such as those in cigarette smoke.

The carcinogens in cigarette smoke can act as both initiators and promoters of breast cancer. Many of these highly toxic carcinogens are fat-soluble substances. They are inhaled through the lungs, absorbed into the circulatory system, and ultimately deposited in fatty tissue, especially the breasts. Once there, they are capable of damaging DNA within the cell. These "initiated" cells transfer the memory of the toxic exposure to new cells during cellular division. Thus, it appears that exposure to indoor, or sidestream, smoke can play a critical role in the initiation of a process that leads to breast cancer approximately twenty or thirty years later.

❧ A Message to Mothers

Mothers, please try to educate your daughters about the dangers of cigarette smoke. And remember, it's not just smoking, it is also associating with smokers that is the problem. Nonsmoking girls exposed to sidestream smoke are at a substantially higher risk for breast cancer. This means that smoke-filled rooms in bars or parties are potentially breast cancer–initiating environments. Teenage girls who ride around in cars with boyfriends who smoke are also in danger. And of course, girls who grow up in households where one or both parents smoke are in a daily deadly, high-risk environment.

And what about you women who either smoked or were exposed to passive sidestream smoke as young girls? If the cells in your breasts received "initiating" insults at parties or in smoke-filled bars one, two, or three decades ago, what can you do to prevent the promotion phase from progressing into breast cancer? The answer lies in the multiple themes that are presented throughout this book. For example, the major antioxidant nutrients have all been shown to decrease the incidence of breast cancers from chemical carcinogens such as those contained in cigarette smoke. Many breast cancers originate in the ductal epithelial cells, and beta-carotene has been shown to actually reverse some epithelial cell cancers.

Healthful low-fat, high-fiber diets, regular exercise, additional antioxidant nutrients, and soy foods can all help to prevent initial "hits" from developing into breast cancer. You obviously cannot eliminate your earlier transgressions, but there are many things you can do to help prevent past mistakes from becoming tomorrow's problems. A healthy lifestyle is your best protection against breast cancer, no matter your history.

◆ Summary

Now we have one more reason to discourage women from smoking; it may increase the risk of developing breast cancer. Recently this issue took on a greater level of significance when research showed that nonsmokers exposed to unfiltered sidestream smoke are also at greater risk. The toxic chemicals in cigarette smoke are capable of causing genetic damage, can initiate destructive free radical chain reactions, deplete levels of antioxidant nutrients, and decrease the amount of oxygen being carried to the cells and tissues. Each of these negative effects of smoke can increase a woman's risk of breast cancer. It is also important to realize that the risk appears to be greater for adolescents whose breast tissue is still in the developmental stage. The answer is pretty simple: Don't smoke, and don't spend time in smoke-filled environments.

Chapter 16

Alcohol Consumption

Alcohol, which is built into the very social fabric of our lives, is a continuing area of controversy with regard to our health. The media tells us on one hand a drink or two a day is great for the heart, and then turns around and informs us the same amount of alcohol can be a risk for breast cancer. In this chapter we will examine the research available on the relationship between alcohol and breast cancer so you may better understand what your risks are.

In 1982 one segment of a large cancer study reported finding that the frequency of alcohol consumption was related to an increased risk of breast cancer.[1] The publication of these findings stimulated a great deal of research, and since then over thirty studies have addressed this issue. Unfortunately, the overall results have been inconsistent and often contradictory.

One of the most important studies is a well-designed, diet-controlled trial in which all of the food and alcohol was measured and provided to thirty-four premenopausal women for a period of six menstrual cycles. In this study Dr. Marsha Reichman and her colleagues reported that regular consumption of 30 grams of alcohol per day (equivalent to approximately two average drinks) resulted in elevated blood levels of estrone and estradiol, and increased levels of estradiol in the urine.[2] You may recall that estrone and estradiol are the forms of estrogen that can be cancer-promoting. Although this study provides strong evidence that alcohol causes a rise in estrogen levels, it does not prove that alcohol causes breast cancer.

The Nurses' Health Study is one of the largest trials that has been conducted. Researchers followed 89,538 women between the ages of thirty-four and fifty-nine, and reported that those who consumed between three and nine drinks per week were 30 percent more likely to develop breast cancer than non-drinkers.[3]

In a comprehensive review of the literature, Dr. Lynn Rosenberg states that the association between alcohol and breast cancer is real, although rather weak.[4] Another literature review reported that five out of six epidemiological studies have found a positive correlation between alcohol consumption and increased risk for breast cancer. In the same review, out of twenty-eight case-controlled studies, eighteen reported a positive association and ten did not.[5] A look at the number of variables in this type of research provides some insight into why there is so much inconsistency.

Some researchers think there may be two distinctly different conditions to evaluate. They feel that alcohol's effect on premenopausal women, who have high levels of estrogen, may be quite different from alcohol's effect on postmenopausal women, in whom estrogen levels are lower and more stable. The type of alcohol consumed (wine, beer, or hard liquor) may also make a difference, as may the amount consumed and the frequency of consumption.

Age is another variable. According to some researchers, the consumption of alcohol is related to an increased risk of both pre- and postmenopausal breast cancer.[6] However, alcohol consumption among postmenopausal women may be more strongly related to breast cancer than is consumption earlier in life.[7]

Another set of variables related to alcohol's effect has to do with whether or not the women were exposed to excess estrogen in the form of oral contraceptives or hormone replacement therapy. Other confounding factors include exercise, smoking, and dietary habits. Recently it has also been suggested that alcohol ingested during the first half of a woman's cycle has a different effect than alcohol ingested during the second half, and this represents another variable that has seldom been addressed.

The significance of the interrelatedness of all these variables can be seen in one of the larger studies on estrogen replacement therapy: an increase in breast cancer was seen only in women who consumed modest amounts of alcohol. The estrogen produced no increased risk in nondrinkers.[8] This means that the ingestion of alcohol in combination with estrogen replacement therapy may increase the risk of breast cancer in postmenopausal women. If this is true, then many earlier studies researching different aspects of breast cancer may be flawed if they did not address alcohol as one of the active variables. However, other studies have failed to substantiate a relationship between alcohol consumption and elevated estrogen levels in postmenopausal women.[9] Thus, the results related to alcohol and elevated estrogen levels in postmenopausal women remain mixed.

One interesting contradiction in the efforts to find a link between alcohol and breast cancer comes from a study reporting that women alcoholics do not have an increased risk to breast cancer.[10]

✒ Summary

Even though there are some inconsistencies, a majority of studies indicate that alcohol consumption causes a slight increase in a woman's risk of breast cancer. One major review article, titled "Alcohol and Breast Cancer Risk—Putting the Current Controversy into Perspective," states that the results of published studies collectively show a weak association of alcohol with breast cancer risk that is found only at relatively high levels of intake (more than one or two drinks daily).[11]

Several studies have now shown that alcohol consumption increases estrogen levels, which suggests a possible explanation for the link between alcohol and breast cancer. At this time it is not possible to predict what level of alcohol ingestion is safe and where increased risk might begin. If you choose to consume alcoholic beverages, we suggest that you do so only occasionally and in moderation, using nutritional supplements and maintaining a healthful lifestyle to protect yourself as much as possible.

Chapter 17

The Benefits of Melatonin

Melatonin is one of the most promising new dietary supplements in recent history. We are devoting a full chapter to it because it may become one of the most important supplements you can take to help prevent breast cancer. In this chapter you will learn what melatonin is, where it comes from, what effects it has on our bodies, and how it can help with breast cancer prevention and treatment.

ᨠ *How Your Body Produces Melatonin*

Melatonin is a regulatory hormone produced by a pea-size region deep within the brain known as the pineal gland. Our bodies manufacture melatonin from serotonin, which is found in highest concentration in the pineal gland. In turn, we synthesize serotonin from tryptophan, an amino acid found in our diet (see Appendix B). Recently, it has been discovered that melatonin is also produced in other parts of our bodies, such as the digestive tract.

Melatonin is secreted by the pineal only at night, since direct sunlight suppresses melatonin secretion. Neural pathways lead from the retinas of our eyes to a pair of small neural "hubs," which, in turn, connect to the pineal. These neural hubs, called the suprachiasmatic nuclei, send out signals that control all of the body's circadian rhythms. Thus, information about duration and intensity of sunlight exposure can be relayed directly to the pineal, affecting its natural rhythms. This retinal neural connection is separate from the visual pathway. Interrupting sleep with very bright light can shut off melatonin production. This light must be five times as bright as normal indoor light. As with many things, melatonin production decreases as we age.[1] Giving melatonin to aging mice, whose own natural melatonin levels are declining, prolongs their survival.

❧ *How Melatonin Functions*

SUPPRESSING BREAST CANCER CELLS

It has been established that melatonin inhibits breast cancer growth in cell cultures of certain estrogen receptor positive (ER+) breast cancer cells. This concentration of melatonin that suppresses the growth of breast cancer cells is found in women during sleep around 2 A.M. It is also known that exposure to a strong electromagnetic field (EMF) suppresses our melatonin production. One of the many theories for our increasing incidence of breast cancers is that of melatonin suppression by our modern environment's ubiquitous electric power and EMFs.[2,3] EMFs alone have no effect on breast cancer cell growth in culture; however, experimentally, EMFs are able to block melatonin's suppression effects upon the breast cancer cells.[4] Through this mechanism the presence of a significant level of EMFs would allow breast cancer cells to proliferate. (EMFs are discussed in depth in Chapter 18.)

AUGMENTATION OF TAMOXIFEN

In breast cancer cell cultures, treatment with tamoxifen, the anti-estrogen agent often used to treat ER+ breast cancers, can be augmented by the presence of melatonin. Experimentally, when breast cancer cells were exposed first to melatonin and then to tamoxifen, there was a significant improvement in the tamoxifen's inhibitory effect. The authors of the experiment stated that tamoxifen is a hundred times more potent as an inhibitor of breast cancer cell growth following the pretreatment of cells with a *physiologic* (normal) concentration of melatonin.[5] On the other hand, if tamoxifen is administered prior to or with melatonin, then the inhibitory effect of melatonin is blocked rather than enhanced. This suggests the tamoxifen is able to tie up or block the estrogen receptors on the breast cancer cells, not allowing the melatonin to do the same.[6] Therefore, though both tamoxifen and melatonin are inhibitors of ER+ breast cancer cell growth, their modes of action appear to be different. The order of their use in future therapy trials would seem to be critical to achieve optimal effects.

EFFECTS OF CHEMOTHERAPY

Interestingly, certain chemotherapy agents used to combat breast cancer are themselves blockers of the anti–breast cancer effects of melatonin. For example, in one study of breast cancer cell cultures, *physiologic* levels of melatonin inhibited the growth of cancer cells 50 percent better than the chemotherapy agent 5-fluorouracil (5-FU). In addition, when 5-FU was present with melatonin, there was a reduction of the inhibitory effect of melatonin. The authors suggest that 5-FU be handled with care for treatment of ER+ breast cancers since it would block the anti–breast cancer effects of what little melatonin the woman is producing.[7]

AUGMENTATION OF IMMUNOTHERAPY

In another study of patients with advanced-stage solid cancers (colon, rectal, stomach, breast, pancreas, liver, and unknown), most of whom had distant metastasis, treatments involved a form of immunotherapy—interleukin-2 (IL-2)—along with melatonin. Standard forms of therapy had not been effective in these patients, and melatonin had previously been shown to have a synergistic action with IL-2. The results of this study showed that the combined therapy was capable of controlling tumor growth in these patients.[8]

CIRCADIAN RHYTHMS IN CANCER PATIENTS

Many patients with cancers, including breast cancers, have no circadian melatonin rhythm owing to loss of nighttime melatonin production by the pineal gland. It is not known at this time whether the abnormal circadian rhythm or the cancer occurs first. It is known that this decline in melatonin is associated with a disturbance in the immune system and subsequent weakened immune response. Furthermore, the lowered melatonin levels may be a predisposing factor that allows a small cluster of malignant cells to develop into a life-threatening tumor with metastatic potential.[9,10]

REGULATING SLEEP CYCLES

Taking an oral supplement of melatonin at bedtime (3 to 9 milligrams) promotes deep, restful, and restorative sleep without side effects. Unlike most over-the-counter and prescription pills, melatonin enables deep REM sleep—the phase of sleep that leaves one refreshed and full of energy upon waking.

Other Conditions Helped Currently, over thirty new melatonin research papers are published every week. Melatonin is currently being tested for treating "winter depression" or seasonal affective disorder (SAD), jet lag, work shift disorders, and other sleep disorders. It is also being investigated for its beneficial effects in treating certain cancers. Its broadest use may stem from this study, and it may be applicable in the actual *prevention* of cancers.

AN IMPORTANT ANTIOXIDANT

Melatonin is an antioxidant, which, as you remember, sops up oxidative free radicals before they can do cellular and intra-

cellular damage. While most antioxidants have difficulty pene-
trating cell membranes and deactivating free radicals within
cells, melatonin easily penetrates not only the cell membrane
but also the subcellular compartments. Melatonin specifically
scavenges hydroxyl radicals, considered the most damaging of
all free radicals. As we learned in Chapter 1, cancers are believed to be formed by "2 hits"—initiation and promotion. Most
methods of decreasing our breast cancer risk act upon the promotion phase, but melatonin acts upon the difficult initiation
phase. If a substance known to produce DNA damage is administered after melatonin pretreatment, there is virtually no
free radical DNA damage.

ENHANCEMENT OF THE IMMUNE SYSTEM

Melatonin has been shown to restore immune function in
aged mice, in which it can more than double the antibody response. It also caused an increase in the vital immune component interleukin-2 (IL-2). In these mice, melatonin was able to
reverse some of the immune-suppressant effects of a
chemotherapeutic agent, which is an important problem of
chemotherapy patients. Recent studies have shown the presence of melatonin receptor sites on lymphocytes, one of the
body's white blood cells. This suggests a direct effect of melatonin on the regulation of lymphocytic immune function.

✺ Who Might Benefit from Melatonin?

Because melatonin is inexpensive and safe, many feel that
after age forty it is wise to supplement the body's declining
melatonin levels to obtain improved overall health and to prevent breast cancer.[11]

❧ Who Should Not Take Melatonin?

Individuals with lymphoma, myeloma, leukemia, or Hodgkin's disease should probably not take melatonin since these diseases originate with the bone marrow's immune cells and further studies are needed to determine if melatonin has a positive or negative effect on regulation of these cells. Women attempting to become pregnant should also avoid melatonin, especially since European scientists are studying high doses of melatonin for its contraceptive possibilities. Individuals with depression usually improve with melatonin; however, if you feel more depressed after taking melatonin, cease taking the supplement.

❧ How Much to Take?

The pineal gland of a healthy young adult produces about 2.8 mg of melatonin nightly. This does not include the melatonin produced by other parts of the body, such as the digestive tract. Under the age of forty, you probably don't need a melatonin supplement. After age forty, though, the body's production begins to drop, and you might consider supplementation. Three-milligram capsules of melatonin are most common, and it is suggested that a starting dose be one capsule at bedtime or an hour before. If you experience no sleepiness from the melatonin, take two 3 mg capsules the next night. You can increase the dose to 9 mg. Sensitivity to melatonin is rare, but it can produce morning lethargy in some individuals. For those so affected, there are 1 mg capsules.

TIMING IS EVERYTHING
The timing of melatonin usage is important. Taking melatonin at random times each day has the potential to interfere with your sleep cycle. Physicians specializing in sleep disorders have discovered that you must first determine your sleep cycle needs before using melatonin. If you have no desire to shift

your sleep period, take the melatonin at bedtime. On the other hand, if you desire to shift your sleep period to an earlier time (termed phase advance), for reasons such as lack of sleepiness at bedtime or travel to a different time zone, take melatonin in the afternoon. Conversely, if you wish to shift your sleep to a later period (termed phase delay), use the melatonin after awakening in the morning.[12] For unresponsive chronic insomnia and treatment or prevention of jet lag or SAD, locate a physician who specializes in sleep disorders and is experienced in the use of melatonin.

BREAST CANCER PATIENTS

If you have breast cancer, you will need to supplement with even higher doses of melatonin. As with all treatments, do this under the care of your physician. He or she can perform computer MEDLINE searches of the recent medical literature to determine the doses and regimen appropriate for your treatment.

~ Summary

Melatonin is a natural antioxidant produced in our bodies which has numerous beneficial effects. It improves the quality of sleep, immune function in older individuals, and breast cancer treatment regimens; prevents free radical damage to our cells and DNA damage; and inhibits the growth of breast cancer cells. Because our melatonin levels decline after the age of forty, it is advisable to use an inexpensive and side effect–free melatonin supplement nightly. As with any product that could make one sleepy, do not take melatonin if you intend to drive or operate machinery. (See Appendix B for information on obtaining melatonin.)

Chapter 18

Electromagnetic Fields

As countries industrialize, there is a tremendous increase in the use of electrical power. In fact, electricity is now such an integral part of our lives that we take it largely for granted. A geographical study showed that the rates of hormone-related cancers, such as those of the breast and prostate, are much higher in industrialized areas.[1] A question that is increasingly being asked is whether or not the enormous increases in our use of electricity in the past century could be partly responsible for these cancers.

Along with the benefits of electrical power have come vast increases in our exposure to certain electromagnetic fields (EMF). These changes have been very recent and abrupt in terms of human evolution. The purpose of this chapter is to examine the possibility that our exposure to various electric and magnetic fields might be causing or contributing to the epidemic of breast cancer.

For millions of years, humans were only exposed to the earth's magnetic field. However, in the last century, the development of commercial electricity has increasingly exposed humans to what is now being referred to as "electronic pollution." There are really two different types of fields to consider: electric and magnetic. Electric fields are measured in volts per meter. They are produced by the voltage, or electrical "pressure," in a wire, which occurs, for example, when an appliance is plugged in but not turned on. By contrast, magnetic fields, measured in milligauss (mG), are created by the current, or flow of electricity, through a wire, which occurs when an appliance is turned on. Electrical fields can be blocked or partially shielded, while magnetic fields can pass through most objects and are much more difficult to shield. Both types of fields can cause potential problems; however, the research that has been done focuses strictly on electromagnetic fields.

During the past two decades there has been a growing concern that exposure to electromagnetic fields can cause an increased risk of certain types of cancer. These fields are generated from electrical installations and/or electrical equipment using the standard 50 to 60 hertz (Hz) alternating current. To date, studies have attempted to evaluate risk from two types of exposure.

❧ Residential Exposure

The first type of exposure concerns people who live in homes located near installations transmitting electrical power. This can include either generating substations or electrical power lines. Two separate studies have reported that children who live in homes with high EMF exposure developed leukemia and lymphomas up to three times more frequently than children living in homes with minimal exposure.[2,3]

More recently, a European study has sent shock waves throughout the world's scientific community. A well-designed, tightly controlled Swedish study reported finding that the rate of childhood leukemia rises with increasing exposure to magnetic fields. Children living in homes with more than 1 mG had twice the rate of leukemia as children in homes where exposure was below 1 mG. Children exposed to more than 2 mG had nearly a three times greater incidence of leukemia, and those exposed to more than 3 mG had almost a four times greater incidence of leukemia.[4]

❧ Occupational Exposure

The second form of exposure occurs in the workplace. A number of studies have reported that people who work either with or near equipment that generates or transmits electricity have slightly increased rates of leukemia.[5]

The debate over this issue continues to draw attention. More recently, several studies have reported a possible link between exposure to electromagnetic fields and breast cancer.

❧ EMF, Melatonin, and Breast Cancer

Melatonin is the primary hormone secreted by the pineal gland in the brain, and one of its effects is the suppression of estrogen. This direct relationship to estrogen has some researchers referring to melatonin as the anti–breast cancer hormone. In fact, research has shown that lower melatonin levels result in higher levels of circulating estrogen and a corresponding increase in breast cancer risk.[6] A detailed discussion of melatonin's association to breast cancer is found in Chapter 17.

Experimental evidence on EMF and breast cancer is limited; however, several animal studies have shown that exposure to 60-Hz electric fields reduces the pineal gland's normal nighttime production of melatonin, which results in increased mammary cancer.[7,8] Other researchers have shown that melatonin, added to the growth medium of a line of actively growing human breast cancer cells, stops their growth. When a small magnetic field was applied to this system, the cancer cells began to grow again.[9]

Four epidemiological studies have reported that men working in various electrical occupations have an increased incidence of the relatively rare disease, male breast cancer.[10,11,12,13] Although breast cancer is obviously far more common in women, evaluation of occupational exposure has been difficult because relatively few women work in trades that subject them to elevated electromagnetic fields.

One study has addressed the incidence of breast cancer among female electrical workers in the United States. This study evaluated data from death certificates containing occupation and industry codes, which enabled researchers to assess potential occupational exposure to electromagnetic fields. Overall, 38 percent more breast cancer deaths were found than would have been expected in a normal population. These women had worked as electrical engineers, electrical technicians, or telephone installers, repairers, and line workers.[14] Because of the small number of participants in this trial, researchers do not consider it a statistically significant study. However, studies like this are drawing increased attention to the potential danger of exposure to electromagnetic fields.

❧ Electronic Pollution

Dr. Luchiano Zaffanella conducted a survey of homes for the Electric Power Research Institute (EPRI). His research showed that problems in the electrical wiring systems in many homes can create dangerously high electromagnetic fields.

International testing agencies suggest that EMF environments in residential buildings should be below 1.0 mG. In his survey of U.S. homes, Dr. Zaffanella found the average magnetic field strength to be 0.35 mG, while homes located near power lines had higher readings, as expected. However, 10 percent of the homes he surveyed had fields measuring 3.7 mG, which is almost four times higher than the suggested limit.

One percent of the homes registered levels as high as 19 mG. The high readings were caused by faulty wiring, grounding problems, unbalanced circuits, or stray currents running along water and gas pipes.

The Environmental Testing & Technology Company of Encinitas, California, has conducted more than 1,000 EMF home surveys, and their work confirms the findings reported by Dr. Zaffanella. In fact, they report finding some homes with house-generated EMF fields higher than fields directly under high-tension power lines. For example, in one home, levels of 18 mG and 0.3 mG were measured in adjacent bedrooms. When a defective electrical circuit was fixed, the 18 mG dropped down to the 0.3 mG background level. In another home, fields fluctuating between 6 and 50 mG were measured in the living room. Extensive investigation finally identified a faulty circuit breaker panel in a house across the street as the source of the stray currents and high magnetic fields. After repairs, the fields normalized.

❧ Swedish Guidelines

Sweden is the first country to officially acknowledge the link between cancer and exposure to elevated electromagnetic fields. In September 1992 the Swedish government announced new guidelines and standards for residential and occupational EMF exposure, based on the assumption that there is a connection between electromagnetic fields and cancer. In Sweden, guidelines now prohibit schools to be built on property where magnetic fields are higher than 2.0 mG and limit the exposure of computer workstations to 2.5 mG.[15]

❧ Testing Their Home

During the process of researching and writing this chapter, Ross and Taffy became so curious and concerned about electromagnetic fields that they decided to have their home tested. It was a very interesting, and somewhat sobering, experience.

Although the entire house was tested, most of the attention was focused on their bedroom. It was pointed out to them that electromagnetic fields often make the bedroom the most dangerous room in your home. Most of us sleep from six to eight hours per night, and spend from one-quarter to one-third of our lives in bed.

Peter Sierck, the director of Environmental Testing & Technology who conducted their tests, emphasized that EMF exposure during sleep is much more harmful than the same EMF exposure during waking hours. During sleep many of our normal defense mechanisms are shut down while the body undergoes rest, relaxation, rejuvenation, and repair. Peter stated, "Nowhere is the impact of environmental stressors more significant than in the hours of sleep." It is generally agreed that undisturbed, relaxed sleep is essential for good health.

❧ Testing Taffy and Ross's Bed

ELECTRIC FIELDS

The tests for electrical fields in their bedroom were a shock to them (no pun intended). While lying in bed, Taffy's body measured 1.8 volts of electricity (a 1.5-volt battery has enough power to run a small radio). Peter explained that with her legs stretched out, Taffy's body actually acted like an antenna which increased the charge on her body. It was very disturbing to realize that while lying in bed, *their bodies built up enough voltage to run a radio!*

To further demonstrate this electrical charge, Peter touched Taffy with an electrician's test pen while she was lying in bed. The LED light on the pen glowed bright red, just as it did when he tested the electrical outlet on their wall.

This experience had a substantial emotional impact on both of them. Peter cautioned them not to be too alarmed, adding that little is known about the physiological or health effects of electrical fields as opposed to magnetic fields. However, Taffy was so disturbed that she refused to sleep in the bed until she and Ross had pulled it out three feet away from the wall. They were able to determine that a strong electrical field emanated from the electrical wiring within that wall.

With no scientific data available on electrical fields, they can only report anecdotally that since they corrected the problem their sleep has improved and they are recalling more dreams than ever. They are led to wonder if sleeping in an electrical field might inhibit dream or dream recall, an important part of healthy sleep patterns.

MAGNETIC FIELDS

Concurrent to testing the electrical fields, Peter was testing the magnetic field strength Taffy and Ross are exposed to when they are in bed. The average safe reading is about 0.35 mG; however, their reading registered a steady 1.1 mG. Although this is about three times higher than average, they were told that the field strength would have to approach 2.0 mG before it could be considered a health hazard. The tests suggested that the source of this magnetic field could be one of the city's underground cables buried beneath the street outside their house.

They also had their computers checked out. The field emanating from Taffy's newer monitor was below 1 mG. Ross's six-year-old monitor measured a magnetic field above 4 mG, which is well into the hazardous zone. From this experience, they would encourage everyone to obtain up-to-date computer equipment, particularly monitors.

Water-bed heaters and electric blankets also generate electromagnetic fields. One small study reported slight, but nonsignificant elevations of breast cancer with continuous nighttime use of electric blankets.[16] Until more evidence is in, it is advisable to turn water-bed heaters and electric blankets on before bedtime to warm things up and then turn them off when going to bed.

Although we have focused our attention on the electrical environment in the bedroom, it should be noted that almost all electrical appliances and devices generate electromagnetic fields. Therefore, appliances like microwave ovens, clothes washers and dryers, electric ranges, fluorescent lights, and television sets all generate EMFs. However, since electromagnetic fields get weaker with distance, the EMFs from these household items do not pose problems from a distance of approximately three feet.

The following chart shows how the magnetic fields from three commonly used household appliances get weaker with distance:

Magnetic Fields Measured in Milligauss[17]

Distance:	1.2 inches	12 inches	39 inches
Microwave oven	750 to 2,000	40 to 80	3 to 8
Television	25 to 500	0.4 to 20	0.1 to 2
Hair dryer	60 to 20,000	1 to 70	0.1 to 3

Note that hair dryers generate powerful magnetic fields. Since hair dryers are used frequently at distances that are relatively close to the body, the general precaution is to use them for shorter periods and to hold them as far away from the body as possible. Parents are also advised not to let their children sit too close to the television set when watching it.

❧ Costs

The cost of professional residential testing for electromagnetic fields is about $500. It cost about $265 to correct the problems in Taffy and Ross's bedroom, but they feel that their health is well worth the expense.

❧ *Summary*

The association between breast cancer and electromagnetic fields should be viewed as a hypothesis that is still in the very early stages of evaluation. To date, only a few small studies have been conducted, and therefore at this time we do not know whether EMFs cause or promote cancer. However, the known effects of EMFs on melatonin levels provide a strong biological rationale for future studies. We need to determine if exposure to electromagnetic fields might be implicated in the increased incidence of several types of cancers, including breast cancer.

For the time being, prudent avoidance is the approach that makes the most sense. Based on the research to date, we feel it is wise to minimize the amount of EMF exposure in homes and occupational environments. This includes identifying sources of EMF exposure, increasing your distance from EMF sources, and changing the amount of time and the way you use common electrical appliances.

Information on how you can have your residential or occupational environment tested for electromagnetic fields is referenced in Appendix B.

Chapter 19

Tamoxifen and Breast Cancer Treatment

An ancient medical expression charges a treating physician to "First do no harm." This is a basic tenet of medical practice and applies as much today as it did thousands of years ago. Physicians must carefully weigh expected benefits against possible risks before making a therapeutic choice. Today we refer to this as a benefit-to-risk ratio. If the risks are too large and/or the possible benefits too small, then the treatment should probably be avoided. In this chapter we will learn about tamoxifen: what kind of drug it is, its approved uses, possible benefits, and risks. We will discuss the federal Breast Cancer Prevention Trial (BCPT), which proposes to place healthy women on a possibly harmful drug. Since this is not a therapy decision but a prevention decision, the notion of first doing no harm to the normal subjects becomes a prime concern.

Tamoxifen, sold in the United States under the name Nolvadex, is an orally administered, potent anti-estrogen drug.

It appears to act by binding to estrogen receptor sites on cells. Depending upon the treatment regimen, one or two ten-mg tablets are taken twice a day, or one tablet three times daily. It has been used for over twenty years and is probably the most prescribed anticancer medication in the world.

APPROVED FOR BREAST CANCER TREATMENT

Tamoxifen is approved only for the treatment of breast cancer and is usually used as an adjuvant agent (an additional therapy, which is added to an existing treatment regimen) in localized, regional, or widespread disease. It seems to have greatest effects with estrogen receptor positive (ER+) tumors in postmenopausal women, or in premenopausal women having both ER+ and progesterone receptor positivity. When used as adjuvant therapy in women with early breast cancer, tamoxifen has increased both "disease-free survival"—meaning survival without clinical evidence of the breast cancer—and "overall survival," or survival regardless of clinical presence of the cancer. It has also reduced the incidence of new breast cancers occurring in the opposite "normal" breast.[1,2] Physicians have the right to prescribe drugs for conditions not listed on the package insert, and tamoxifen is no exception. As a result, tamoxifen is being used as a part of treatment protocols with other malignancies, such as melanoma.

⮞ *Tamoxifen Breast Cancer Prevention Trial*

One of the most controversial "prevention" studies of our time is the Breast Cancer Prevention Trial, a massive $68 million trial studying 16,000 healthy women with a "high risk" for breast cancer. *Prevention*, in this instance, means giving a potentially harmful drug to normal healthy women in an attempt to prevent breast cancer. Because of the known decreased incidence of new primary breast cancers in the opposite "normal" breasts of women being treated for breast cancer with tamoxifen, the National Cancer Institute designed and funded a clinical experiment. Its four objectives are to determine if tamoxifen is effective in (1) reducing the incidence of invasive breast cancer, (2) reducing breast cancer mortality, (3) reducing deaths from cardiovascular disease, and (4) reducing bone fractures. In addition, the study will evaluate side effects, toxicity, and the quality of life of the women in the trial. Both pre- and postmenopausal women aged thirty-five and up will be included in the experiment. Women over sixty years of age may be entered into the study, even without risk factors other than age. For a ten-year period, one-half of the women will receive tamoxifen, the other half a placebo.

Many medical critics say the study may do more harm than good.[3,4] Others emphasize the importance of performing such a needed study while involving such little risk.[5,6] Based on epidemiological data from the past, tamoxifen may prevent 30 to 40 percent of the breast cancers in high-risk women. Since tamoxifen acts as an estrogen with regard to serum cholesterol, the drug's effect on osteoporosis and coronary heart disease is also being studied. The statistical prediction is that of the women given tamoxifen, 124 will develop breast cancer, compared to 186 breast cancer cases in the group not receiving the drug. However, this drug is not innocuous, as it produces an increase in the number of hot flashes and vaginal discharges, as well as additional risks for premature menopause, blood clots, blindness, birth defects, liver failure, cancer of the liver, and endometrial cancer.

Of special concern is the impact of tamoxifen on ovarian function in premenopausal women and the potential risks to the fetus if pregnancy occurs. Tamoxifen has been previously used only in women who have had a personal history of breast cancer, never in those who were simply at "high risk." This study is somewhat unusual because it is using people who are not sick rather than individuals whose only other alternative is to die. Past studies with breast cancer patients showed that the tamoxifen appeared to decrease the incidence of breast cancer in the remaining breast and was most effective in postmenopausal women. Studies done in Sweden suggest that tamoxifen *increases* mortality in postmenopausal women who developed cancer in the other breast, since these cancers were very aggressive and treatment-resistant. Even in rat experiments, the drug decreases the rate of breast cancer, but the breast cancers that do develop are highly malignant. For the 124 women with breast cancer receiving the tamoxifen, this could mean that their cancers could be much more deadly than those of the 186 women with breast cancer in the control group.

A recent critique of the trial by the Johns Hopkins School of Public Health notes that the results showed a negative to slightly positive benefit. If the eye complications, such as blindness, are included, then certainly "more harm than good will result from the [tamoxifen] intervention." The authors go on to say: "The lack of significant benefit to participants . . . may raise the question of whether the trial should continue as designed." They conclude that "the fundamental philosophical question of whether large numbers of healthy women should be 'treated' with a *toxic drug* [emphasis added] for the primary prevention of a rare event remains."[7] The authors of this book would remind the scientists involved in the prevention trial to follow the "First do no harm" axiom.

HOW DOES TAMOXIFEN WORK?

In some instances, tamoxifen can act as an antioxidant. (We discussed antioxidants in Chapter 9.) It does not have the same activity as the antioxidant vitamin E, but can enhance vitamin E's protectant effects on fatty tissues. It is this free radical-scavenging ability that may be in part responsible for preventing breast cancer.[8] One recent study found measurably lower levels of free radical damage to fatty tissues in postmenopausal women taking tamoxifen for breast cancer than normal women, as well as significantly increased levels of antioxidant vitamins A, C, and E.[9] Remember that an antioxidant is "used up" when it scavenges a free radical. It sacrifices itself for the cause, so to speak. So when tamoxifen scavenges free radicals, this allows the antioxidant vitamins to remain in an active state, since there are fewer free radicals to "use" them up. Keeping these levels higher is beneficial for many reasons, as we learned in Chapter 9.

TAMOXIFEN'S ESTROGENIC AND ANTI-ESTROGENIC EFFECTS

Even though tamoxifen is anti-estrogenic, it has some estrogenic properties. Just as estrogen improves the cholesterol profile and protects against cardiovascular disease, tamoxifen decreases total serum cholesterol by lowering the "bad" LDL form without changing the "good" HDL form.[10,11,12] Tamoxifen has also been found to lower another potent risk factor for cardiovascular disease, a substance in the blood called lipoprotein (a), in the same manner as estrogen.[13] Yet another estrogenic effect is protection against osteoporosis in estrogen-deficient states. Tamoxifen treatments may result in increased or stabilized bone mineral density in the spine and pelvis regions, together with a stabilization in the bones of the arms and legs.[14,15,16,17] It may also alleviate symptoms of so-called fibrocystic disease of the breasts.[18]

✦ Side Effects of Tamoxifen

Tamoxifen's adverse effects include hot flashes and nausea and/or vomiting in up to 25 percent of patients. Less frequent problems include vaginal dryness, bleeding or discharge, menstrual irregularities, and skin rash. There may also be a decrease in the number of circulating white blood cells and platelets. Platelets, tiny circulating blood elements, are very important in preventing excessive bleeding. When tamoxifen is used by a woman who is also taking certain forms of anticoagulants, over-anticoagulation can occur, and bleeding results. Furthermore, certain blood fat levels can become elevated, and fertility may be impaired. Women with breast cancer having adjuvant tamoxifen therapy have a dropout rate of 4 percent as a result of side effects. Interestingly, in a series of men with breast cancer, the dropout rate was almost 21 percent, owing to decreased libido, weight gain, hot flashes, insomnia, and blood clots in deep veins of the legs.[19] There have even been a few rare reports of acute arthritis involving multiple joints (similar to rheumatoid arthritis) in women taking tamoxifen.[20] And if that's not enough, eye toxicity has been reported, causing cataracts, abnormalities of the cornea or retina, visual symptoms such as blurred vision, and rarely, blindness.[21,22]

LIVER ABNORMALITIES

An extra-disturbing side effect concerns the liver. Animal studies have shown that tamoxifen can cause liver cancers at many dose levels, not just at unreasonably high concentrations. In one experiment, a single dose of tamoxifen in rats produced multiple changes in liver cells, including chromosome damage. All cancers begin with chromosome damage, either inherited or developed. The authors of this study state that the "risk versus benefit of tamoxifen treatment should be very carefully evaluated."[23] Another group that demonstrated liver cell DNA damage related to tamoxifen stated that "further studies may be required to establish the safety of tamoxifen treatment of women for purposes other than chemotherapy."[24,25]

PELVIC TUMORS

The list of negatives grows longer. Studies have shown that tamoxifen (acting as an estrogen) causes women to have a significantly increased number of gynecological tumors and cancers.[26] For one thing, endometrial carcinomas are a well-known complication of tamoxifen therapy. Women using tamoxifen will have a larger uterus with more blood flow through uterine arteries. Thirty-five percent have evidence of abnormal cells lining the inside of their uterus (endometrium), compared with 10 percent in a control group. This study showed that tamoxifen caused premalignant changes in the endometrium of postmenopausal women, and that transvaginal ultrasonography should be used to screen these women. If ultrasonography is positive, those women would undergo more definitive tests for endometrial cancer.[27] Studies have estimated this risk of endometrial carcinoma to be from 2.2 to 7.5 times greater than for women not taking tamoxifen. The aggressiveness and prognoses of these tamoxifen-induced endometrial cancers vary. Some studies have shown the type of endometrial cancer and prognosis to be no worse than the typical endometrial cancer found in women not using tamoxifen,[28] or the cancers can be much more deadly.[29] One study found that women who have used tamoxifen for longer than two years had a risk of endometrial cancer twice that of those who had never used the drug, and there was a trend of increasing risk with longer duration of use.[30]

Cancers of the fallopian tubes have also been associated with tamoxifen therapy.[31] Less common are uterine fibroids (leiomyomas) caused by tamoxifen.[32,33] In premenopausal women, tamoxifen can cause paradoxical elevation of estrogen levels. This can stimulate endometriosis, a condition in which endometrial cells grow in abnormal locations, such as the abdominal wall and pelvic organs, often producing masses of tissue. This produces painful nonmalignant masses, including ovarian masses.[34,35]

ᴥ How Does Tamoxifen Affect Breast Cancer Cells?

This topic is very important to "normal" women without known breast cancer. If this group is to be given tamoxifen for possible breast cancer prevention, the effects of the drug on preclinical, undiscovered breast cancers hidden deep within these women's breasts should be considered. What are the beneficial and possibly dangerous effects of tamoxifen on breast cancer cells?

EFFECTS ON ESTROGEN RECEPTORS

Tamoxifen can reduce the amount of detectable estrogen receptors (ERs) in breast cancers. In one study, ERs were measured in biopsy specimens of women's breast cancers prior to treatment with tamoxifen; then, eight weeks after tamoxifen treatments, a second biopsy was performed. A significant de-

238 •ꞵ How to Prevent Breast Cancer

crease in ER content was observed.[36] What effect this change has on prognosis is unknown at this time. In general, ER + breast cancers are easier to treat and have a more favorable prognosis. So theoretically, tamoxifen could worsen the prognosis.

LESSENING THE INVASIVENESS OF BREAST CANCER

Past experiences had shown that tamoxifen inhibits the invasiveness of certain breast cancer cells. This ability to reduce the invasiveness of breast cancers is one of the known therapeutic benefits of tamoxifen in cancer therapy. Recently, it has been demonstrated that tamoxifen has the ability to activate a site on the surface of some breast cancer cells that increases the clumping of cancer cells. Clumping, or aggregated, cells have more difficulty invading normal tissue. Therefore, tamoxifen's ability to "turn on" this site may reduce tumor invasion.[37]

POTENTIAL CREATION OF LETHAL TUMORS

Most estrogen receptor positive (ER+) breast cancers are suppressed by tamoxifen therapy. Sometimes, ER + cancers, while at first being suppressed by tamoxifen, are later not affected by the drug, and may begin growing again. Oncologists have termed these ER + breast cancers "resistant."

We now know that the cells of a single breast cancer are typically heterogeneous in many ways, meaning each is unlike another. Each cell may behave differently with exposure to different drugs such as tamoxifen. In a single malignant breast tumor, some of the cells could be stimulated by tamoxifen, while others might be suppressed.[38,39,40,41]

Just as long-term antibiotic therapy can lead to major problems with the development of antibiotic-resistant strains of bacteria, long-term tamoxifen exposure can create similar pitfalls. While suppressing sensitive cells, tamoxifen can cause the generation of a population of resistant cells. In an example of the process of "survival of the fittest," breast cancer cells that are tamoxifen-resistant will survive the treatment. In fact, these cancer cells may even have their growth stimulated by the tamoxifen, leading to potentially fast-growing and *lethal* tumors.[42]

This scenario is important to consider since investigators are placing so-called normal women on tamoxifen for prevention trials, when it is possible that any one of these women could harbor occult, or undiscovered, breast cancer. Some scientists believe that tamoxifen given to healthy women could cause aggressive and lethal breast cancers to develop.

In a published medical paper, scientists from the University of Colorado Health Sciences Center have issued a warning regarding the use of tamoxifen in a chemopreventive role: "Our data suggest that its use as a chemopreventant in women at high risk of developing breast cancer should be viewed with caution, since in the presence of tamoxifen subpopulations of cells may arise that are stimulated, rather than inhibited by the drug."[43]

✦ Tamoxifen Therapy for Breast Cancer

In a recent review of all randomized clinical trials dealing with adjuvant therapy for early breast cancer, it was found that when older or postmenopausal women having breast cancer used tamoxifen, the annual death rate declined by 25 percent. This was especially true for ER+ tumors. The absolute survival rate of those with positive lymph nodes who are taking tamoxifen is 8 to 10 percent at the end of ten years. This amounts to an average survival of an extra two years. The adjuvant tamoxifen will result in greater survival for women with many positive nodes than for those with negative nodes. Therefore, tamoxifen seems to be very useful in this group of postmenopausal women with ER+ breast cancers, especially if lymph nodes were positive.[44] Some studies have indicated the value of conservative surgery in conjunction with tamoxifen for older women, producing a five-year relapse-free rate of 82 percent and avoiding the risks of major surgery.[45] In some frail elderly women who cannot undergo surgery, tamoxifen therapy may represent a desirable alternative approach. Such treatment can result in complete and partial response rates of 50 to 80 percent, often resulting in local control of the tumor within the patient's lifetime.[46] It is important to consider the physiological rather than chronological age of the elderly patient before deciding upon appropriate therapy. Older women with younger physiologies, for instance, do well under standard therapy usually reserved for younger women.

⁂ Summary

Tamoxifen represents a double-edged sword. While it has demonstrated excellent results when used as adjuvant breast cancer therapy, there are many risks associated with its long-term use. In women with breast cancer, the risks of recurrent or metastatic breast cancer easily outweigh the risks of tamoxifen therapy. However, its use in women who *do not* have breast cancer poses a predicament. Questions remain as to whether its benefits outweigh its risks when used as preventive therapy. Experts differ in their assessment of risks of tamoxifen when used in normal women. Dr. Paul P. Rosen, a physician at the Sloan-Kettering Cancer Center, has recently written in the medical journal *Cancer* about the futility of attempting so-called prevention of breast cancer only in women who are considered high risk. "Intervention to prevent breast carcinoma, even if highly effective and targeted among so-called 'high risk' women ... may have little effect on the overall frequency of and mortality due to breast cancer unless additional indications for preventive treatment that apply to a *much larger number of individuals* can be identified and highly effective nontoxic therapy becomes available."[47] Taking a circumspect approach, it is premature at this time to recommend that normal healthy women take tamoxifen to prevent breast cancer. Remember, the theme of this book is avoidance of breast cancer through effective, nontoxic methods that can be used on the *entire* female population.

Chapter 20

Treatment for Early Breast Cancer

❦

While this book is written to empower women in *preventing* breast cancer, many of you will already have the disease or have a friend or relative who does. Empowerment involves knowledge. What options are available to a woman who is told she has breast cancer? It is beyond the scope of this book to attempt to detail all the treatment regimens available to women with breast cancer, so we have chosen to focus on the *newer* treatment for the *earliest, most common* stages of breast cancer. If proper mammographic screening is performed, up to 78 percent of all breast cancers will be detected in these early stages. It is in these stages that newer breast-conserving treatment is most valuable. When is radiation therapy or chemotherapy appropriate in early-stage breast cancer treatment? Let's find out.

THE BIOPSY SHOWS CANCER

The Multidisciplinary Team Okay, you are diagnosed with a breast cancer. To whom do you go for your care? In the best of situations you should be evaluated by a multidisciplinary medical "breast cancer team" composed of a breast surgeon, medical oncologist, radiation oncologist, mammographic radiologist, and surgical pathologist. This team will examine you, your medical reports and tests, your mammograms, other imaging studies, your biopsy specimen, and specimen tests. Subsequently, members themselves meet in formal conference to discuss their opinions and recommendations with one another. Following this conference, the physicians are able to provide the patient with all of her available options, along with recommendations.

When such a multidisciplinary medical team approach is used, significant advantages include more therapeutic options for the patient. In this setting, women receive more breast-conserving therapy and newer treatment regimens.[1] According to a very prominent surgical journal, "The practice of multidisciplinary breast cancer treatment has become the standard of care for the majority of breast cancer patients."[2,3,4]

When There is No Multidisciplinary Team If you live in an area where there are no multidisciplinary breast-cancer treatment programs, beware and be informed! Know your alternatives! Only eighteen states have enacted statutes of some type requiring that breast-cancer patients be informed of treatment options. (See Appendix B for a list of these states.) But beware! There is a lot of variation in the thoroughness and effectiveness of these requirements among those eighteen. Only fourteen require the development and publication of a standardized summary on medically acceptable treatment alternatives for breast cancer; however, four of these states place no explicit duty on the physician to have the brochure distributed (Georgia, Illinois, New Mexico, and Texas). In two states, the information is limited to a brief general sentence on the preoperative consent form (Pennsylvania, Virginia).

The ideal statute is rare, because in only five states (California, Kansas, Kentucky, New Jersey, and New York), the physician must personally provide a standardized brochure to his or her patient.[5] This is very important, for as more screened women are diagnosed with early breast cancer, there should, and will be, more patient participation in medical decision-making. If you have been diagnosed as having breast cancer and you live in one of the states having weak or no statutes, demand a full explanation of *all* current treatment options with appropriate risks and benefits. If your physician cannot or will not provide this, see another who will.

• *Your prognosis*
Breast cancer prognosis is determined from information regarding the makeup of the cancer cells themselves, involvement of axillary (armpit) lymph nodes, and tumor size. For example, patients with tumors smaller than 5 millimeters (size of a small pea, or 3/16 inch) have a recurrence rate of less than 2 percent, compared to 20 to 25 percent for tumors ten times that size. This is why physicians use the patient's node status and tumor size in the clinical staging system described in Chapter 2.

In the future, there will be many refinements in analyzing the biochemical and genetic makeup of cancer cells, and this information will be used to individualize treatment regimens and provide prognostic information.[6,7] The future will also no doubt bring new classes of chemotherapeutic agents, such as Taxol, the newly discovered agent originally derived from the bark of the western yew tree.[8,9,10,11]

❧ Dietary Habits in Breast Cancer Patients

No matter what the clinical stage of the breast cancer or the treatment options chosen by the patient, her dietary habits will enhance her survival. A low-fat diet is especially valuable for women with estrogen receptor positive (ER +) tumors. Studies have shown more treatment failures in women with higher intakes of both saturated and total fats.[12] Healthful dietary habits, exercise, supplements, and other lifestyle changes will benefit women with breast cancer.

❧ Menstrual Cycle and Breast Cancer Surgery

Does it make a difference when you schedule your lumpectomy or other breast surgery? Yes, if you are premenopausal. Specifically, you should consider your menstrual cycle stage when planning or scheduling surgery because it does seem to affect the outcome. A recent study of premenopausal patients with breast cancer and positive axillary lymph nodes showed that those operated on when they were in their second half of the cycle had a significantly better prognosis than those operated on in the first half of the cycle. The explanations for this are unclear. It may be due to the dominant estrogenic effect of the first half of the cycle or a reduction in certain immune system cells.[13] Another explanation could be that breast cancer cell proliferation is suppressed by the dominant progesterone levels during the second half of the cycle. Unfortunately, not all investigations have demonstrated this effect of menstrual cycle upon outcome.[14] But if you have a choice, choose a surgical date during the second half of your cycle. Postponing surgery for a couple of weeks will not worsen your outcome, and it may improve it.

❧ Stage 0 Breast Cancer

Stage 0 breast cancers, the earliest forms, are those types that are termed ductal carcinoma *in situ* (DCIS). Stage 0 breast cancer is determined by the noninvasive appearance of the cells under the microscope, not upon size; however, sizes can vary from that of a pinhead to more than an inch. The key to the excellent prognosis of DCIS is the lack of invasion (penetration) outside the duct. Of all breast cancers detected by modern screening mammography, 25 percent will be Stage 0, carrying with it a five-year survival rate of 95 percent. (As we discussed in Chapter 2, lobular carcinoma *in situ* does not represent a true cancer and will not be discussed in this chapter.)[15]

• *Treatments*
The currently recommended treatment for ductal carcinoma *in situ* is lumpectomy followed by radiation therapy. This combination of treatments is known as breast-conservation therapy (BCT).[16,17] Adjuvant systemic chemotherapy is probably not warranted.

❧ Stage I Breast Cancer

Stage I is a clinical stage of the disease in which there is only local involvement. It is a tumor less than 2 centimeters in diameter (size of a grape, or about 3/4 inch), no involved lymph nodes, and no distant spread; however, some degree of invasion (penetration outside the ducts) is present. When a biopsy shows invasive cancer, some of the lymph nodes in the armpit must also be surgically removed to evaluate for local metastases. This "lymph node sampling" operation is important for distinguishing Stage I invasive disease from the more advanced clinical stages, which, in turn, determines prognosis and therapy. The overall five-year survival rate for Stage I patients is 85 percent. Stage I breast cancers are the most common stage detected by modern mammography. Over half of all screen-detected cancers will be in this stage.

• *Treatments*
There are many synonyms for lumpectomy, including tumorectomy, tylectomy, segmental resection, subtotal mastectomy, partial mastectomy, tumor resection, and quadrantec-

tomy. In this chapter we will use the commonly accepted term *lumpectomy* to refer to the surgical procedure that removes the primary tumor plus a minimal amount of surrounding normal tissue.

Today in the United States, mastectomy (radical or modified) should rarely be performed with Stage I patients, since it has been proven many times to offer no increased survival rate over lumpectomy.[18,19] While one multicenter trial included a small amount of falsified data from one investigator, this trial proved lumpectomy plus radiation therapy (BCT) equal to mastectomy in terms of survival rates, even after removal of this false data. There was no statistical change in the overall results. The trial stands as proper and valid.

Small Stage I cancers, 10 millimeters or less in size, have an excellent prognosis, even without adjuvant chemotherapy. In a European prospective study, the average seven-year survival rate (without distant metastases) was 98.7 percent in node-negative patients and 79.3 percent in node-positive patients. Mammography played an important part in improving patient survival, as lymph nodes were involved in only 9 percent of the cancers detected by screening mammograms, compared to 20 percent of the cancers detected by clinical exam.[20]

An additional benefit of BCT to women is that it can produce an acceptable cosmetic result and helps provide greater psychological adjustment and acceptance of the treatment program.[21]

RADIATION THERAPY

Among the options most currently chosen for Stage I breast cancer are lumpectomy and/or chemotherapy and/or radiation therapy. Radiation therapy (XRT) continues to be the most effective adjunct to surgery to achieve long-term local control of breast cancer. It is more effective in doing so than both adjuvant chemotherapy and adjuvant tamoxifen.[22] In a recent study of Stage I patients, lumpectomy alone was compared to lumpectomy with XRT. While the two groups did not differ in overall survival rates, women not receiving XRT had eight times the local recurrence rate as the XRT group, as well as a local recurrence rate of almost 20 percent after five years.[23] Similar studies have shown the same results.[24] Thus, XRT is highly recommended.[25]

CHEMOTHERAPY

Two large studies demonstrated that breast cancer is basically a systemic disease, and that simply directing treatment at prevention of recurrent disease in the breast or metastasis to regional nodes had little effect on survival. In Stage I and II node-negative women, both chemotherapy given for ER− disease and tamoxifen given for ER+ disease produced increased patient survival rates. It follows that adjuvant therapy, which in early node-negative disease is of value, is becoming more commonplace.[26,27,28]

For women with node-negative tumors smaller than one centimeter, adjuvant therapy is not needed, as prognosis is excellent with BCT alone.[29,30]

We look forward to the time when a scientific study of Stage I breast cancer patients will compare the benefits of adopting a lifestyle based on all the breast cancer avoidance techniques discussed in this book to traditional therapies to see if adopting a new lifestyle provides longer survival and better quality of life than chemotherapy.

MASTECTOMY

With the proper emphasis on BCT, is there a role for mastectomy? Who should undergo mastectomy? Mastectomies, either radical or modified, are not being performed as much as in the past, especially in progressive modern, multidisciplinary cancer centers. A woman should not undergo a mastectomy only because her surgeon talked her into the operation. Mastectomy should be reserved for women who cannot or do not wish to undergo the intensive radiation therapy schedule. The patient must go for XRT five days a week for six to seven weeks. Some women who cannot or do not wish to have follow-ups of their treated breast every six months by mammography and clinical exam will choose mastectomy. One advantage of the mastectomy is that immediate reconstruction can be carried out.[31] For some women who have considered all factors, mastectomy may be the appropriate treatment.

BCT VERSUS MASTECTOMY: PSYCHOLOGICAL STRESSES

One recent study indicates that in newly diagnosed women with Stage I or II breast cancer, those choosing BCT over mastectomy had experienced no difference in psychological parameters of uncertainty, quality of life, and functional status. Both groups responded to the original diagnosis in similar ways, experienced the same amount of distress, and used similar coping strategies to equal degrees. The testing was performed prior to the surgery and eight weeks afterward.[32] We suggest that this similar psychological reaction of the two groups of women may have occurred because the "shock" of the diagnosis of breast cancer was equal, no matter which treatment option was selected. Unfortunately, psychological testing was not performed in these two groups beyond two months, when possible differences might be seen after the initial "shock" had worn off.

Other BCT patients, however, have found a psychosocial advantage in preserving the configuration of the body. They maintain the sensation of female identity and body image to a better extent than their counterparts who chose mastectomy. In the end, though, BCT does not seem to reduce the high frequency of anxiety phenomena, mental instability, and depression.[33] Studies are needed which would compare the long-term psychological functioning of BCT patients to mastectomy patients. One of the authors, Taffy Pelton, feels that the psychological benefits of BCT are indeed much greater than previously reported in medical journals.

• Alternative Cancer Therapies

Ross Pelton's book *Alternatives in Cancer Therapy* (Simon & Schuster, 1994) is an important resource for anyone diagnosed with cancer, including women with breast cancer. Every year thousands of cancer patients seek therapies in foreign countries because potentially lifesaving therapies are withheld from them in the United States.

❧ *Summary*

Earlier diagnosis and treatment has led to the beginning of a decline in breast cancer mortality in this decade, including that of women in their forties.[34,35] However, before a woman can make her decision on treatment, her multidisciplinary medical breast cancer team must inform her about the nature of her individual cancer, her clinical stage, and the current treatment options for that stage. Her physicians should be available to comfort, then inform, make medical recommendations, and aid in the woman's decision-making process. If in doubt, obtain a second or third opinion. Empowered by this knowledge, it is your right to choose the therapy appropriate for your personal situation.

Chapter 21

Breast Implants:
An Increased Risk?

There is no established link between breast implants and breast cancer, but substantial controversy exists about the other health hazards, including immune system disorders. When we realize that approximately 2 million U.S. women currently have implants, the subject becomes a substantial woman's health issue.

Approximately 80 percent of implant procedures were performed for cosmetic reasons to increase breast size, and 20 percent of the implants were for reconstruction reasons (surgery for cancer or deformity). What do we really know about breast implants?

Implants are silicone-based envelopes usually filled with saline or silicone gel. Current controversies include the effect silicone gel or the silicone envelopes have on a woman's body in the long term. Prospective investigations of this sort were not performed in women before the widespread use of implants and still have not been completed. To date, implantation of silicone-based products has given no indication of potential health risks. In fact, cardiac pacemakers, small joint replacements, penile implants, and catheters have all been placed in humans for decades without significant problems. As a consequence, almost all current studies regarding silicone breast implants are retrospective; in other words, we are studying the health of women who already have implants, not performing preimplant studies. Despite the lack of scientific evidence for physical harm from implants, the FDA (for political and legal reasons) has banned the use of silicone gel implants, except in cases of postcancer reconstruction.

Testing of a new type of nonsilicone gel implant has recently begun in this country. These implants are filled with a nontoxic vegetable oil, through which mammogram X-rays can penetrate more easily than they can through saline or silicone gel. In contrast with other implant patients, a woman with the new implants, along with eliminating the risks of silicone gel, may receive more accurate mammography. The risks of these implants are not known, but are not believed to be significant, because the vegetable oil is not toxic to tissues. Full test results are pending.

❧ What Are the Complications?

The most controversial aspect of implants is the complications and their possible effects upon your health. Let's look at the sorts of complications that can occur.

HARDENING AND RUPTURING OF IMPLANTS
The most common complications of implants are implant rupture (leakage) and implant envelope hardening, termed capsular contracture. When a saline implant ruptures, it deflates rapidly. Saline, essentially a saltwater solution, is naturally absorbed by the woman's breast tissues without consequence. The empty silicone envelope must then be surgically removed.

If rupture or leakage occurs in a silicone gel implant, the more viscous gel may ooze out so slowly the woman is unaware that she has a problem. Dr. Vint has seen mammograms on women who had small gel leakages that had not changed for years. While mammograms and ultrasound can detect larger implant leakage, the best technique currently in use for detecting possible small leaks is breast MRI (see Chapter 3).[1,2] Many cases of implant silicone gel leakage cannot be detected by any other technology, making MRI the testing method of choice.

Both types of implants can develop surface hardening, which occurs when a woman's body interacts with the silicone envelope, causing an inflammatory reaction called capsular contraction; however, this occurs much less frequently with saline implants. The tissue surrounding the implant can become calcified, which appears eggshell-like on a mammogram. The capsular contraction can be painful and cause the implants to harden and occasionally crack with minimal trauma. If cracking occurs, the implants will rupture and leak.

Leakage can also present problems. Long-standing silicone gel that has leaked into surrounding breast tissue can cause a localized inflammation, leading to the development of a palpable mass that may be painful. This is known as a silicone granuloma, and while not premalignant, it can sometimes be mistaken for a tumor during clinical exam or on a mammogram. If palpable, a needle biopsy (FNA) can be used to confirm the condition.[3,4]

IMPLANTS AND AUTOIMMUNE DISEASE

Implant "Bleeding" Silicone gel implants have been known to leak microscopic particles of the gel through the *intact* envelope and into the surrounding breast tissues. Physicians call this silicone "bleeding." These particles can then be carried to distant regions of the body by the lymph and blood systems. Particles have been microscopically identified in such distant sites as joint lining tissue, lung cells, and skin, as well as in inflammatory tissue surrounding the implants.

A scientific investigation from the University of Maryland Hospital, using an ultrasensitive method to measure the element silicon in tissues taken from different parts of the body, showed that patients with implants had five times the silicon levels of patients who had never had implants. Significantly, the silicon level was elevated in the implant patients *whether or not the implants were ruptured.*[5] In another study of three implant patients, inflammation was associated with these silicone particles wherever they were found. Connective tissue disease was present, as diagnosed by clinical exam, blood tests, and biopsies. The condition of each patient improved after implant removal.[6]

In another medical report, a woman developed typical capsular contraction and had her implants removed. Her fibrous tissue capsules, which are usually not removed with the implants, had formed numerous inflamed cysts. The patient, who was suffering breast pain and swelling, joint aches, fever, and enlarged axillary lymph nodes, and whose blood tests showed abnormalities, did not show improvement until after removal of the capsule itself.[7]

Autoantibodies: We Attack Ourselves   A recent pathology article notes that breast implants may act like vaccinating devices, causing the body to produce abnormal antibodies.[8] Along with similar cases as these, over the past ten years instances of autoimmune connective tissue diseases such as scleroderma, systemic lupus erythematosus, rheumatoid arthritis, and other similar diseases have been found in women with implants.[9]

In our bodies, natural antibodies are present to recognize and attack foreign invaders, such as bacteria and viruses, thus keeping us healthy. These normal antibodies are genetically "programmed" not to attack the body's normal cells. In the case of autoimmune diseases, our bodies generate autoantibodies (abnormal antibodies) that attack normal cells. According to some investigators, 5 to 30 percent of women with implants will develop autoantibodies.[10] Conflicting evidence comes from a study done in Toronto, where 200 patients with silicone gel implants were compared to 200 age-matched controls who did not have implants. Implant patients tested positive for auto-antibodies in 26.5 percent of the cases, but the controls were similarly positive, with 28 percent developing autoantibodies. The positivity for implant patients *with ruptures* was only 17.2 percent.[11] These results indicate that the presence of low levels of autoantibodies is more common in "normal" women than we previously believed, and that at these levels "abnormal" antibodies may not be associated with clinical disease.

While the medical literature contains anecdotal reports such as the ones we just mentioned, no research studies connect an increase in connective tissue disease with the presence of implants.[12] A large literature review of the subject published in 1994 indicates that while the behavior of silicone gel implants in the human body is compatible with the *theory* of inducement of connective tissue disease (especially scleroderma), there is inadequate epidemiological data to show a definite cause and effect.[13,14] The Mayo Clinic recently reviewed their thirty-year experience with implants. Of all their patients who had had implant failures (through leakage or rupture), none had developed a clinically evident health problem.[15] Some investigators have gone on to hypothesize that silicone from implants provokes an autoimmune response only in women who have a genetic predisposition.[16]

In general, autoimmune diseases are much more frequent in women than men. In fact, 75 to 90 percent of patients with these illnesses are women. Consequently, among the 2 million U.S. women who have had implant surgery, a number of these women would logically be expected to develop autoimmune diseases for no other reason than that they are female. That is to say, we should expect many women with implants to develop autoimmune disease strictly because they are female— not because they have implants. Statistically, we would expect about another 1,000 of these implant patients to develop such a disease by pure coincidence; however, we find a much lower number than this reported in the literature.[17] Consequently, we encourage more research in this area.

IMMUNE SYSTEM SUPPRESSION

Our bodies have specific types of large white blood cells, termed natural killer cells, whose primary job is to seek out and destroy abnormal cells. These natural killer cells are especially important in our early immune response against viral infections and cancer cells. Recent research has demonstrated that silicone breast implants can suppress the activity of these killer cells. It has not been shown that this phenomenon is linked to an increased incidence of cancer, but theoretically, this suppressive effect could place women at increased risk for future breast cancer development or recurrence. The natural killer cell suppression is not permanent and is reversed when the implants are surgically removed.[18]

❧ Implants and Mammograms

When a woman has breast implants, the breast tissue is more difficult to image because the implants tend to block the view of the tissue. Therefore, two additional views per breast are required; however, even these views do not allow the same level of visualization as do breasts without implants.[19,20,21,22] On the positive side, this limitation may not be that significant because in a study of forty-one women with implants who developed breast cancer, it was found that the presence of implants did not have a detrimental effect on breast cancer detection and survival. The women with implants did not suffer later diagnosis than their nonimplant counterparts. In fact, the five- and ten-year survival rates for the implant patients were the same as for the nonimplant women.[23]

Proper mammography compression *very slightly* increases the chance for implant rupture and leakage during the exam; for this reason, an increasing number of centers require women with implants to sign an informed consent or release form. Naturally, such legal concerns cause increased anxiety in these women. However, it is important to remind ourselves that the possible risk of not detecting a potentially curable breast cancer on an "undercompressed" mammogram is *enormously greater* than the very slight risk of implant damage from a correctly performed exam.

❧ How Do Breast Cancer Patients Feel About Their Implants?

Many women who choose to have a mastectomy also choose to have breast reconstruction using implants. How do women who have had this surgery for breast cancer feel about their implants? In a Duke University survey of 174 women, participants were questioned about both their experiences with surgery and their feelings on the implant controversy. Seventy-six percent stated that the implants helped them cope with their cancer, while only 16 percent had regrets about reconstruction. Because of the controversy over the implant safety, 55 percent of the women were worried, yet only 13 percent were considering having the implants removed. Reflecting the debate over types of implants, only 27 percent stated they would choose silicone implants again. Not surprisingly, the vast majority of patients in the survey, were they to choose again, would not be willing to accept the risks of complications from silicone implants.[24]

❧ Summary

Much is yet to be learned about the effects of silicone implants on a woman's body. While federal law no longer allows such implants for augmentation, 2 million women are living with some form of augmentation, or implant. Complications of leakage and encapsulation are well known; what is not well understood is what effect the mere presence of the implant will have on the woman's immune system. There have been indications of a possible relation to connective tissue disease, but this causal relationship has not been proven. Our conclusion is that while there are probably some women who form a genuine immune response or "allergic reaction" to the implants, many more develop autoimmune diseases only coincidentally. The issue is further blurred because we cannot discern one group of women from the other. Clearly, much more research needs to be conducted in this area.

One study has shown immune suppression with implants, thus representing a warning flag requiring further confirmative research on the subject. With regard to breast cancer detection and prevention, although implants make detection of small breast cancers through mammography more difficult, they have never been implicated in causing breast malignancy. Regardless of whether or not you have breast implants, however, remember to have annual mammograms after you turn forty.

Chapter 22

The Latest on Nonsexual Breast Massage

Breast massage and stimulation of the nipple is a ground-breaking concept in breast care. While only hypothetical in nature, it could be a technique that provides a measure of protection against breast cancer, and at the very least, it is a practice that will contribute to healthy breasts. The benefits of breast massage are both physical and psychological, bringing a new level of energy and awareness into a part of our bodies that is often either ignored or considered a site of potential hazard.

Since there is scant scientific data on this topic, we will be taking a slight departure from our usual style of relating information. This chapter, therefore, will be presented from the perspective of personal experience and subsequent conjecture. Before we continue, know that this is a serious topic—one that is not meant to be sensationalized or treated insensitively.

The concept of breast massage and stimulation of the nipple came to our attention from two different sources concurrently.

First, Taffy had been receiving therapeutic massage from a highly skilled massage therapist who was working on the periphery of her breasts. It was extraordinarily painful, particularly in the area where a bra underwire would sit against the ribs. As the therapist continued to work around her breast, Taffy cried out in pain, thinking the therapist was hurting the breast tissue. In fact, she was working the pectoral muscles under the breast that probably had never been touched before. Knowing the value of massage in stimulating blood flow and oxygen to an area, as well as the movement of the lymph fluid, Taffy began to realize the implications this might have regarding the health of her breasts. After the session Taffy experienced a new kind of relaxation and a greater connection with her breasts. Recognizing that she had stored years of tension in this area, she decided to ask her husband, Ross, if he would massage around and under her breasts on a regular basis.

Concurrently, Ross was working in a hospital that treated many breast cancer patients. While finishing *Alternatives in Cancer Therapy* and working on the proposal for this book, he contacted a medical researcher to obtain some information. Upon learning about Ross's projects, the researcher showed Ross a scientific paper written by Dr. T.G.C. Murrell of Australia, entitled "Epidemiological and Biochemical Support for a Theory on the Cause and Prevention of Breast Cancer," which had been published in the journal *Medical Hypothesis* (1991).[1] In short, Dr. Murrell was making the case that the encouragement of regular nipple erections through breast massage may prevent breast disease, specifically fibrosis and cancer. This will be discussed in greater depth later.

The medical researcher who gave this paper to Ross proudly announced he liked to think that the health of his wife's breasts was in part due to his consistent and loving attention to them. This paper stimulated a host of new thoughts for Ross, and thus he and Taffy began the new technique of breast massage and stimulation of the nipple for nonsexual purposes.

A few months after they began this practice, a family member noticed that Taffy appeared to have larger breasts. Sometimes it is hard to see gradual changes in oneself, but Taffy did notice that her breasts felt more full, robust, and youthful, and that she enjoyed touching them more. The only variable in her life was that her breasts were getting lots of attention and non-sexual stimulation (this is not meant to diminish the sexual aspects in any way, of course). Taffy had begun to be less fearful about her breasts and was feeling proud of them. Both Ross and Taffy found this ritual to be nurturing, relaxing, fun, and healthy. Subsequently, they have heard numerous anecdotes of similar experiences between couples.

With some hesitancy they share the side benefit of larger, fuller breasts. This result may not be enjoyed by everyone, and in any case should not be considered the goal for this practice. They would instead like to focus on the hypothesized health benefits of breast massage, so that this topic may be understood and appreciated in the spirit with which it was introduced.

✿ *Murrell's Hypothesis*

Dr. Murrell proposed that lack of oxygen in localized breast tissue would induce biochemical events that could produce free radicals. These unstable substances could, in turn, damage breast tissue, leading to the development of breast cancer. He reasoned that regular nipple erections would drain away the products of free radical production, thereby decreasing the risk to breast cancer.

For Ross, who has been studying and teaching the free radical theory of aging for over ten years, this hypothesis made immediate sense. It is well known in the scientific community that conditions of low oxygen (hypoxia) result in the increased production of free radicals in the affected tissues. Furthermore, it is a well-accepted notion that free radicals cause damage to tissues, which can then lead to cancer.

Ross took Dr. Murrell's hypothesis and advanced it one more step. It seemed to him that breast massage and nipple stimulation would accomplish several things. First, stimulation of the breast and nipple would result in an increased flow of blood supply to the breast, which means the breast tissue would be receiving both more oxygen and nutrients. It seemed, then, that this process could serve only to enhance the overall health of the breast tissue. Secondly, the increased oxygenation from massage and stimulation would decrease hypoxia, thereby lessening free radical damage and cancer risk (see Chapter 9). And finally, since massage is an effective method of detoxification and moving pooled fluids out of tissues, it seemed natural to assume that massage and stimulation would increase lymphatic drainage from the breast, thereby detoxifying the tissue within.

Ross reasoned that for millions of years of evolution, most women were nursing a child during most of their reproductive years. Thus, for millions of years, women's breasts were being stimulated by nursing for much of their adult lives. It is only within the last fifty years, with the advent of birth control pills and other forms of contraception, that women have started to have children later, fewer children, or no children at all. Another reason that breasts are not as stimulated as before is that breast-feeding has declined for a number of generations. Recently, new mothers have become increasingly more enlightened about its benefits, yet many still cannot or choose not to breast-feed.

For these and other reasons we suspect the breasts of most Western women today receive far less stimulation than those of premodern women. The question then becomes whether a lack of stimulation is a contributing factor in the tremendous rise in breast cancer. Furthermore, could regular breast massage help increase breast health and reverse this trend? The fact that breast massage would increase tissue oxygenation, stimulate lymph flow, and reduce hypoxia presents a biochemical rationale to support this hypothesis.

In his article, Dr. Murrell also suggested that nipple stimulation might protect against breast cancer by raising and lowering levels of the breast hormones, oxytocin and prolactin. However, when we began to research the effects of prolactin and oxytocin on both the lactating and nonlactating breast, we found we were delving into a fascinating area filled with confusion and contradiction.

Prolactin is the hormone that causes milk to be produced in the female breast. Oxytocin is the hormone that causes milk to be discharged from the breast during suckling. Most of the research on these two hormones has been done in relationship to pregnancy and nursing after childbirth. Very little research has been done on these hormones in nonlactating women, and much of the research that has been done is contradictory.

For example, some studies say that higher prolactin levels indicate an increased risk to breast cancer while others do not.[2,3] Some papers say that massage of the breast in nonlactating women increases blood prolactin levels, others say it does not.[4,5]

The best we can report is that the hormonal response to massage of the breast and stimulation of the nipple in normal nonlactating women is not well researched or well understood at this time.

❧ Our Case for Breast Massage

We had hoped to find some scientific studies which showed that breast massage actually increased oxygenation and removed toxins from the breast tissue. Unfortunately, it appears that scientific validation of this hypothesis has not been attempted yet. However, in the process of researching this chapter, we connected with the Executive Director of a reputable massage therapy school in Canada, Ms. Debra Curties, who is currently writing a textbook on massage techniques. It will be published in early 1996.[6] She has devoted one chapter to breast massage, as it is a mandatory part of the curriculum in Canada.

Ms. Curties feels that breast massage has been banned because our society is uncertain whether breasts can ever be touched in a nonsexual manner. She states, "Given the incidence and seriousness of breast disease in North America and the large number of breast surgeries, the massage profession cannot justify overlooking he necessity for preventive and case-specific treatment. In fact, I think it is important to be aware that our society's inability to consider breasts neutrally from the point of view of tissue-needs has probably contributed substantially to what could be considered one of our most underrated health crises." She further states that "we should strive to accord breasts the status of body tissues with specific health-care requirements, as legitimate as those of other body parts."[7]

Ms. Curties agrees that "longstanding conditions of poor circulation and drainage jeopardize breast health." Some of the conditions that contribute to breast congestion (and would therefore indicate the need for breast massage) are tight breast clothing, use of antiperspirants, poor posture, surgical scarring, and implants.[8]

✤ Too-tight Bras

In support of Ms. Curties's view that tight breast clothing may lead to conjestion, two medical researchers, Sydney Ross Singer and Soma Grismaijer, found that wearing too-tight bras may be implicated in breast cancer. They interviewed 4,730 Caucasian American women between the ages of thirty and seventy-nine about their bra wearing habits. They found that "women are wearing bras too tightly for too long, and women with breast cancer tend to do that more than other women."[9] Their research showed that twice as many women in the breast cancer group reported that their bras made red marks on their skin and six times as many breast cancer patients had regularly worn bras or breast-supporing garments to sleep. Furthermore, only 1 percent of the breast cancer patients reported that they wore their bras fewer than twelve hours per day compared to 20 percent of women in the general population. This analysis indicates that women who wear a bra fewer than twelve hours per day may decrease their risk of breast cancer nineteenfold.

In their book, *Dressed To Kill: The Link Between Breast Cancer and Bras*, Singer and Grismaijer theorize that tightly contained breasts experience longer exposure to toxins, due to decreased lymph drainage from the constrictive clothing. (See following section on the lymphatic system.) The authors admit that their research is not a rigorously designed double-blind scientific study; however, their purpose is to inform women about the potential hazard of tight breast clothing and to call for further research on the relationship between bras, the lymphatics, and breast cancer.[10]

In our search, we also learned about a wonderful European massage technique called Manual Lymph Drainage (MLD). Manual Lymph Drainage is a gentle, rhythmical massage technique developed in the 1930s by two Danish masseurs, Dr. Emil Vodder, Ph.D., and his wife Estrid.[11] This highly regarded form of therapeutic massage, which is routinely used in hospitals and clinics throughout Europe, is the fourth most prescribed physical therapy and is covered by health insurance.[12] MLD was introduced in North America in 1982, and although it is being taught widely in the United States, Canada, and Mexico, it has yet to be recognized by our health-care delivery system for the important therapeutic effects it offers.

Upon discovering that the largest population of patients treated by licensed MLD therapists are former breast-cancer patients who had been treated with radiation and/or surgery, we were eager to learn more about this method in the hope that it would support our hypothesis on breast massage. So that you will understand how this type of massage can be important to breast health, we would like to diverge briefly and explain the importance and function of the lymphatic system and what happens when it is damaged.

❧ The Lymphatic System

Almost everyone who has had the flu, a cold, or other common illness has experienced swollen lymph glands on the neck or under the arm. These swollen glands (actually nodes, often referred to erroneously as glands) are the result of the body's attempt to filter and purify a fluid called lymph. Lymph is comprised of excess fluid, protein, waste products, bacteria, viruses, and foreign material deposited into the spaces between cells from porous blood capillaries. To maintain balance, this fluid is picked up by lymphatic capillaries which then converge to form larger lymphatic vessels. These vessels are as thin as silk threads and are found throughout the body. The lymph flows through the vessels in one direction only. Unlike blood which is pumped by the heart, the lymph is moved primarily by contractions of the skeletal muscles and secondarily by movements of the diaphragm during breathing. This is one important reason why exercise is so crucial to maintaining good health. Movement of the lymph is also stimulated by the pulsation of the arteries adjacent to lymph vessels and peristalsis of the intestines.[13]

Located along the lymph vessels are more than 600 lymph nodes which act as purifying stations. Here antibodies and killer immune cells (lymphocytes, macrophages) respond to carry away and render harmless bacteria, viruses, dead cells, and inorganic material such as dusts, dyes, inks, and tar from cigarettes. Sometimes during a cold or other illness, the lymph nodes become overwhelmed with bacteria, viruses, or toxic substances, which results in swelling and soreness. The cleansed lymph then rejoins the blood circulatory system at two points at the base of the neck where two major veins meet, called the "venous arch." As you can see, the lymphatic system is one of the most important detoxifying systems in the body.

✒ Lymphedema

Surgery, radiation, injuries, or removal of lymph nodes can seriously damage the effectiveness of the lymphatic system. The loss of lymph nodes under the arm coupled with lymph vessels damaged during breast surgery or radiation therapy impairs the fluid drainage mechanism of the arm, creating a condition called lymphedema. Variable estimates range as high as 62 percent of women treated for breast cancer with surgery and/or radiation as likely to develop this uncomfortable and often disfiguring ailment.[14]

The difficulty lies in the fact that lymphedema may not occur right after treatments. It can happen up to twenty years after surgery, when the afflicted side sustains an injury, receives an injection, or suffers any other physical trauma. It is for this reason that we strongly recommend that every woman who has had surgery or radiation contact the National Lymphedema Network's 800 number (see Appendix A) to obtain information on how to avoid or control lymphedema, to join the organization, or to find a licensed MLD or lymphedema therapist in your area.

Many women who develop lymphedema are angered that they were not warned sufficiently of this possibility and were therefore robbed of the benefit of the simple preventive measures which could have helped them avoid it. Women report not only distress in dealing with the physical aspects of lymphedema (pain, swelling, disfiguration, risk of severe or chronic infection), but also serious psychological consequences such as depression, social isolation, fear, and lowered self-esteem.[15]

&* Manual Lymph Drainage

There have been a variety of protocols developed to address lymphedema which primarily include compression bandaging, therapeutic exercises, meticulous hygiene, and Manual Lymph Drainage. The Manual Lymph Drainage therapists we spoke with reported having excellent results working with former breast cancer patients. The gentle pressure from the MLD massage technique reportedly causes the tiny lymphatic capillaries to repeatedly open and close, thus siphoning away excess water, proteins, bacteria, and other unwanted or used materials from the cells. The therapist uses MLD to shunt excess fluid to those areas where lymph vessels are healthy and will resorb the fluid.[16]

Since MLD appears to effectively improve cellular health in tissues where lymphatic drainage has been compromised, we feel this type of massage has great potential to enhance the health of normal breast tissue. Breasts that don't get regularly stimulated with either nursing or massage will probably have less than optimal lympathic drainage. We think that this gentle MLD massage technique accomplishes what Ross and Taffy intuitively envisioned in their nonsexual breast massage program, namely improved circulation, oxygenation of tissues, and removal of toxins and waste materials, resulting in healthier breasts.

❧ Breast Energetics

When they first began massage therapy, Taffy was uncomfortable. In fact, it was a bit frightening for her, thinking that Ross might discover a lump. Additionally, simply having all this attention focused on her breasts was part of the discomfort. One day they were sharing their experience with a friend, who, while fascinated by what they were doing, was appalled at the suggestion that she might have her husband massage her breasts. "I can't even stand to touch them myself!" she exclaimed. We have heard many such responses since. Are we ashamed of our breasts? Has there been so much sexual emphasis on them that we want to hide them or even disregard them unless they are "perfect"? It is important to know what happens when we voluntarily and energetically distance ourselves from this delicate and lovely part of our anatomy.

Biofeedback, which offers a way to measure and change unconscious bodily activity, provides concrete evidence that our thoughts and intentions can affect the body. Norman Cousins, in an attempt to increase mind/body awareness in his students, instructed them to relax and focus their minds on their hands, using their consciousness like an intense beam of light. Invariably, his students' hands would become as much as ten to fifteen degrees warmer, making them instant believers in their ability to control the autonomic (automatic) functions of their bodies.[17]

Understanding this power to bring blood supply and heat to an area of our bodies, we wondered what would happen to a region that is ignored. It stands to reason that most things neglected do not flourish. What would happen to my plants and pets if I didn't constantly tend to them? It is well documented that babies who get no attention often simply die. We believe that a woman's breasts, just like any other part of the body, need attention in a *nourishing* manner.

Give some thought to how your breasts get care. If they are not receiving regular loving attention and energy, ask your mate to join you in a practice that will provide it. If you are not in a relationship, you can provide it yourself. Taffy often massages her breasts when she is in the shower or putting on lotion. Remember that this is not a sexual act, but one of healing and nurturance. Visualize the increased levels of oxygen and nutrients going to the tissues and toxins flowing out. Create a time of self-nourishment.

✒ *How Is Breast Massage Done?*

Since there is not an exact and published protocol for the type of breast massage we practice, and since it is illegal in most U.S. counties for a massage therapist to touch breasts, we will share a technique created by MLD therapist Dana Wyrick, R.M.T., director of the Wyrick Institute in San Diego, California. This is based upon her training with Drs. John and Judith Casley-Smith of Australia, who are among the leading world authorities on the lymphatic system and lymphedema. The technique we describe is a self-massage, but it can be easily adapted for use with a partner. This can be accomplished in a sitting or lying position. Use gentle, but deliberate stroking motions, similar to the pressure you would use when petting a cat firmly.

Before you begin to massage the breast, it is important to

first activate and prepare the lymph nodes and vessels which will be receiving and purifying the lymph. Of the 600–800 lymph nodes in the body, 160–200 are in the neck and throat area. We recommend the following procedure (see illustrations below):

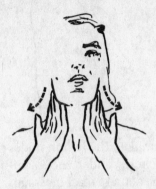

1. Beginning under the ears and using both hands, stroke down the neck and throat area into the hollow top of the shoulders. Do this stroke fifteen times.

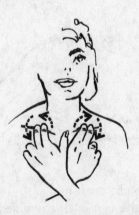

2. Cross your arms; press your index and middle finger into the hollow behind the collar bone at the base of the neck (the venous arch). Move your fingers in circles, the right hand moving clockwise and the left hand counterclockwise. Do this fifteen times.

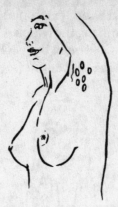

3. In order to stimulate the lymph nodes under the arm (the axila), massage in circles under each arm fifteen times. Now you are ready for the actual breast massage.

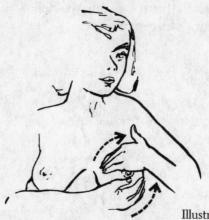

Illustrator: Dick Sorel

4. Using both hands, push and pull the breast tissue from the breast bone in the center of the chest across towards the axila. Using a gentle, firm motion, stroke up and around the breast tissue, always ending the stroke in the armpit. Intermittently massage the armpit following the stroke. Pay special attention to the upper outer-quadrant where 50 percent of all

breast cancers develop. Do this for both breasts for a minute or more.

In her aforementioned textbook, which includes breast massage techniques, Ms. Curties suggests that treatment of the pectoral muscles through standard Swedish-massage techniques is also necessary to facilitate circulation and drainage. She also mentions several other techniques, which would be done more appropriately by a trained massage therapist. If you plan to work with a professional, we suggest that you encourage her/him to consult Ms. Curties's new text.[18]

The important thing about breast massage is not that you concern yourself with exact technique, but that it becomes a regular part of your regimen for good health. These techniques are meant to serve as guidelines and can be incorporated into your life in ways that work for you. Simply bear in mind that you want to stimulate circulation in your breasts in a very gentle way.

We do not recommend breast massage for women with active breast cancer. In fact, active cancer of any kind is considered a contraindication in Manual Lymph Drainage massage therapy. The mechanisms of metastasis are still not fully understood, and the question remains unanswered whether massage therapy, which stimulates blood and lymph flow, might promote metastasis under some conditions.[19] If you are a previous breast-cancer patient, we urge you to consult with your doctor or a trained massage therapist before beginning this practice.

❧ Summary

Although we have few scientific answers to explain what biological mechanisms occur during breast massage, we feel that we have uncovered enough support from the massage community to suggest that breast massage is a beneficial practice for healthy women. Furthermore, it can be a practice that stimulates greater bonding and connection between couples, creating an increased sense of well-being. Finally, breast massage can reconnect a woman in a nonsexual way with a part of her body that has previously been associated primarily with sex or disease. We strongly encourage women to try these techniques and develop a healthy new relationship with their breasts.

Chapter 23

The Mind/Body Connection

Modern medical science has slowly begun to acknowledge a fact that has been observed and instinctively known for centuries: a person's state of health or disease cannot be explained solely in terms of physical mechanisms. However, as scientific methods are applied to studying the complex interactions among emotions, behavior, the neuroendocrine system, the immune system, and ultimately disease, we find ourselves in a maze of conflicting findings, flawed studies, and a call for more research.

Despite the controversy there appears to be some general consensus that people who remain healthy and live longer in the face of disease have certain qualities in common. These qualities include the ability to express emotions, a sense of control regardless of stressful events, an ability to view problems as challenges, a joy in living, and an emotional connection with others. While many researchers with positive findings conclude that these attributes *may* contribute to health and healing, the researchers admit they do not understand with certainty the mechanisms of action.

The newest thinkers are proposing that, in our attempt to apply the scientific method to the mind/body question, the mechanisms of action may be beyond what is measurable and quantifiable by current scientific methods. Embracing new knowledge from the respected field of physics, cutting-edge medical theorists are talking about consciousness, spirit, soul, and the broadly defined notion that while the mind and body are now viewed as one inseparable unit, so are we inseparable from our environments, other people, and the universe in general.

✒ Historical Perspective

"I would rather know what sort of person has a disease than what sort of disease a person has," recounts Hippocrates, one of the fathers of medicine from the fifth century B.C. The mere need to make such a statement indicates the eternal phenomenological struggle in medicine about the relationship of the mind, body, and spirit. Although clinical observations have related illness to certain psychological states since ancient times, there has also been a concurrent need to separate, bisect, dissect, and understand nature from the perspective of its parts.

The era of medicine spawned by this quest can be considered "mechanistic" or "physical" in nature. It is based upon the classical laws of matter and energy from the seventeenth century, which perceived the body and the entire universe as a great machine that functioned according to predetermined principles.[1] This paradigm was supported by the philosophy of René Descartes, who viewed the mind and the body as separate entities. This view is commonly referred to as the Cartesian split. As this idea gained acceptance, physicians and scientists were able to perform invasive procedures on people and animals without having to worry about harming the soul.

The accomplishments of this era have been so great that this mechanistic view still dominates modern medicine. In fact, benefactors from this model have enjoyed such esteem, power, control, and wealth that proponents of new ideas and methodology have found it difficult to introduce their concepts without creating serious opposition and polarization.

While it is important to acknowledge the powerful impact of conventional medicine upon our lives, it is also critical to recognize that this model is only one part of the picture. In the last thirty years we have witnessed the emergence of another aspect of the health and healing puzzle, now referred to as mind/body health or behavioral medicine. The premise of this new field of study is that our thoughts and emotions can influence the physiology of the body, the implication being that we can gain control of our health through the proper utilization of the mind. This concept, though certainly not new, became so popular and accepted in many circles that it led to a new branch of science, most commonly referred to as psychoneuroimmunology (PNI).

≈ Psychoneuroimmunology

PNI is the study of the relationship of the psyche (the mind), emotions, the neuroendocrine system (hormones and the nervous system), and the immune system. Although PNI is in its infancy, the evidence continues to mount in favor of a strong and intimate relationship within the major systems of the body and mind. One of the most important breakthroughs made by neuroscientist Candace Pert is the discovery of neuropeptides and their receptor sites.[2] A neuropeptide, which can be created by a thought, is a chemical that transfers information from nerve cells to other cells in the body. Endorphins, the morphinelike substances that the body creates under stress or intense physical activity (the "runner's high"), are an example of a commonly known neuropeptide.

A receptor site is a place on a cell that is the right size and configuration to receive the message from the neuropeptide. Pert found that there are forty times the number of receptors for neuropeptides in the limbic system, the part of the brain known as "the seat of emotions," as in any other part of the brain.[3] Furthermore, receptor sites were also found on the cells of the immune system, explaining the connection of emotions to immune system function. To complete the loop, it has been recently discovered that cells in the immune system have the capacity to generate neuropeptides.[4] In essence, we now know that the immune system can learn, recall, and initiate, as well as receive messages from the brain. In fact, neuroscientists suggest that there are sixty to a hundred powerful informational biochemicals such as neuropeptides and other hormonelike substances that carry messages back and forth among the endocrine systems, the central nervous system, and the immune system.[5]

Why is this information so significant? It means that the mind is actually a part of the body, and vice versa. We have a thinking body. We can no longer separate the mind from the body.

As PNI hypotheses, theories, and research findings make their way into the media, the potential for oversimplification and extrapolation is high, and in fact not uncommon. Well-meaning health professionals, therapists, authors, and patients will adopt new philosophies or therapies based on findings from one study or from one aspect of knowledge on the mind/body continuum. Many myths are born this way, usually followed by a reactionary backlash. This has frequently been the case with any reference to cancer. Let's examine the mind/body issues as they pertain to breast cancer.

◆ Is There a Cancer Personality?

The concept of a cancer-prone personality, as introduced by psychotherapist Lawrence LeShan, has stimulated much controversy and research. LeShan noted a life pattern during his many years of studying cancer patients. This pattern has three stages. In stage one, a person begins life poorly bonded with a parent and/or parents, resulting in an impaired ability to make healthy intimate connections. As an adult, during stage two, this individual may find external sources of satisfaction in a relationship or career that allows for some creative expression of self. The third stage represents the loss of this source of expression. The key to this pattern, one that may promote a health risk, is the ensuing coping style. If the earlier conflicts (or impaired developmental phases) have not been resolved in adult life, one might be inclined under severe stress to regress emotionally. In the described pattern, the individual would revert to isolation, lack of connectedness, and eventually a sense of hopelessness. In addition to outlining this general pattern, LeShan noted in cancer-prone individuals the traits of passivity, despair, and suppression of emotional expression.[6]

LeShan's research gave rise to more research and eventually the coining of the term *Type C,* or *cancer personality.* Central to this personality is the aforementioned suppression of emotional responses, particularly anger. Other characteristic qualities include conformity, compliance, unassertiveness, and passivity. This individual also holds to the belief that it is useless to express one's needs, promoting a state of chronic helplessness and hopelessness.[7,8]

The attempt to connect breast cancer patients with Type C personality traits has resulted in conflicting evidence. Part of the problem is that studies of this nature are fraught with methodological problems. Many of the studies are retrospective—that is, conducted *after* the appearance of breast cancer. Under these circumstances, researchers have to rely on patients' self-reports in highly subjective areas, as well as deal with the confounding issue of the psychological changes that occur after a life-threatening diagnosis. However, one personality attribute is consistent throughout most controlled studies. It is this pattern of emotional suppression we have cited, specifically the withholding of anger and a repressed or suppressed style of dealing with stress.[9,10,11,12] For clarification, suppression is a conscious choice not to express an emotion of which you are aware. Repression, on the other hand, is more of an unconscious process, usually learned early in life and often a result of habitual suppression.

Unfortunately, these concepts have become popularized in self-healing books, and messages that have been well intended have become disastrous for many women and their families in their search for the whys of breast cancer. A recent unpublished study reports that 40 percent of all women diagnosed with breast cancer believe they are to blame for their cancer through a personality trait or behavior.[13] One can only imagine the emotional burden of this belief while dealing with a diagnosis of this frightening, life-threatening disease.

This is a real double-edged sword. To protect women from this problem of guilt, many health professionals, and women themselves, want to minimize the role of personality characteristics, emotional problems, issues of the past, or anything different from "positive thinking." This is a natural response and no doubt quite appropriate during the initial adjustment to a diagnosis. However, for women interested in taking control of their healing process, avoidance in dealing with these areas can represent a lost opportunity. It could mean bypassing the chance to learn about their inner world and make the kind of profound internal transformations known to be so important to the healing process.

A disease sometimes is the only way our beings know how to express unconscious conflicts, stress, or destructive lifestyles. Given proper attention, illness can be the great teacher for bringing important aspects of our personal growth into consciousness, WITHOUT *blaming ourselves for what we did not know before.*

It is also important to realize that even for women who had conscious knowledge about areas of health and yet for some reason were unable—or chose not to—follow a healthful path, self-blame is still not appropriate to inflict. There are usually habit patterns, lifestyle issues, or unfulfilled needs that drive these detrimental behaviors. While it may be important to examine these areas, it can be detrimental to healing to inflict self-blame.

✒ Can Stress and Depression Cause Cancer?

It is commonly feared that acute or chronic stress and depression can lead to a major illness such as breast cancer. In visiting several breast cancer support groups, we found that most women blamed the stress in their lives for their cancer. Jobs, family difficulties, finances, deaths, and other losses were felt to be out of their control. While this is a widely held belief, there are no studies that definitively support this notion. What accounts for this discrepancy?

There are many studies that support a correlation among psychosocial factors (family, work, societal pressures, relationships), lowered immunity, and disease. A correlation is only evidence that *suggests* a relationship between the topics being studied. Let us review these and see how they may relate to the risk of breast cancer.

STRESS AND IMMUNITY

Research abounds indicating the role of stress in lowered immunity. In fact, numerous pathways and mechanisms explaining how psychological processes influence immune function have been identified and understood. These complex mechanisms can be mind-boggling for the nonscientist to grasp. However, if you are serious about gaining a deeper understanding of your physiological processes, it might prove beneficial to wade through a little simplified science.

The existence of a potential stressor (a thought or event perceived as a threat) is processed in the cortex of the brain. The limbic system (the lower or most primitive part of the brain) communicates the emotional information to the hypothalamus gland, which keeps our systems balanced. This balance is termed homeostasis. The hypothalamus sends neuropeptides to the pituitary gland (the master gland) and other parts of the brain, mobilizing one or both of the two main stress systems that affect immunity: the sympathetic adrenal-medullary (SAM) system and the hypothalamic-pituitary-adrenocortical (HPAC) system. The SAM is associated with fight-or-flight, fear and anger, and other acute emotional states such as excitement. Activation of the SAM stimulates release of a class of hormones known as catecholamines, which include epinephrine (adrenaline) and norepinephrine (noradrenaline).

The HPAC system is activated by circumstances that are appraised to be overwhelming or beyond the control of the individual. Chronic stress, clinical depression, and the states of helplessness and hopelessness are often associated with the activity of this system. The activated HPAC system releases adrenocorticotropic hormone (ACTH) and corticosteroids. The fact that both systems could be activated at any given time adds to the complexity inherent in trying to understand the stress response.[14,15]

It is generally agreed that ACTH, corticosteroids, and catecholamines can suppress the immune system. Now it starts to get really complex. Do specific emotional states tend to lower immunity? What does it mean that a person has a compromised immune system? What types of immune cells are affected? Does lowered immunity lead to disease? If so, how long does it have to be lowered and how serious does the disease have to be? A brief discussion of the immune surveillance theory is necessary here to begin to address these questions.

IMMUNE SURVEILLANCE THEORY

The immunological surveillance theory is based on the premise that when abnormal cells with proliferative potential arise in the body, they develop a substance called an antigen.[16] Antigenic material stimulates cells of the immune system to engulf, poison, or otherwise kill the abnormal cell. Most of you have heard that this process goes on constantly in the body, with our immune system destroying potential cancerous cells daily. One might be tempted to draw the conclusion that if our immune system is strong and functioning optimally, we are not at risk for cancer. Or for that matter, one might be worried that if one's immune system is compromised, cancer may flourish unchecked.

A survey of the PNI literature indicates that such a direct causal relationship cannot be confirmed. A review published by the *Journal of the National Cancer Institute* on the topic of the immune system and cancer states there are different categories of tumors. Some are not recognized by the immune system and therefore do not receive the benefit of surveillance. Among these are tumors developed through exposure to chemical carcinogens. Only part of the time will the immune system recognize these cancerous cells as something to be eliminated.[17] To further complicate matters, recent evidence suggests that there is no way the surveillance system can detect the very earliest malignant cell, which must go through significant change before it can be recognized and destroyed.[18] Moreover, some tumors can produce immunosuppressive substances, disabling the immune system's interaction with the tumor.

Some scientists suggest that the immune system need not be impaired for cancer to occur and progress.[19] This assertion may explain why thousands of women who contract breast cancer exclaim that they never considered themselves candidates for cancer. They were healthy and required few sick days in their lives, leading them to believe they had a strong immune system.

The next question to pose, then, is whether fears that a compromised immune system can cause cancer are founded. Once again, a direct causal relationship cannot be substantiated. It *is* known that when immunity is lowered, a person is more susceptible to infectious diseases. However, as we have discussed earlier, the development of cancer is more complex, requiring an initiation and a promotion phase. Lowered immunity may predispose you to a greater risk in one or both phases, but bear in mind it is only a risk factor, not a direct cause.

The point here is not to downplay the importance of the immune system in cancer, but to recognize that the interactions between the two are highly complex, variable, and difficult to predict. The efficiency of the immune system is influenced not only by the state of the psyche and the neuroendocrine system, but also by the type, origin, and stage of tumor involved. These variables may explain the wide variation seen in tumor progression and regression in cancer patients.[20]

❧ Findings in PNI Research

As mentioned earlier, findings in PNI literature are a mixed bag, with the bulk of the research supporting some correlation between psychosocial factors and lowered immunity. However, attempts to link alterations in immune function to actual clinical outcomes, including breast cancer, have been few.[21] Nonetheless, we can still learn something from preliminary results.

Bereavement and major loss-related events appear to be the most significant psychosocial predictors of breast cancer. A prospective British study of 2,163 women demonstrated that women predisposed to breast cancer were more likely to have lost a loved one or experienced some other major loss-related event. It was also found that the severity of the event correlated significantly to breast disease. Women who were unable to externalize their emotions about the event were at greater risk. Women with the least risk were exposed to stressful events on a consistent basis as opposed to one catastrophic event.[22,23]

As correlation, an American study of 1,052 women reported that the only critical life events that correlated to breast cancer incidence represented a major loss. Interestingly, the English study indicated that the loss was most often focused on friendships, whereas the loss for American women centered around jobs. The suggested explanation for this difference was that American women have more social support and counseling available for bereavement issues.[24] A Finnish study also found that breast cancer patients had significantly more important losses and difficult life situations prior to the discovery of breast cancer than the control group.[25]

Many studies investigating bereavement and social disruption actually measure the activity of certain cells of the immune system. Natural killer (NK) cells, a type of lymphocyte, appear to be the most common immune markers studied. The natural killer cell is thought to have an innate ability to recognize and kill cancer cells even though the cancer cells do not possess an antigen. The proficiency of these cells is recognized as being especially important in the control of metastasis.[26,27,28,29] One researcher who has studied bereavement, depression, and NK cells found that loss events themselves did not predict NK cell activity. It is, instead, severe depression that correlates to reduced NK cell function.[30] While numerous other studies confirm this association,[31,32,33,34] it is important to note here that these findings are consistent only in the presence of severe and acute symptoms of depression.

While the focus of this book is on breast cancer prevention, we clearly also have much to learn from the PNI research being done with women who have already been through diagnosis and treatment for breast cancer. Recurrence and metastasis of early-stage breast cancer is often studied in the context of psychosocial factors and natural killer cells. The earliest studies reported that recurrent breast cancer patients who were rated hostile and unpleasant by their doctors lived significantly longer than patients who reported milder moods. Nonmetastatic breast cancer patients with a "fighting spirit" and "positive avoidance" (in which they pay little attention to their disease) had better survival rates than women who showed stoic acceptance or a hopeless/helpless response.[35,36]

A research team from the National Cancer Institute has reported that low NK activity was significantly associated with the spread of cancer to the lymph nodes, and conversely, high NK activity was related to less metastases to nodes. The team also found that they could account for 51 percent of the difference in NK activity through psychological factors. Among these factors was the perception of outstanding emotional support from a spouse or intimate other, additional social support factors, and a beneficial coping style. The team was able to replicate these findings at a three-month follow-up, at which time they noted that the extent of the tumor was clearly associated with NK activity.[37,38] A seven-year follow-up of this study found that patients who reported feelings of sadness, hopelessness, and worthlessness tended to live less than two years postrecurrence. Conversely, they found that a positive mood and joyful feelings predicted longer survival.[39]

One researcher reported that breast cancer patients in remission who used humor as a coping style had higher NK cell activity than others in his sample.[40] Another study showed that severely threatening life events were significantly correlated to the first recurrence of breast cancer, while life difficulties rated less severe were not related to relapse.[41] In a fifteen-year follow-up of nonmetastatic breast cancer patients, the researcher concluded that the psychological stance patients adopt toward their disease can affect the course of certain breast cancers. Additionally, he finds that passive and helpless/hopeless responses are consistently related to poor outcome, while the "fighting spirit" appears to be correlated with a longer duration of survival.[42]

The studies reported in this section represent only a few of the more commonly cited ones. You can see that there are many variables and a variety of findings. It is also easy to see how certain "truths" can be extracted from these studies and popularized in nonscientific literature. In attempting to assess the bottom line here we can arrive at the following conclusion: Severe life events can be predictive of breast cancer incidence or recurrence, but only if they are loss-related and the event is interpreted or perceived by the woman as beyond her control and coping abilities, thus fostering the possibility of severe depression. By the same token, better health outcomes may be predicted for women who, regardless of life events, have and can utilize social support, can mobilize their abilities to express grief and anger, and enjoy a sense of personal control.

✒ Behavioral Medicine

As we understand that psychosocial and psychological factors may play a role in the onset of breast cancer, is it logical and safe to assume that these factors can help reverse the disease process? In other words, can the mind heal the body? These questions have stimulated much controversy and a growing body of research. Again, while our focus here is on altering our behavior before the appearance of disease, the efforts and discoveries women have made in their attempts to put cancer into remission can teach us much about how to make ourselves healthier now.

In the early 1970s studies in biofeedback indicated that certain bodily processes, such as heart rate and blood pressure, could be mentally influenced. Since these autonomic processes were once thought to be out of our conscious control, this information began a major shift in our thinking about the mind/body relationship. At the same time, the surveillance theory (the ability of the immune system to recognize and destroy cancer cells) was becoming popular. It made sense to investigate the possibility that the mind could also affect the activity of the immune system, thereby enhancing the remission of cancer.

Dr. Carl Simonton and Stephanie Matthews-Simonton, authors of the best-selling book *Getting Well Again,* were among the pioneers in this research. They are most noted for creating a program that teaches cancer patients visualization as an adjunct to traditional medical treatment. The Simontons developed a method of using mental images to influence healing mechanisms, such as augmenting the action of the immune system. Although their work was heavily criticized by medical traditionalists, they were able to advance a new approach to healing and help many terminal patients extend their lives well beyond average expectancy. In fact, the Simontons reported a doubling in survival time.[43]

Dr. Bernie Siegel, through his books *Love, Medicine and Miracles* and *Peace, Love and Healing,* popularized the Simontons' work. He also popularized conclusions drawn from some of the research reported in the previous section. This wide dissemination of findings gave rise to the concept of the "exceptional cancer patient," one who has a fighting spirit, the will to live, and a positive outlook. Dr. Siegel's work was misinterpreted by many to mean that if you heal your life (change negative thinking, find meaning in life, resolve conflicted relationships), you can heal your body, too. While Dr. Siegel posed this idea as a possibility and provided anecdotes to support it, his central message was the instillation of hope and an exhortation to live life to the fullest, regardless of the outcome.[44,45]

Dr. Siegel's work has inspired many cancer patients to take control of their own healing program and express themselves more fully. Concurrently, it has also created some difficulties. Many cancer patients who are aware of the documented cases of spontaneous remission (healing that cannot be explained medically) tend to blame themselves if they are unable to effect their own physical healing through mental processes. This self-flagellation serves to compound the already difficult psychological issues facing those with a life-threatening illness.

Although there has been a conservative backlash in some circles, the field of behavioral medicine continues to grow by leaps and bounds. Mind/body clinics and wellness centers have sprung up all over this country. They teach and utilize techniques such as meditation, visualization, biofeedback, goal setting, new problem-solving techniques, restructuring of thinking and attitudes, music, yoga, acupuncture, psychotherapy, and group therapy.

Evidence that these healing techniques and practices can alter the course of disease is meager. However, most agree that they can offer some physiological benefits and enhance the quality of life. For example, physiological changes can be measured in most activities that engage the relaxation response. Meditation, yoga, hypnosis, and self-hypnosis decrease heart rate and respiratory rate.[46] There is no question that we can think our bodies into a state of relaxation. Doesn't it follow that if stress can diminish the competence of the immune system, a continuous practice of relieving stress could normalize immune function and improve health? Support for this contention is plentiful from anecdotal literature.[47] Additionally, a research team studying the effects of relaxation, imagery, and biofeedback training on the immune systems of breast cancer patients found that these behavioral interventions significantly increased lymphocyte and natural killer cell activity.[48] Another researcher reported that psychological therapy for cancer patients resulted in significant improvement in anxiety, depression, fighting spirit, anxious preoccupation, and helplessness.[49] These results were confirmed in a following study.[50]

Social support, especially group therapy, is the area of behavioral medicine that has received the most attention in medical circles. While it is commonly reported that married people enjoy better health, one study found specifically that married cancer patients lived longer than unmarried cancer patients, all other things being equal.[51] Furthermore, owning a pet, particularly for senior citizens who are often at risk of being isolated and lonely, has been shown to increase longevity.[52] A long-term population study in Alameda, California, found that individuals who were the least socially connected were twice as likely to die as those with strong ties. Women who were isolated were particularly vulnerable to cancer.[53]

Epidemiologists from Berkeley, California, studied the amount of social interaction of cancer patients. They report that women with the least amount of social contact were 2.2 times more likely to die of cancer over a seventeen-year period than those with a high degree of contact. They also note that this correlation is strongest among women with hormone-related cancers, such as breast cancer.[54] One research reviewer concluded that from a statistical point of view *it may be as important to your health to have good social support as it is to lower your cholesterol or quit smoking!*[55]

Only a few studies address the issue of behavioral intervention and survival, and those that do have mixed results. An analysis of Dr. Bernie Siegel's ECAP groups (Exceptional Cancer Patients) yielded small, but not statistically significant increases in survival time compared to nonparticipants. This study took the wind out of the sails of many who were convinced intuitively that enhancement of the quality of life through group support would increase longevity.[56] However, as is typical with these back-and-forth scenarios, a following study did show a survival benefit for patients participating in psychotherapy. Investigators reported that women in a randomized group who were sent to psychotherapy survived 18.6 months following diagnosis, as opposed to 12.6 months for women not receiving psychotherapy.[57]

The landmark study that changed the tide, conducted by Dr. David Spiegel, examined the effects of group therapy on metastatic breast cancer patients. Dr. Spiegel initiated this study with the intent of disproving the notion that psychological support could affect the course of disease. Analysis of the data nine years later showed a 36.6-month average survival time for women in the therapy group, compared to 18.9 months for women receiving no psychological intervention. In effect, the women in the therapy group lived twice as long. What is remarkable about these results is that both groups received the same standard medical treatment of surgery, chemotherapy, and radiation. The only difference was that one group of women got together once a week to talk. We are unaware of any drug or other therapy that can claim such phenomenal results: a doubling of survival time! Dr. Spiegel has since written a book and many articles, and he is traveling the country speaking about group therapy and cancer.[58]

We think it is important to note that these results were based on group therapy, which should be distinguished from support groups. Support groups, often led by seasoned patients, are generally designed to help people with their adjustment to cancer, treatment issues, and a chance to be heard and understood by others in the same situation. Group therapy, led by a professional, creates an environment that allows for the expression of deep emotions, negative and positive feelings alike, with feedback and help from other members. It is mostly a closed circle, and participants commit to regular attendance, giving rise to an almost familial bond between participants. "Positive thinking," while important in the proper context, is not the central tenet, so women have a chance to rail against their disease and directly confront death and loss. This kind of freedom in a group environment can do wonders for one's ability to cope with difficult situations. It can lighten a heavy burden and create a special kind of joy. Social connectedness is central to these benefits.

Clearly, to disregard the psychological and psychosocial aspects of healing would be as foolish as to ignore the need for physical therapies. We think it is safe to say that our mind and emotions, among other factors, play a very important role in healing. Advances in mind/body health and behavioral medicine can only benefit us in our quest for health and longevity. *However, it is important that we are mindful not to mechanize the mind into a tool to control the body and forget the component of spirit.* Dr. Rachel Naomi Remen, medical director of the Commonweal Cancer Help Program, says, "The real questions of health may not be questions of mechanism but questions of spirit. . . . Something in us participates in our humanness, but has its source and its connection far beyond it, and in that connection may lie the hope of healing."[59]

✖ The Role of the Spirit in Healing

Long overlooked and even scorned by Western medicine and science, the concept of spirit in healing is now finding a new acceptance in our society. In fact, the dramatic popularity of alternative medicine underscores the desire for the inclusion of the spiritual aspects of medicine. There are two primary ways the spirit plays a role in healing. One is a personal sense of connection to the transcendent, which serves as a type of coping mechanism, providing a buffer for illness and loss. The other is spiritual healing, an encounter in which one or more people have the intention of effecting a physical change to benefit another. We will define and examine both these areas, demonstrating the importance of this dimension in healing.

SPIRITUALITY DEFINED

There are numerous definitions of spirituality which reflect the biases of religion, personalities, and society. To synthesize these definitions, let us say that spirituality appears to be an essential aspect of human awareness and existence that encompasses the physical but also extends beyond the physical domain, including all that is concerned with life-meaning and purpose. Clifford C. Kuhn states: "Spiritual elements are those capacities that enable a human being to rise above or transcend any experience at hand. They are characterized by the capacity to seek meaning and purpose, to have faith, to love, to forgive, to pray, to meditate, to worship, and to see beyond present circumstances."[60] It is important to note that the spiritual dimension is distinct from religious doctrine or dogma.

Spirituality is intangible and cannot be measured. While spirituality is reported in all human cultures, modern Western society views the material realm as being more important and valid than the spiritual. What cannot be measured is dismissed and considered "immaterial."[61] Yet 70 percent of all Americans report that spirituality is central to their lives, with 95 percent avowing a belief in a greater power.[62] Considering that the fathers of medicine, Hippocrates, Galen, Aristotle, and Paracelsus, applied a holistic (whole person) approach in diagnosis and treatment, it seems as though Western man has made a giant digression into the material, objective, and biomedical realms. We have forgotten our roots. The loss of the psychosocial well-being often achieved by spirituality is showing up in increased rates of depression, anxiety, and alcohol and drug abuse. This is especially evident in the baby boomer generation and the generation following it, despite unprecedented economic prosperity.[63]

With this in mind, we know that approaching healing from only the material side of existence is extremely limiting, especially in light of the latest research in quantum physics. Physicists have confirmed that matter can be understood as very dense energy; hence, the body may be perceived as energy rather than matter.[64] The current medical paradigm views consciousness as a byproduct of the extraordinary complexity of our nervous systems, while the new paradigm considers matter (all things appearing physical) as arising from consciousness. Mind, according to the traditionalists, is associated with the brain, whereas the new model relates the mind to consciousness and spirituality. While this is a very complex issue stated simply, what is important to understand is that these are completely opposite worldviews. It is no wonder that these two approaches to medicine are polarized. However, there is a growing body of research pointing to the need to redefine our biomedical model to provide a comprehensive bio-psycho-socio-spiritual model of health and illness.[65]

Research has begun to confirm reports of out-of-body experiences (projecting awareness outside the physical body)—that the mind extends beyond the body via telepathy, projects beyond time (precognitions), and can interact with matter (psychokinesis). It has been shown that near-death experiences (NDE) are transformative. However, those who are proclaimed clinically dead but do not recall an NDE have no experience of transformation. Deathbed experiences, bereavement apparitions, reincarnation, and spiritual healing are all being researched, with reports that challenge Western society's most basic assumptions about life and death.[66]

Twice as many studies assessing the role of spirituality on mental health show positive results as report no correlation or a negative one. A review of 250 studies on the role of spiritual commitment in health outcome also shows positive results.[67] It is important to note here that these studies all used religious affiliation or denomination as the spiritual variable. Attendance at a religious gathering and the resulting social connectedness would no doubt account for part of these positive results. However, it is in this connectedness that an important aspect of spirituality can be expressed.

Spirituality is shown to be particularly important in the aged or people dealing with a life-threatening disease. Beliefs about origins and meanings of symptoms, often in spiritual terms, have implications for the way patients may be healed. Spiritual assessment can bring forth growth and transformation that might otherwise be lost by addressing only the physical dimension. Prayer and meditation are also shown empirically to be powerful coping tools for maintaining well-being in the face of illness and impending loss.[68] John B. Ellis says, "Spiritual well-being is the affirmation of life in a relationship with God, self, community, and environment that nurtures and celebrates wholeness."[69]

The Spiritual Healing Encounter

Spiritual healing, an area often thought to be the domain of shamans, evangelist faith healers, psychic healers, or those with special healing capacities, is actually something that we all experience or can perform. Theorist D. Benor says, "Healing is the direct influence of one or more persons upon another living system without using known physical means of intervention."[70] Healer intention, unconditional love, and compassion are primary facilitators of this process.

In his provocative book *Meaning & Medicine*, Larry Dossey takes the position that spiritual healing occurs anytime someone's self-healing capacity is made more effective by another. Hippocrates states, "Nature heals; the physician is nature's assistant." This kind of healing cannot be explained away by the mere power of suggestion or the placebo effect, because it can bypass the conscious mind of the patient. In other words, healing can be mediated by the unconscious, unaware part of the mind.[71]

No one knows exactly what occurs during a spiritual healing encounter. However, four theoretical models attempt to explain this phenomenon: (1) Electrical, electromagnetic, or another type of energy is exchanged between the practitioner and the patient, although some theorists think the energy is strictly from the healer to the patient. (2) There is an altered state of consciousness within the practitioner or patient, or both. (3) There is a communication by direct or intuitive processes between the two, creating a synergistic event. (4) According to theorists with religious affiliations, healing occurs through the grace of God.[72]

There are two general modes of spiritual healing: hand contact or near contact, and healing at a distance. There are 155 published studies, with over one-half showing significant results. Some are seriously flawed, but the majority that show significant results are not.[73]

Well-controlled and experimental trials were done by nurse researcher Dr. Dolores Krieger, who developed Therapeutic Touch (TT). This noncontact healing technique, similar to the "laying on of hands" from some religions, consistently produced beneficial changes in blood chemistry, as well as anecdotal evidence that the well-being of patients improved. TT is now being taught to thousands of registered nurses in the United States. One doctoral dissertation demonstrated that Therapeutic Touch using actual hand contact significantly alleviated anxiety in patients hospitalized in a cardiovascular intensive care unit. Another dissertation corroborated this finding, this time using noncontact TT, and showed that anxiety reduction was possible without touch.[74]

One researcher, attempting to evaluate whether healing can take place with noncontact TT, designed a double blind study in which the participants had no idea they were recipients of the technique. The wounds of the group being administered TT healed significantly sooner and more completely than those of the control group, indicating that noncontact TT is an effective technique even when the patient is unaware of its application.[75]

In a landmark double-blind controlled study, Dr. Randolph Byrd, a cardiologist, studied 393 patients who were admitted to a coronary care unit. These patients were divided into two groups who both received state-of-the-art medical treatment. However, various Protestant and Catholic prayer groups throughout the United States prayed for only one of the groups. The purpose of the prayer was for rapid recovery and the prevention of complications and death. None of the attendant health professionals knew which patients were the objects of prayer. The results were that the group receiving prayer had a better course of treatment than the control group. They were less likely to develop congestive heart failure, five times less likely to require antibiotics, and three times less likely to need diuretics. None of these patients required a breathing tube, fewer developed pneumonia, and none died.[76] While critics claim that the statistics are open to interpretation, they nonetheless highlight a healing method that defies the beliefs of modern medicine and builds the case for spiritual healing from a distance. It is interesting to note that in the seven years that followed, no one has attempted to replicate this study.

One theorist said that since there are no known deleterious effects, if spiritual healing were a drug, it would be on the market.[77] Another said that it offered one of the best risk-to-benefit-ratio therapies available.[78] Couple these findings with those mentioned in PNI research which link social support to stronger immune function, and you will quickly see that the presence of a compassionate, loving health professional with clear intent to activate the healing response could definitely enhance a patient's overall emotional and physical health.

❧ Summary

The connection between the mind and body, an idea once relegated to ancient wisdom or intuition, is now being documented scientifically and therefore stimulating new treatment directions. While it is unfair to say that a certain constellation of personality traits predicts breast cancer, it should be noted that certain qualities can be protective of good health. Expressing emotions, maintaining good social connections, and experiencing a sense of control in one's life, regardless of the severity of life events, all contribute to a cancer-free life. While it is known that stress and depression can affect immune system function, the direct relationship between these psychological states and breast cancer is not fully understood owing to the complexity of all the interconnected systems. However, the role of emotions in protecting or threatening health is being acknowledged as new treatment protocols that include the psychological, emotional, and spiritual well-being of breast cancer patients are being instituted in hospitals and healing centers throughout the country. These treatments focus primarily on social support and stress reduction. The spiritual element in health and healing is beginning to command research attention and is considered an important aspect in the recovery from illness and maintenance of good health. The following chapter will show you how you can utilize this information in your quest to prevent breast cancer.

Chapter 24

On Health, Healing, and Empowerment

One year ago Taffy got hit by what she calls the "universal two by four." Her dearest friend, who was barely forty, came to visit for the holidays with her husband and six-month-old son. She had a small lump in her breast and a huge walnut-size lump under her arm. On the day before Christmas, she was diagnosed with Stage II breast cancer with positive lymph node involvement.

It was Taffy's worst nightmare. This was too close to home and to her own fears. Her friend, whom we shall call Sandra, went through the various phases of shock and disbelief, yet traveled through the initial stages of the experience with strength and aplomb.

One day Taffy arrived home to find Sandra consoling her distraught husband over her disease. Taffy was furious. Sandra had often placed others before herself, playing the role of the "support" person, working hard to please, and maintaining a happy, cheerful personality. Furthermore, she often had difficulty expressing anger and other negative emotions. Taffy saw in that moment the extent of the healing process Sandra would need to undertake, but she also knew that she would have to put into practice all that she knew and taught about the healing process. Sandra's cancer shocked Taffy into realizing how important it is to institute all of the changes necessary for good health today, not tomorrow.

* It Can't Happen to Me

It never occurred to Sandra that she would get cancer. It was the sort of thing that happens to someone else. Not one of us is immune to the possibility of contracting this disease. We may live healthy lifestyles (the definition of which is certainly open to interpretation), we may have no cancer in our families, we may have positive attitudes, express our feelings, get our exercise, and think we have "cancer-proofed" our lives. But what if we were raised in an industrially polluted town, unknowingly drank contaminated water as a child, or grew up breathing secondhand smoke from a parent's cigarette? How many of us are unknowingly walking around with the first "hit," the irreversible initiation phase of cancer, already established in our bodies?

It is not our intention to make breast cancer seem random and uncontrollable; however, too many women are getting breast cancer, and the medical establishment says they haven't a clue about its origin in 70 to 80 percent of the cases! It is time to take your head out of the sand and acknowledge that it could just as easily be you with breast cancer as your best friend, mother, or sister. It is time to ask what you can do *now* to give yourself maximum protection. And now is the time to act.

❧ *The Healing Begins Before Disease*

Most people don't think much about healing until they have a disease. Seldom does a woman seek therapy unless she is feeling emotionally upset or some aspect of her life isn't working. Crisis and illness are the prime movers. Healing, which implies change, can be hard work, and it is not usually in our natures to take on such a task unless we have to. While researching and thinking about this book, we often wondered, What will it take for women to want to make changes before a disease develops? We have asked many breast cancer patients this question, and most reply that nothing but a disease this critical would have forced the types of changes they have had to make. Nonetheless, for those of you who have been startled by the previous chapters, and for those of you who can use this book as the "crisis," rather than waiting for the real thing, we want to share the psychosocial areas many of our courageous sisters with breast cancer have had to address in order to engage in the healing process. Perhaps those of us free from cancer today can integrate this information into our lives, creating a greater possibility for a cancer-free future.

❧ *Health, Illness, and Disease*

Before we begin to explore healing, it is important to examine how we view health, illness, and disease. On a practical level, we can consider disease as a malfunctioning or breakdown in physiological and biological processes. It is a material process that is confined to the body. Hence, treatment for disease is also focused totally on the physical and its goal is a "cure." Conversely, according to many writers in the mind/body field, illness refers more to the whole person, including physical, social, psychological, and spiritual factors. Treatment approaches for illness take into consideration all these factors, with the focus on "healing" or "making whole."

In the West, health is something we become concerned

about only when we develop disease or illness. In these terms, we often view health as the absence of disease. We strive for long and materially comfortable lives, while we try to ignore death and disease.

Many of you may be familiar with the concept of the "shadow" introduced in the late nineteenth century by the famous psychiatrist Carl Jung. The shadow is the part of our natures that is often hidden from conscious view, yet still can be a strong driving force in our personalities. It is part of our unconscious mind, referred to by some as the "denied self." Many therapists seek to help their clients bring this unconscious part into consciousness, so that these individuals can make new choices in areas that seemed previously out of their control. Essentially, the same concept applies to the way we view disease, illness, and death. In order to experience true health, which is often defined as being "whole," the experience of illness, disease, and death must be acknowledged, embraced, and understood rather than ignored, suppressed, and abhorred.

Health is an experience rather than something that can be acquired or possessed.[1] Health involves the expression of the whole person and a sense of "internal congruence." This means there is a strong alignment of what we feel, say, and do. It means *not* saying yes when we feel no.

Health also means being in balance. As mentioned in the previous chapter, feedback loops and chemical messengers help the regulatory systems sustain a dynamic inner balance. These elements combine in a state referred to as homeostasis. When we become ill, there is a breakdown in or disconnection among these built-in repair mechanisms. Abuses from external sources such as food, destructive chemicals, polluted air, continual physical injury, or hostile relationships can overload this system. When this breakdown occurs, the imbalance expresses itself through the symptoms of disease. Naturally, we can also create imbalances internally through vehicles such as continual negative thinking, unexpressed anger, hopelessness, helplessness, and depression. Imbalances that spring from these sources can also create physical symptoms. Such symptoms, then, are warning signs that some part of you is out of balance and needs *attention, not suppression.*

🗠 Healing Defined

Healing can be defined as the process of restoring balance and bringing into focus the parts of your life that are disowned and neglected. It also means taking action or making decisions based on new information and insights.

Sometimes healing requires you to leave relationships. Sometimes it requires that you open communication in order to enhance faltering or disconnected relationships. Other times it calls for a change in your diet. Alternately, it may mean changing jobs, moving to a new environment, or simply incorporating meditation and exercise into your life. This diversity of responses or conditions is what makes healing so different for everyone. And because it is different for everyone, it is inappropriate for well-meaning friends or even professionals to offer simple answers for any individual's situation. While it is advised that you take advantage of all resources available, ultimately it is very important that your healing journey becomes self-generated.

🗠 Stories of Healing Journeys

Let us recount the stories of two brave young women, Lisa and Sandra, who were diagnosed with breast cancer in the prime of their lives. These stories will give you an intimate look into the methods each used to cope with a life-threatening disease and their subsequent healing journey.

One day Lisa, a lovely young woman in her mid-thirties, noticed a dimpling in her breast and an inverted nipple. She was diagnosed with infiltrating ductal carcinoma, a kind of cancer that may not be detectable on breast exam and sometimes does not show up on a mammogram. With little prior consciousness on maintaining personal health and very few sick days in her entire life, this news came as a devastating shock to her. Heeding the oncologist's warning, believing medical therapies to be her only options, Lisa submitted to a modified radical mastectomy, followed by the most potent type of chemotherapy available. As might be expected, she was not prepared for the overwhelming grief and psychological devastation that resulted from the loss of her right breast. Being young and unmarried, she found that the loss precipitated a change in her view of her own femininity. She was vaguely aware that chemotherapy might result in the cessation of her menstrual cycles. Well into the treatment, she fully realized that her chemotherapy treatments had rendered her sterile. She felt betrayed by the medical community for their casual disregard of the necessity and importance of making very clear to her, a childless woman, the possibility of infertility when they were explaining the effects of chemotherapy prior to her receiving her first treatment.

Lisa, who experienced deep depression and suicidal thoughts following these losses, began to realize that it would be extremely difficult to fight her illness unless she could gain control over her emotions and seething anger toward herself and the physicians. She sought the help of a well-reputed healer, therapist, and naturopathic physician, who offered adjuvant treatments as Lisa completed her chemotherapy. Today Lisa is in remission and has been symptom-free for four years. Despite these positive signs, her healing journey continues.

To understand this journey in its entirety, we have to backtrack into Lisa's past. She had been involved in several destructive relationships over the years, always believing that if she were to try harder things might work better. Thus she remained in relationships that were harmful to her health. She was on overload all the time, feeling that her value lay in how well she served others. She grew up very disconnected emotionally from her parents and was ultimately unable to connect to her peers. She remembers the desperate longing to "belong," yet she felt defeated and hopeless most of the time. Lisa recalls the intense grief she used to feel for her beloved grandmother, who continually expressed her disappointment in life, particularly for her unachieved dreams. Lisa feels, in retrospect, that much of the grief she carries was transmitted down through generations of family members who felt unfulfilled.

The first order of business for Lisa in her healing process was to begin to ask for support. Her family and friends responded, and she began to learn how to receive their love and attention. She became very angry about having cancer, which mobilized her into a mind-set that denied cancer any power to take away her life. Utilizing imagery as a technique to enhance her treatments, she visualized a tractor going across her chest, with little farmers planting seeds of good health. She joined support groups and began to understand the joy of belonging for the first time. In therapy she began her inner work, focusing on concurrently building self-esteem and tearing down the obstacles in the path to achieving self-love and communicating her truths. She meditated, changed her diet, and left her relationship.

After the death of her mother, Lisa moved home to be with her father. Herein lay the most significant aspects of her healing. Acknowledging that she had never been able to have a successful relationship with a man, Lisa initiated new levels of communication with her father. This exercise forced Lisa to practice things she needed most to learn: staying in the present moment even under stress, removing the blocks to self-love and gaining the ability, for the first time in her life, to communicate her truths. She felt, for the first time, that she had a good, yet challenging, relationship with a man—her father. At this point, Lisa's next greatest challenge will be to integrate the understanding she has gained into a relationship with a potential partner, as she simultaneously faces considerations about her sexuality, femininity, loss of fertility, and a reconstructed breast that cannot take the place of the one lost. Through it all, Lisa maintains a deep belief that she will not have to face a recurrence of cancer.

Sandra, meanwhile, took a different treatment path from Lisa. She agreed only to a lumpectomy, refusing radiation and chemotherapy. While not a popular decision from a traditional perspective, Sandra did not need to face disfiguration, loss of fertility, and other often debilitating side effects. Yet her challenge was equally difficult. She had to maintain her faith in the decisions she made, against the protests of those who feared she would die because she chose not to follow standard protocol.

Sandra was highly influenced by David J. Frahm's book *A Cancer Battle Plan* which encouraged her to take whatever approach was necessary to get her body to a level of normal functioning.[2] Sandra instituted a radical diet change from standard American fare to a menu of organic, whole foods. To her routine she added cleansing fasts, colonics, and vitamin supplementation, and she revived her practice of Transcendental Meditation. She searched for alternative health practitioners in the United States and Europe, and read as much information on cancer, treatments, health, and healing as she could, while still maintaining a balance of her other interests. Sandra feels that the educational part of her healing was one of the most important aspects. As she says, "The more I know, the more I am able to utilize my own personal power and strengths to help heal myself. In fact, all this new knowledge and the resulting insights have helped me function better in all areas of my life."

Psychotherapy has also been instrumental in Sandra's healing. She found a therapist who was a proponent of healing the whole person and who understood the mind-body connection. Together they dealt with the emotional aspects of having breast cancer, as well as all the other aspects of her life. Sandra also attended breast cancer support groups, and although she received little support for her treatment path, she still felt emotional support from being able to connect with women who shared the experience of breast cancer.

During the initial phases of Sandra's healing path, she pulled back from many of her relationships to address her pattern of being "other directed." This enabled her to go more deeply inward, creating a more solid inner core. As a result, she feels she is much better at assessing her own needs, setting boundaries, saying no, and asking for what she needs and wants in her relationships.

Facing the possibility of an early death stimulated deep soul-searching in Sandra, as it does in many people who face a life-threatening disease. She realized she needed to come to terms with her Catholic upbringing, which led her to evaluate her spiritual, social, and personal belief systems. Wanting to face death in a fully conscious way, she decided to become a hospice volunteer. This experience helped Sandra gain a deeper understanding of the process of dying. She says that it has helped her become much better equipped to deal with this eventuality, whenever it may come, and she has developed peace of mind.

While Sandra continues to grapple with her ability to express negative emotions, and continues to stand vigilant against negative self-talk, she has become more involved socially and more available emotionally, and she has much less difficulty stating her positions and beliefs. To date, it is unknown whether Sandra is "cured"; however, she carries the belief that as long as she remains dedicated to the healing process, the harmony within her body will correct the biochemical imbalances that allowed cancer to grow. She expects to live a long life free from cancer recurrence.

Although the healing journeys of Lisa and Sandra have different features, there are some common threads in their stories that coincide with our original definition of healing. They have both assessed their lives in the physical, spiritual, psychological, and social realms, and have made major transformations in each area. Both women acknowledged the necessity of physical treatments, however different, and embraced them fully. Each turned to loved ones for support and established new relationships with others on the same path. Both Lisa and Sandra chose to look within themselves for answers and understanding, utilizing meditation and therapy. They examined their relationships and began to take control of the directions of their lives. Both recognized the critical aspect of self-love and view the continuing enhancement of self-esteem as central to their healing. Sandra and Lisa remain dedicated to expressing themselves fully, although they recognize this as a lifetime challenge. They both continue to search for greater spiritual connection, while maintaining a strong belief in their own abilities to heal.

❧ Your Own Healing Journey

There are hundreds of such inspirational stories throughout popular cancer literature about women taking their healing into their own hands. The reason it is so important to pay attention to these women's journeys is that, beyond medical treatment, their healing processes contain many of the components we recommend for breast cancer prevention. There are wonderful books written in all these areas, and we encourage you to peruse Appendix C, Supplemental Reading. Following is a brief overview of the areas we believe to be most important, with the hope that you will be inspired to expand your knowledge and embark on your own healing journey. These topics are not listed in any order, as each is inextricably interconnected to the others.

FORM SUPPORTIVE RELATIONSHIPS

Good, healthy social connectedness appears to be a primary determinant of health and healing. By social connectedness we don't mean knowing the "right" people and being seen in the "right" places. Instead, we are referring to a level of contact with others in which you have the freedom to fully express yourself and be accepted for who you are, are willing to accept others for who they are, and have the ability to share your thoughts, fears, triumphs, and everyday details of your life. That level of contact is called love.

Does this sound a little idealistic? Many people in therapy

find that the therapeutic relationship is the only one in which they experience this kind of freedom and acceptance. While we are realistic about the fact that this kind of connectedness has not been the focus of many people's upbringing, it is a bit disappointing. It requires courage, self-confidence, and diligence to express your thoughts and show your vulnerabilities in a society that rewards competitiveness, stoicism, emotional restraint, and "niceness."

Many people find connectedness in an intimate relationship with one other person. While we don't want to downplay the importance of such a relationship, it is not the full answer. One-to-one bonding can create a closed system, so that when there is a disturbance in the system there is no buffer from the full impact of the disturbance. A support group, family members, or a therapist can help absorb the tensions and anxieties that may result from this type of relationship.

Assess your social connectedness. If you feel isolated, misunderstood or ignored, it might be worth your while to seek out a therapy or support group. We generally favor therapy groups because they are run by professionals and are feedback-oriented. Such a group can give you a chance to expose your fears and vulnerabilities and still be accepted for who you are. On the other hand, support groups are great for connecting with people who may be experiencing similar difficulties; you will find it is easier to bond with people with whom you share common experiences. Support groups are usually inexpensive or free.

If you are not "therapy" oriented, joining clubs or organizations with people who share your interests can be of immense value, not to mention just plain fun. Be patient with yourself since it can take time to explore and form connections. The important thing is to challenge yourself in some way to open your heart to the potential of loving relationships. If this feels impossible, we strongly recommend that you find a good therapist, one who is capable of forming a bond with you and can help you set the stage for a new way of relating to others.

LEARN TO EXPRESS EMOTIONS

You may recall from the previous chapter that suppressed emotion—particularly the inability to express anger and other negative emotions—is a trait often associated with breast cancer. Frankly, most of us struggle with the expression of emotion. In particular, women have a difficult time with anger since its expression goes against society's notion of femininity.

We either under- or overexpress anger. Neither way is healthy for our bodies. When we underexpress, the stress hormones from the autonomic arousal caused by this emotion have no place to go except to harm our bodies. Panic and depression often result from holding in these strong emotions. When we overexpress, besides having an overload of stress hormones on a continual basis, we either get called a bitch or end up hating ourselves for thinking we are out of control. Very few of us have had good models for the expression of anger. Unfortunately, this is something we have to get a handle on on our own, usually as adults.

We suggest as supplemental reading *The Dance of Anger* by Harriet Goldhor Lerner, Ph.D.[3] It is easy to read and quite insightful. Then *practice* what you learn. In almost every women's therapy or support group there is much talk about anger, but when it comes down to actually releasing it, most women are terrified. The expression of anger triggers enormous fear of loss and abandonment, and challenges our self-esteem to the very core. We think it is important to understand and accept that anger is frightening for us, but we must risk its expression to find balance. From a psychosocial perspective, discovering this balance is one of the more important keys in the breast cancer prevention program.

EXPERIENCE JOY

Joy is the other emotion we would like to address here. In the previous chapter we learned that the experience of joy was a predictor of longer survival time in breast cancer patients. Using this information, we suggest that being joyful can aid in activating good health for those without the disease. How many of us live joyful lives? Or how many even experience joy on a regular basis?

Joy may come to us from a variety of sources; however, overall it is the rapturous feeling we experience when we acknowledge how wonderful life is. In her book *A Woman's Worth*, Marianne Williamson explains that we are blocked in our experience of total joy because "we're unconsciously afraid of a reaction against us if we dare to shine fully, embrace joy, and permit ourselves to have too great a life."

Do you recall being embarrassed or downplaying the moment when you won a contest, felt beautiful, or accomplished something important? An unconscious mechanism tells us that our success may limit someone else's possibilities, or that others will dislike us for being too great.[4] Perhaps you yourself have rejected someone else who seemed "too full of herself."

As an exercise, try examining how often you feel proud of yourself, and how willing you are to express this pride. Ask yourself how much you enjoy your life. What are your simple pleasures? How often do you allow yourself these pleasures? Do you feel it is okay to feel happy?

One of the most important components in experiencing the state of joy is the extent to which you live life with a sense of purpose. Dr. Jean Shinoda Bolen, during her speech at the conference "Cancer as a Turning Point," discussed the "soul's journey." She said that certain life events, such as illness or midlife, can sharpen consciousness and force such questions as "Am I doing what I came here to do?" and "Am I healing what I came here to heal?"[5] This aspect is also central to the healing therapy of Lawrence LeShan in his book of the same title, *Cancer as a Turning Point*.[6] He talks about finding your own "song" as the road to health and joy. When we are engaged in our "soul's purpose," we are offering our talents to the world for the betterment of ourselves and others (this kind of service is distinguished from "sacrifice"), and we are living the greatest experience of joy. It is in this state of joy that we experience the most benefit in health and the prevention of disease.

Here is a trick to create an immediate experience of joy. Go into a childhood state and hold your hands together up to your chest as if you are clutching something very special given to you by someone you love. Squeeze tightly and look up with a smile on your face, basking in the energy of joy. Such an exercise can sometimes reverse the most unhappy emotions and allow the "joy" chemicals to rush through your body. If this particular visualization doesn't work, use the power of imagery to find your own memory of joy, and practice the feeling every day.

Although we have only discussed in detail the emotions of anger and joy, it is important that you learn to establish a good balance in the expression of all emotions. In part, this means giving voice or physical release to strong feelings. As a counterpoint, you should learn to shift your thinking, to establish a new, constructive focus that may serve as an antidote to your painful feelings.

ENHANCE YOUR SELF-ESTEEM

This is the big one. Unless we had unusual parents with exceptionally high self-esteem, most of us sustained some injury to this very important part of our persona in the early stages of development. It is our common bond, and the very thing we try the hardest to hide. Many of us are terrified others will see our imperfections and our wounds, and we are all too eager to believe the seeming self-confidence others project. Such barriers we create for ourselves!

Most authors and practitioners in the mind/body health field agree that good self-esteem is the primary key to the healing process. A strong self-concept is the underlying issue in all the areas previously mentioned: social contact, expression of emotion, and experience of joy. It is the central aspect of Lisa's and Sandra's healing process. Without a strong degree of self-love it is hard to feel good about oneself, and it is hard to pursue a life with deep purpose, confidence, joyousness, and laughter.

If you find your self-esteem significantly lacking, develop a plan to address the problem. We heartily recommend Marianne Williamson's A *Woman's Worth*[7] and Gloria Steinem's *Revolution from Within.*[8] If Jack Canfield offers a seminar in your area, take it. He is a wonderful expert on self-esteem. There are many other resources to help you enhance your self-concept, some of which are listed in the appendices. Remember, *good self-esteem is the strongest psychological component in developing good health and preventing breast cancer.*

PRACTICE MEDITATION

Meditation, while gaining acceptance in many circles as central to the healing process, is still largely misunderstood. While meditation may be connected with religion in some societies, the way in which we recommend using this technique has nothing to do with religion per se. This technique, in fact, can enhance the spiritual lives of people who have a variety of religious convictions.

When we speak of meditation, we are referring to a quiet time that allows you to sit with yourself. This may be a time to clear your thoughts and be still or a time of observing, without attachment, the thoughts and feelings that arise in the moment. Briefly, the technique is as follows: Sit comfortably in a quiet place and focus on a mantra, devotional phrase, word, or your own breath. You should become consciously aware of each moment and permit your thoughts to go by freely without your involvement. The chatter in your mind should quiet down, allowing the body to come into balance.

Why do so many people who attempt to heal utilize this technique? The reasons range from the physical and practical to the spiritual and intangible. The most practical is that meditation serves as an antidote to the stress response. Muscles relax, the heart rate slows, blood pressure decreases, and the body goes into a deep state of relaxation. It is in this state that our natural repair and healing mechanisms function optimally.

On a psychological level, meditation gives us the time to become aware of our thoughts and helps us recognize problem areas in our lives which need attention. Meditation can help us increase our self-knowledge, gain a greater sense of our inner core, and build self-esteem. Once we have reached that point, new levels of communication are possible in our relationships, generating an upward cycle of growth and personal power.

On a more esoteric or spiritual level, meditation can help us connect with our Source, Higher Power, God, or however you may define the mysterious aspect of life. During meditation we can let go of our earthly concerns and commune with the essence of life. We can achieve a moment at which we experience a feeling of "oneness" or interconnectedness with all of life. Many people who are ill find tremendous relief in these moments, knowing that while their bodies may be sick, their spirits are still vital and connected. At this level, meditation and prayer are quite similar.

Although it offers wonderful benefits, meditation is not easy to incorporate into one's life on a regular basis, and many people experience great resistance sitting still and shifting from an external to an internal focus. The busyness of our lives, as we attempt to cope with the ever-increasing demands of survival in this society, also makes daily practice very challenging.

Meditation can be one of the most challenging aspects of one's healing journey. It is too much like doing nothing, and most of us were raised to accomplished things. Our self-concepts are tied intimately to how well we do, and less to who we are. Our society reinforces this every step of the way. We must be competitive to survive, and we end up constantly comparing our achievements to those of others.

It is also hard to stop and listen to the chatter in our minds. The busier we stay, the less we have to deal with the nagging hurts of the day, the relationships that are not working, the stupid things we said, resentments, and unfinished business. Sitting still for thirty minutes is a guarantee that all those things will surface! Joan Borysenko, in *Minding the Body, Mending the Mind*, calls this the "anxiety parade."[9]

Dr. Borysenko says that meditation is a form of martial arts.

She suggests that you "move gracefully aside and let the thoughts speed by without engaging them in a struggle. In that way, the mind will tire itself out as you hold the centered position of witnessing your own thoughts." She also says that the primary goal of meditation is not relaxation but awareness. It is through awareness that we eventually get the mind under control. Relaxation is a side benefit.[10]

There are many ways to meditate, and like your healing journey, your technique must be tailored to suit your needs in order to be fully effective. This issue is not about how you meditate, or how well you meditate—rather it is *that* you meditate. If you have no experience in this type of endeavor, first see what types of meditation exist and what instruction may be available in your area. We have listed some first-rate books on this topic in Appendix C, but any bookstore will have numerous offerings. It is important that you approach meditation not as another thing you *have* to do, but rather as a chance to enhance the *experience* of health and healing.

❧ *Simplify Your Life*

In the previous chapter, we discussed at length the effects of stress on health and ultimately, its impact on the prevention of breast cancer. You may also recall that the breast cancer patients we met with almost universally blamed the stress in their lives as a significant reason for their disease. Unfortunately, most of us, sick or healthy, can relate to this problem. It is the age of stress. The crux of the problem is that so many of us feel as though there is nothing we can do about the excessive demands made on our lives today. Also, it appears to be very difficult to make different choices which could serve to make our lives more simple. This fast-paced age of information provides endless seductive ways to stay stimulated and busy. It is easy to forget about what is really meaningful in our lives.

One important thing that we have learned by working with

breast cancer patients over the years is that cancer forces them to reexamine their values, and ultimately simplify their lives. We consider this process crucial in the maintenance of health and thus in the prevention of breast cancer. We urge you not to wait until an illness forces you to make new choices in favor of a less stressful lifestyle.

We have discovered two wonderful, easy-to-read books by Elaine St. James entitled *Simplify Your Life*,[11] and *Inner Simplicity*,[12] that can be of great assistance in this process. Each book offers 100 ways to slow down, enjoy things that matter, to regain peace, and nourish your soul. These kinds of changes take time, commitment, and discipline, but each little step you take can be one large step away from breast cancer.

❧ Words of Wisdom from Breast Cancer Victors

We have asked many breast cancer victors, "What would you like to communicate to other women who do not yet have breast cancer to help them prevent this terrifying disease?" We received a wide range of responses, many of which we have woven throughout this book and will undoubtedly be familiar to you. They are:

1. Do not delay seeing a doctor if you find a suspicious lump.
2. Pay attention to your own instincts if you have a lump in your breast, even if you are told it is "nothing." Get second and third opinions until you are fully satisfied you have the most complete diagnosis.
3. You have to love yourself to be disease free.
4. Learn to communicate and express yourself. Stop believing you have to be nice to everyone all the time.
5. Pay attention to the stress in your life and know it is harmful to your health. To reduce stress, simplify your life. Learn to say no.

6. Educate yourself about breast cancer, focus on prevention, be willing to change harmful habits, and take responsibility for your own good health.
7. Create a sanctuary that is yours, then spend time there and get to know yourself.
8. Find God or a spiritual connection.
9. Realize what is important in life. Spending time with loved ones and having open loving relationships are infinitely more meaningful than any amount of money or material goods.
10. Life is very precious, and none of us ever knows when it may be taken from us. Live each day to the fullest in as much peace and joy as you can.
11. Feed yourself and treat yourself as though you are the most special person in the world. Honor your body.
12. Be willing to take a stand, and live your life according to your beliefs.

☞ Summary

Remember that breast cancer is not only a personal disease, but a social, political, and economic disease as well. In this book we have placed a great deal of emphasis on personal healing; however, unless we jump-start political, environmental, and economic healing, it will be very difficult to maintain any semblance of good health among the female population of this country. *We can no longer afford to be silent!! It is killing us!*

Stir the activist within you. Hundreds of cancer victors have found new meaning in their lives by joining other women in the fight to eradicate breast cancer. They are not only fighting for their lives but for the rest of ours as well. *We need to join them.* We include in Appendix A the names and addresses of various political action groups. Find one in your area and offer your services or a donation.

As we began to network among the women who run political action groups and support groups for breast cancer, we have been met with mixed reactions. "Women with cancer" in many ways have formed a very private club. Many feel, and often rightly so, that no one except other breast cancer patients can possibly understand their experience. More than once we have been asked with suspicion, "Why are you interested in this topic?" If you encounter this experience, understand that these women, no matter how hard they are trying to be "positive," are hurting and angry. They have a right to these feelings. It is our sincerest hope that you, too, will be mobilized by feelings of outrage to take personal and political action in fighting the tragedy of breast cancer.

Finally, we have condensed the main topics of this book into a Twenty-three–Point Plan for the prevention of breast cancer, and we urge all women to incorporate as many of these points as possible into their lives.

HOW TO PREVENT BREAST CANCER
A TWENTY-THREE–POINT PLAN

1. Increase joy and happiness and minimize stress.
2. Reduce your exposure to estrogen.
3. Exercise regularly.
4. Reduce fat intake to 20 percent or less.
5. Increase intake of fresh fruits and vegetables.
6. Lower intake of animal protein.
7. Consume certified organic produce.
8. Increase fiber intake.
9. Increase the use of soy food products.
10. Drink purified or filtered water.
11. Take nutritional supplements.
12. Use alcohol sparingly, if at all.
13. Don't smoke.
14. Take melatonin.
15. Use natural progesterone.
16. Reduce exposure to electromagnetic fields (EMF).
17. Reduce exposure to environmental toxins.
18. Practice regular nonsexual breast massage.
19. Get proper mammograms.
20. Get proper breast exams performed by a physician.
21. Do a monthly breast self-exam (BSE).
22. Develop a daily meditation, prayer, or relaxation practice.
23. Develop positive relationships and social support.

Appendix A

BREAST CANCER ORGANIZATIONS

National Alliance of Breast Cancer Organizations (NABCO), 9 East 37th Street, 10th floor, New York, NY 10016. 212-719-0154; Fax: 212-689-1213. This is the umbrella organization for all breast cancer groups. It publishes the *Breast Cancer Resource List,* 1994/95 edition.

American Cancer Society Hotline: 1-800-ACS-2345.

Breast Cancer Action, 1280 Columbus Avenue #204, San Francisco, CA 94133. 415-922-8279; Fax: 415-922-3253. Political advocacy with highly recommended newsletter.

Foundation for a Compassionate Society, 227 Congress Avenue, Austin, TX 78701. 512-472-0131. Environmental issues.

The Komen Alliance, Occidental Tower, 5005 LBJ Freeway, Suite 370, LB74, Dallas TX 75244. 1-800-I'M AWARE; 214-450-1777. Research, education, diagnosis, treatment.

National Black Leadership Initiative against Cancer: 510-652-3256.

National Breast Cancer Coalition, P.O. Box 66373, Washington, DC 20035.

National Cancer Institute Hotline: 1-800-422-6237 or 1-800-4 CANCER.

National Latina Health Organization: 510-534-1362.

National Lymphedema Network, 2211 Post Street, Suite 404, San Francisco, CA 94115. 1-800-541-3259.

National Women's Health Network, 1325 G Street, NW, Washington, DC 20005. 202-347-1140. General health issues.

National Women's Health Resource Center, 2425 L Street, NW, Washington, DC 20037.

Pesticide Action Network, 116 New Montgomery Street, Suite 810, San Francisco, CA 94105.

The Wellness Community, 2716 Ocean Park Boulevard, Suite 1040, Santa Monica, CA 90405. 310-314-2555. Support and education programs.

Women's Environment & Development Organization (WEDO), 845 Third Avenue, 15th floor, New York, NY 10022. 212-759-7982.

Y-Me National Organization for Breast Cancer Information and Support. 212 West Van Buren Street, Chicago, IL 60607. 1-800-221-2141; 312-986-8228. Support, education, political advocacy, newsletter.

Appendix B

OTHER RESOURCES

Eighteen states with statutes on informing breast cancer patients of alternative therapies:

California, Florida, Georgia, Hawaii, Illinois, Kansas, Kentucky, Maine, Maryland, Massachusetts, Michigan, Minnesota, New Jersey, New Mexico, New York, Pennsylvania, Texas, and Virginia

Environmental Testing & Technology Company, P.O. Box 230369, Encinitas, CA 92024. 619-436-5990; Fax: 619-436-9448.

Greenpeace, 1436 U Street, Washington, D.C., 20009. 202-462-1177.

Haelan Products, Inc., 3200 Severn Avenue, Suite 120, Metaire, LA. 504-885-2776.

There are several different schools that teach Manual Lymphatic Drainage massage. The following resources are provided for women seeking a therapist who has been trained and certified in this type of specialty:

Educating Hands Massage School
　　Contact: Joachim Zuther
　　Phone: 800-999-6991
The Henry Thomas Laboratory (Micro-Circulation Research)
　　Contact: Dr. Judith R. Casley-Smith
　　University of Adelaide
　　Adelaide, S.A. 5005, Australia
　　Phone: 08-271-2198; Fax 08-271-8776
　　U.S. Contact: Dayna Wyrick, 619-273-9764
Lymphedema Services
　　Contact: Guenter Klose
　　Phone: 800-882-9498
North American Vodder Association of Lymphatic Therapy (NAVALT)
　　Contact: Kathryn Thrift, President
　　Phone: 214-243-5959; Fax: 214-243-3227

Source for melatonin: Most health food stores do not stock melatonin. An excellent source for high-quality, pharmaceutical-grade melatonin, as well as for many other important dietary supplements, is The Life Extension Foundation, P.O. Box 229120, Hollywood, FL 33022-9120. Phone: 1-800-841-5433. Membership is $75 per year and includes significant discounts on supplements, as well as an informative monthly magazine.

Resources to purchase natural progesterone and other natural hormones:

College Pharmacy, Colorado Springs, CO. 1-800-748-2263.
Madison Pharmacy Associates, Madison, WI. 1-800-558-7046; 608-833-9102.
Professional and Technical Services/Transitions for Health, Portland, OR. 800-888-6814.
Women's International Pharmacy, Madison, WI. 1-800-279-5708; 608-221-7800.

To order the Sensor Pad, send a personal check for $25 to Transocean Trading Company, P.O. Box 46, Nottingham NG1 4GS, England.

Tryptophan: An amino acid that was formally available in health food stores to aid in sleep. It had been used for decades with complete safety and effectiveness. People who had difficulty falling asleep or staying asleep could take this inexpensive, reliable amino acid, without resorting to expensive, sometimes addicting, potentially dangerous prescription sleeping pills. The sale of tryptophan was prohibited by the FDA because of a problem with a single manufacturer, whose error led to a residual impurity in its tryptophan that could cause serious health problems. The remainder of the manufacturers were prohibited from selling their products in the United States, although they had never experienced problems with impurities.

Appendix C

SUPPLEMENTAL READING

DIET AND NUTRITION

Bliznakov, Emile, and Gerald Hunt. *The Miracle Nutrient CoEnzyme Q10* (New York: Bantam, 1986).

Clouatre, Dallas. *Anti-Fat Nutrients: How Fat-Burning Vitamins Can Help You Lose Weight (and Cholesterol Too)* (San Francisco: Pax, 1993).

Erasmus, Udo. *Fats That Heal, Fats That Kill* (Burnaby, B.C., Canada: Alive Books, 1986).

Gittleman, Anne L. *Beyond Pritikin: A Total Nutrition Program That Goes Beyond the Pritikin Principles by Adding Essential Fats for Rapid Weight Loss, Longevity, and Good Health* (New York: Bantam, 1988).

Haas, Robert. *Eat Smart: How to Use Nutrients and Supplements to Achieve Maximum Mental and Physical Performance.* (New York: HarperCollins, 1994).

McDougall, John, and Mary McDougall. *The McDougall Plan* (Piscataway, NJ: New Century, 1983).

Messina, Mark, et al. *The Simple Soybean and Your Health* (Garden City Park, NY: Avery, 1994).

Pearson, Durk, and Sandy Shaw. *Life Extension: A Practical Scientific Approach* (New York: Warner, 1982).

Pelton, Ross, and Taffy Clarke Pelton. *Mind Food and Smart Pills* (New York: Doubleday, 1989).

Robbins, John. *Diet for A New America* (Walpole, NH: Stillpoint, 1987).

Rudin, Donald O., M.D., and Clara Felix. *The Omega-3 Phenomenon* (New York: Rawson 1987).

Walford, Roy. *The 120-Year Diet: How to Double Your Vital Years* (New York: Simon & Schuster, 1986).

Wysong, Randy. *Lipid Nutrition: Understanding Fats and Oils in Health and Disease* (Midland, MI: Inquiry, 1990).

HORMONE REPLACEMENT
Kamen, Betty. *Hormone Replacement Therapy: Yes or No?* (Novato, CA: Nutrition Encounter 1993).

Lee, John. *Natural Progesterone: The Multiple Roles of a Remarkable Hormone* (Sebastopol, CA: BLL Publishing, 1993). P.O. Box 2068, Sebastopol, CA 95473.

Sheehy, Gail. *The Silent Passage* (New York: Pocket Books, 1991).

ENVIRONMENTAL FACTORS
Epstein, Samuel. *The Politics of Cancer* (New York: Anchor, 1979).

Levenstein, Mary. *Everyday Cancer Risks and How to Avoid Them* (Garden City Park, NY: Avery, 1992).

Rogers, Sherry. *The E.I. Syndrome: An Rx for Environmental Illness* (New York: Prestige, 1986).

———. *Tired or Toxic?: A Blueprint for Health* (New York: Prestige, 1990).

Sugarman, Ellen. *Warning: The Electricity Around You May Be Hazardous to Your Health* (New York: Simon & Schuster, 1992).

EXERCISE, STRETCHING, AND YOGA
Carter, Albert. *The New Miracles of Rebound Exercise* (Scottsdale, AZ: A.L.M., 1988).

Christensen, Alice, and David Rankin. *Easy Does It Yoga: Yoga for Older People* (New York: Harper & Row, 1979).

Evans, William. *Biomarkers.* (New York: Simon & Schuster, 1994).

Hittleman, Richard. *Yoga: 28-Day Exercise Plan* (New York: Bantam, 1973).

Iyengar, B.K.S. *The Concise Light on Yoga* (New York: Schocken, 1982).

Serman, Miriam. *Yoga for the Absolute Novice, Yoga for Advanced Beginners, Yoga Athletic Stretch* (Home Video Tapes). Miriam Serman, P.O. Box 43, Redondo Beach, CA 90277.

POLITICS

Batt, Sharon. *Patient No More: The Politics of Breast Cancer* (Gynergy, 1994).

Brady, Judy. *1 in 3: Woman with Cancer Confront an Epidemic* (Pittsburgh: Cleis, 1991).

Morgenthaler, John, and Steven Fowkes. *Stop the FDA* (Menlo Park CA: Health Freedom, 1992).

Pearson, Durk, and Sandy Shaw. *Freedom of Informed Choice: FDA versus Nutritional Supplements* (Neptune, NJ: Common Sense, 1993).

BREASTS AND BREAST CANCER

Agency for Health Care Policy and Research. *Things to Know About Quality Mammograms* (booklet). Publications Clearinghouse, P.O. Box 8547, Silver Spring, MD 20907. 1-800-358-9295.

Austin, Steve, and Kathy Hitchcock. *Breast Cancer: What You Should Know (but may Not Be Told)* (Rocklin, CA: Prima, 1994).

Kradjian, Robert. *Save Yourself from Breast Cancer* (New York: Berkley, 1994).

Love, Susan M. *Dr. Susan Love's Breast Book* (Reading, MA: Addison-Wesley, 1990).

EMOTIONAL HEALING IN CANCER

Frahm, David J. *A Cancer Battle Plan* (Colorado Springs, CO: Pinon, 1992).

Kay, Ronnie. *Spinning Straw into Gold: Your Emotional Recovery from Breast Cancer* (New York: Simon & Schuster, 1991).

LeShan, Lawrence. *Cancer as a Turning Point* (New York: Plume, 1990).

———. *You Can Fight for Your Life: Emotional Factors in the Causation of Cancer.* (New York: M. Evans, 1977).

Siegel, Bernie. *Love, Medicine and Miracles* (New York: Harper & Row, 1986).

———. *Peace, Love and Healing* (New York: Harper & Row, 1989).

Simonton, Carl, D. et al. *Getting Well Again* (New York: Bantam, 1978).

Soffa, Virginia. *The Journey Beyond Breast Cancer* (Rochester, VT: Healing Arts Press, 1994).

MIND/BODY MEDICINE

Achterberg, Jean. *Imagery in Healing: Shamanism and Modern Medicine* (Boston: Shambhala, 1985).

Benson, Herbert. *The Mind/Body Effect* (New York: Simon & Schuster, 1979).

Chopra, Deepak. *Quantum Healing: Exploring the Frontiers of Mind/Body Medicine* (New York: Bantam, 1989).

Dossey, Larry. *Meaning & Medicine: Lessons from a Doctor's Tales of Breakthrough and Healing* (New York: Bantam, 1991).

———. *Space, Time & Medicine* (Boston: New Science Library, 1982).

Goleman, D., and J. Gurin, eds., *Mind/Body Medicine* (New York: Consumer Reports Books, 1993).

Kabat-Zinn, Jon. *Full Catastrophe Living: Using the Wisdom of Your Body and Mind to Face Stress, Pain and Illness* (New York: Delta, 1990).

Rossman, Martin. *Healing Yourself* (New York: Pocket Books, 1987).

WOMEN'S PSYCHOLOGY AND SELF-ESTEEM

Beane Rutter, Virginia. *Women Changing Women: Feminine Psychology Reconceived Through Myth and Experience* (San Francisco: HarperCollins, 1994).

Chernin, Kim. *Reinventing Eve: Modern Woman in Search of Herself* (New York: Times Books, 1987).

Claremont de Castillejo, Irene. *Knowing Woman: A Feminine Psychology* (New York: Harper & Row, 1973).

Edelman, Hope. *Motherless Daughters: Legacy of Loss* (Reading, MA: Addison-Wesley, 1994).

Goldhor Lerner, Harriet. *The Dance of Anger: A Woman's Guide to Changing the Patterns of Intimate Relationships* (New York: Harper & Row, 1985).

Miller, Alice. *For Your Own Good: Hidden Cruelty in Childrearing and the Roots of Violence* (New York: Farrar, Straus and Giroux, 1983).

Moore, Thomas. *Care of the Soul* (New York: HarperCollins, 1992).

Shinoda Bolen, Jean. *Goddesses in Everywoman: A New Psychology of Women* (New York: Harper Perennial, 1984).

Steinem, Gloria. *Revolution from Within: A Book of Self-Esteem* (Boston: Little, Brown, 1992).

Williamson, Marianne. *A Woman's Worth* (New York: Random House, 1993).

MEDITATION AND RELAXATION

Benson, Herbert. *The Relaxation Response* (New York: Avon, 1976).

Borysenko, Joan. *Minding the Body, Mending the Mind* (New York: Bantam, 1987).

Goldstein, Joseph. *The Experience of Insight: A Simple and Direct Guide to Buddhist Meditation* (Boston: Shambhala, 1983).

LeShan, Lawrence. *How to Meditate* (New York: Bantam, 1974).

Levine, Stephen. *A Gradual Awakening* (New York: Anchor, 1979).

Pennington, M. Basil. *Centering Prayer: Renewing an Ancient Christian Prayer Form* (New York: Image Books, 1982).

NEWSLETTERS

Whitaker, Dr. Julian. *Health & Healing: Tomorrow's Medicine Today.* 1-800-777-5005.

Williams, Dr. David. *Alternatives: For the Health Conscious Individual.* 1-502-367-4492.

Nutrition Action. 202-332-9110.

MAGAZINES

Eating Well: The Magazine of Food and Health. 1-800-678-0541.

Health Freedom News: The Natural Health Magazine That Dares Tell the Truth! 818-357-2181.

Life Extension Magazine. 1-800-841-5433; 305-966-4886.

Longevity: A Practical Guide to the Art and Science of Staying Young. 1-800-333-2782.

Natural Health: The Guide to Well-Being. Customer Service, P.O. Box 57320, Boulder, CO 80322. 617-232-1000.

Vegetarian Times. 1-800-435-9610.

COOKBOOKS

Bauer, Cathy, and Juel Andersen. *The Tofu Cookbook* (Emmaus, PA: Rodale, 1979).

Bienenfeld, Florence, and Mickey Bienenfeld. *The Vegetarian Gourmet* (Beverly Hills, CA: Royal House, 1987). More than 200 low-fat, low-cholesterol, low-salt, sugar-free recipes.

Bricklin, Mark, and Sharon Claessens. *The Natural Healing Cookbook* (Emmaus, PA: Rodale, 1981).

Brody, Jane. *Good Food Book: Living the High-Carbohydrate Way* (New York: Norton, 1985).

Estella, Mary. *Natural Foods Cookbook: Vegetarian Dairy-Free Cuisine* (New York: Japan Publications, 1985).

Madison, Deborah. *The Greens Cook Book* (New York: Bantam, 1987).

———. *The Savory Way* (New York: Bantam, 1990).

Moosewood Collective. *Sundays at Moosewood Restaurant: Ethnic and Regional Recipes from the Cooks at the Legendary Restaurant* (New York: Simon & Schuster, 1990).

Shulman, Martha Rose. *Mediterranean Light* (New York: Bantam, 1989).

Thomas, Anna. *The Vegetarian Epicure* (New York: Vintage, 1972).

MISCELLANEOUS
(Re: melatonin research) Pierpaoli, Walter; Regelson, William; and Fabris, Nicola; eds. *The Aging Clock, the Pineal Gland and Other Pacemakers in the Progression of Aging and Carcinogenesis* (New York: New York Academy of Sciences, 1994).

Appendix D

POLITICAL ACTION: HOW TO WRITE TO YOUR CONGRESSPERSON

A 1993 survey of congressional staff members revealed that personal letters are far more important than phone calls, postcards, or form letters. Eighty percent of the aides surveyed indicated that in most cases, phone calls and postcards are simply tallied and then forgotten. On the other hand, personal letters are set aside for response and sometimes even forwarded to the boss.

When you write to your political representative, staff members advise you to (1) keep your message brief, (2) relate how the issue affects you personally, and (3) avoid making threats to enhance your point.

We hope every woman will take the time to send either a typewritten or handwritten letter to her elected representatives in both the Senate and the House of Representatives. If you do not know the names and mailing addresses for those elected officials, ask directory assistance for the telephone number of the specific local politician or for the local office of the Democratic or Republican party. Staff people there will be able to give you the necessary information.

If you cannot find the time or inspiration to write a letter, then we urge you to pick up the phone and call Washington. The White House Hotline is 202-456-1111. The House and Senate Main Capitol switchboard is 202-224-3121.

Sources Cited

CHAPTER 1: FIGHTING THE EPIDEMIC

1. American Cancer Society, *Cancer Facts & Figures—1993* (Atlanta, 1993).
2. E. Feuer, "NCI Cancer Statistics Review 1973-1989," *Journal of the National Cancer Institute* (June 2, 1993).
3. NABCO, *Facts About Breast Cancer in the USA* (New York, 1994).
4. Dede Alpert, assemblywoman, state of California. *Breast Cancer: the best prevention is early detection* (Sacramento, Calif., 1992).
5. W. D. Dupont, "Evidence of Efficacy of Mammographic Screening for Women in Their Forties," *Cancer* 74 (1994): 1204-1206.
6. D. B. Kopans, "Screening for Breast Cancer and Mortality Reduction Among Women 40-49 years of age," *Cancer* 74 (1994): 311-22.
7. L. Tabar, S. W. Duffy, et al., "New Swedish Breast Cancer Detection Results for Women Aged 40-49," *Cancer* 72 (1993): 1437-48.
8. L. H. Baker, "Breast Cancer Detection Demonstration Project: Five Year Summary Report," *Cancer* 32 (1982): 194-225.
9. J. B. Buchanan et al., "Tumor Growth, Doubling Times, and Ability of the Radiologist to Diagnose Certain Cancers," *Radiology* 21 (1983): 115-26.
10. L. Laurence, "Women Aren't Just Scared, We're Mad," *McCall's*, November 1991, pp. 24-30.
11. R. E. Scott et al., "Mechanisms for Initiation and Promotion of Carcinogenesis: A Review and a New Concept," *Mayo Clinic Proceedings* 59 (1984): 107-117.

12. American Cancer Society, *Cancer Facts & Figures—1993.*

13. P. Kelly, "Breast Cancer Risk Analysis in Breast Care Management," *Cancer Bulletin* 35 (2) (1983): 53–57.

14. G. A. Colditz and W. C. Willett, "Family History, Age, and Risk of Breast Cancer," *Journal of the American Medical Association* 270 (3) (1993): 338–43.

15. M.C. Pike et al., "Oral Contraceptive Use and Early Abortion as Risk Factors for Breast Cancer in Young Women," *British Journal of Cancer* 43 (1981): 72–76.

16. J. L. Kelsey and N. G. Hildredth, *Breast and Gynecologic Cancer Epidemiology* (Boca Raton, Fla.: CRC Press, 1983): 138–40

17. B. MacMahon et al., "Age at First Birth and Breast-Cancer Risk," *World Health Organization Bulletin* 43 (1970): 209–221.

18. H. Seidman et al., "A Different Perspective on Breast Cancer Risk Factors: Some Implications of the Nonattributable Risk," *American Cancer Society Professional Education Publication* (New York, 1983).

Chapter 2: Breast Structure, Function, and Abnormalities

1. T. J. Anderson, "Genesis and Source of Breast Cancer," *British Medical Bulletin* 1991 (47): 305–318.

2. K-Y Yoo, K. Tajima, et al., "Independent Protective Effect of Lactation Against Breast Cancer: A Case-control Study," *American Journal of Epidemiology* 135 (1992): 726–33.

3. G. Kvale and I. Heuch, "Lactation and Cancer Risk: Is There a Relation Specific to Be?" *Journal of Epidemiology and Community Health* 42 (1987): 30–37.

4. A. Glasier and A. S. McNeilly, "Physiology of Lactation," *Baillière's Clinical Endocrinology and Metabolism* 4 (1990): 379–97.

5. Anderson, "Genesis and Source of Breast Cancer."

6. R.V.P. Hutter et al., "Consensus Meeting. Is "Fibrocystic Disease" of the Breast Precancerous?" *Archives of Pathology and Laboratory Medicine* 110 (1986): 171–73.

7. J. L. Connolly and S. J. Schnitt, "Clinical and Histologic Aspects of Proliferative and Non-proliferative Benign Breast Diseases," *Journal of Cellular Biochemistry Supplement* 17G (1993): 45–48.

8. W. D. Dupont, F. F. Parl, et al., "Breast Cancer Risk Associated with Proliferative Breast Disease and Atypical Hyperplasia" [see comments] , *Cancer* 71 (1993): 1258–65.

9. P. P. Rosen, "Proliferative Breast 'Disease'" [comment], *Cancer* 71 (1993): 3798–807.

10. R. D. Bulbrook, "Endocrinological Aspects of Benign Breast Disease," *Cancer Detection and Prevention* 16 (1992): 21–23.

11. R. J. McKenna, Sr., "The Abnormal Mammogram Radiographic Findings, Diagnostic Options, Pathology, and Stage of Cancer Diagnosis," *Cancer* 74 (1994): 244–55.

12. P. C. Stomper and F. R. Margolin, "Ductal Carcinoma In Situ: The Mammographer's Perspective," *American Journal of Roentgenology* 162 (1994): 585–91.

13. J. T. Holt et al., "Histopathology: Old Principles and New Methods," *Cancer Surveys* 18 (1993): 115–33.

14. F. E. Gump, "Lobular Carinoma In Situ (LCIS): Pathology and Treatment," *Journal of Cellular Biochemistry* 17G (1993): 53–58.

15. E. R. Frykberg and K. I. Bland, "Management of In Situ and Minimally Invasive Breast Carcinoma," *World Journal of Surgery* 18 (1994): 45–57.

16. M. Dollinger, E. H. Rosenbaum, et al., *Everyone's Guide to Cancer Therapy* (Kansas City, MO.: Andrews and McMeel, 1991).

17. American Cancer Society, *The Staging of Cancer*, Publication 89-12M—No. 3485.01.

CHAPTER 3: MAMMOGRAPHY

1. L. Tabar, "Control of Breast Cancer Through Screening Mammography," *Radiology* 177 (1990): 655–56.

2. A. G. Haus, S. A. Feig, et al., "Mammography Screening: Technology, Radiation Dose and Risk, Quality Control, and Benefits to Society," *Radiology* 174 (1990): 627–56.

3. K. C. Chu et al., "Analysis of Breast Cancer Mortality and Stage Distribution by Age for the Health Insurance Plan Clinical Trial," *Journal of the National Cancer Institute* 88 (1988): 1195.

4. A. B. Miller et al., "Canadian National Breast Screening Study: 2. Breast Cancer Detection and Death Rates Among Women Aged 50–59 Years," *Canadian Medical Association Journal* 147 (1992): 1477–88.

5. D. B. Kopans, "Mammographic Screening for Women 40–49: A History of the Guidelines Controversy and the Screening Facts" [guest commentary], *Radiology Today* 1994;11.

6. "ACR Criticizes Mammography Study—Canadian Study Is 'Seriously Flawed'," *American College of Radiology, Bulletin* 48 (12) (1992): 1, 6–7.

7. R. E. Tarone, "The Excess of Patients with Advanced Breast Cancer in Young Women Screened with Mammography in the Canadian National Breast Screening Study." *Cancer* 75 (4) (1995): 997–1003.

8. L. Nystrom, L. E. Rutqvst, et al., "Breast Cancer Screening with Mammography: Overview of Swedish Randomised Trials," *Lancet* 341 (1993): 973–78.

9. W. D. Dupont, "Evidence of Efficacy of Mammographic Screening for Women in Their Forties," *Cancer* 74 (1994): 1204–1206.

10. C. J. Rosenquist and K. K. Lindfors, "Screening Mammography in Women Aged 40–49 Years: Analysis of Cost-Effectiveness," *Radiology* 191 (1994): 647–50.

11. D. B. Kopans, "Breast Imaging and Breast Cancer Prevention," *Journal of Cellular Biochemistry* 17G (1993): 92–95.

12. L. Tabar, S. W. Duffy, et al., "New Swedish Breast Cancer Detection Results for Women Aged 40–49," *Cancer* 72 (1993): 1437–48.

13. D. B. Kopans, "Screening for Breast Cancer and Mortality Reduction Among Women 40–49 Years of Age," *Cancer* 74 (1994): 311–22.

14. Rosenquist and Lindfors, "Screening Mammography in Women Aged 40–49 Years."

15. J. King, "Mammography Screening for Breast Cancer" [letter to the editor], *Cancer* 73 (1994): 2003–2004.

16. N. Bjurstam et al., "Mammography Screening in Women Aged 40–49 Years at Entry. Results of the Randomized, Controlled Trial in Gothenburg, Sweden," presented to the 26th National Conference on Breast Cancer in Palm Desert, California, May 8–13, 1994.

17. S. Moss et al., presentation to the International Union Against Cancer (UICC) meeting on breast cancer screening in premenopausal women in developing countries, Geneva, Switzerland, September 29–October 1, 1993.

18. R. J. McKenna, Sr., "The Abnormal Mammogram Radiographic Findings, Diagnostic Options, Pathology, and Stage of Cancer Diagnosis," *Cancer* 74 (1994): 244–55.

19. D. M. Radford, D. T. Cromack, et al., "Pathology and Treatment of Impalpable Breast Lesions," *American Journal of Surgery* 164 (1992): 427–31.

20. P. A. Newcomb and P. M. Lantz, "Recent Trends in Breast Cancer Incidence, Mortality and Mammography," *Breast Cancer Research and Treatment* 28 (1993): 97–106.

21. D. Reintgen, C. Berman, et al., "The Anatomy of Missed Breast Cancers," *Surgical Oncology* 2 (1993): 65–75.

22. McKenna, "Abnormal Mammogram Radiographic Findings."

23. S. A. Feig and R. E. Hendrick, "Mammography's Upside Outweighs Possible Risks," *Diagnostic Imaging*, March 1993: 121–25.

24. National Safety Council, "Transportation Accident Passenger Death Rates 1987" (Washington, D.C.: NSC, 1988).

25. S. A. Feig and S. M. Ehrlich, "Estimation of Radiation Risk from Screening Mammography: Recent Trends and Comparison with Expected Benefits," *Radiology* 174 (1990): 638–47.

26. C. E. Land, "Estimating Cancer Risk from Low Doses of Ionizing Radiation," *Science* 209 (1980): 1197–1203.

27. BEIR V Committee on Biological Effects of Ionizing Radiation, "Health Effects of Exposure to Low Levels of Ionizing Radiation" (Washington, D.C.: National Academy Press, 1990).

28. A. B. Miller, "Mammography in Women Under 50," *Hematology/Oncology Clinics of North America* 8 (1994): 165–77.

29. S. Shapiro, P. Strax, et al., "Periodic Breast Cancer Screening in Reducing Mortality from Breast Cancer," *Journal of the American Medical Association* 215 (1971): 1777–86.

30. G. D. Dodd, "American Cancer Society Guidelines from the Past to the Present," *Cancer* 72 (1993): 1429–32.

31. G. D. Dodd, "Screening for Breast Cancer," *Cancer* 72 (1993): 1038–42.

32. A. B. Miller, C. J. Baines, et al., "Canadian National Breast Screening Study: 1. Breast Cancer Detection and Death Rates Among Women Aged 40 to 49 Years," *Canadian Medical Association Journal* 147 (1992): 1459–76.

33. A. B. Miller, "Mammography: Reviewing the Evidence. Epidemiology Aspect," *Canadian Family Physician* 39 (1993): 85–90.

34. C. J. Baines, "The Canadian National Breast Screening Study: A Perspective on Criticisms," *Annals of Internal Medicine* 120 (1994): 326–34.

35. L. J. Burhenne and H. J. Burhenne, "The Canadian National Breast Screening Study: A Canadian Critique," *American Journal of Roentgenology* 161 (1993): 761–63.

36. A. B. Miller, "Mammography Screening Guidelines for Women 40 to 49 and Over 65 Years Old," *Annals of Epidemiology* 4 (1994): 96–100.

37. S. Eckhardt et al., "UICC Meeting on Breast-Cancer Screening in Premenopausal Women in Developed Countries," *International Journal of Cancer* 56 (1994): 1–5.

38. Shapiro, Strax, et al., "Periodic Breast Cancer Screening."

39. C. J. Mettlin and C. R. Smart, "The Canadian National Breast Screening Study. An Appraisal and Implications for Early Detection Policy," *Cancer* 72 (1993): 1461–65.

40. C. J. Mettlin and C. R. Smart, "Breast Cancer Detection Guidelines for Women Aged 40 to 49 Years: Rationale for the American Cancer Society Reaffirmation of Recommendation," *A Cancer Journal for Clinicians* 44 (1994): 248–55. (American Cancer Society, California.)

41. D. B. Kopans, "Mammography Screening for Breast Cancer" [editorial; comment], *Cancer* 72 (1993): 1809–1812.

42. Mettlin and Smart, "Canadian National Breast Screening Study."

43. D. B. Kopans, "Breast Cancer Detection in an Institution. Is Mammography Detrimental?" *Cancer* 72 (1993): 1457–60.

44. J. H. Frischbier, "Controversial Attitude to Mammography Screening in Asymptomatic Women Between 40 and 50 Years of Age," *Geburtshilfe Frauenheilkd* 541 (1994): 1–11.

45. Kopans, "Mammographic Screening for Women 40–49."
46. Ibid.
47. *American College of Radiology Bulletin* 50 (1994): 30.
48. M. Moskowitz, "Breast Cancer: Age-Specific Growth Rates and Screening Strategies," *Radiology* 161 (1986): 37–41.
49. Kopans, "Mammographic Screening for Women 40–49."
50. S. Shapiro et al., *Periodic Screening for Breast Cancer: The Health Insurance Plan Project and Its Sequelae, 1963–1986* (Baltimore: John Hopkins University Press, 1988).
51. Moskowitz, "Breast cancer."
52. L. Tabar et al., "What is the Optimum Interval Between Screening Examinations? An Analysis Based on the Latest Results of the Swedish Two-County Breast Cancer Screening Trial," *British Journal of Cancer* 55 (1987): 547–51.
53. H. Seidman et al., "A Different Perspective on Breast Cancer Risk Factors: Some Implications of Nonattributable Risk," *Cancer* 32 (1982): 301–313.
54. Kopans, "Mammographic Screening for Women 40–49."
55. S. V. Cocca, "Who's Monitoring the Quality of Mammograms? The Mammography Quality Standards Act of 1992 Could Finally Provide the Answer," *American Journal of Medicine* 19 (1993): 313–44.
56. R. McLelland, R. E. Hendrick, et al., "The American College of Radiology Mammography Accreditation Program," *American Journal of Roentgenology* 157 (1991): 473–79.
57. J. R. Paquelet, "Medicare, Mammography, and the Mammography Quality Standards Act of 1992," *Radiology* 190 (1994): 47–49.
58. R. E. Hendrick, "Mammography Quality Assurance. Current Issues," *Cancer* 72 (1993): 1466–74.
59. T. G. Langer and E. S. de Paredes, "Breast Disease: The Radiologist's Expanding Role," *Current Problems Diagnostic Radiology* 22 (1993): 190–227.
60. F. J. Keefe, E. R. Hauck, et al., "Mammography Pain and Discomfort: A Cognitive-Behavior Perspective," *Pain* 56 (1994): 247–60.
61. B. Neilsen, C. Miaskowski, et al., "Pain with Mammography: Fact or Fiction?" *Oncology Nursing Forum* 20 (1993): 639–42.
62. M. K. Fine, B. K. Rimer, et al., "Women's Respnoses to the Mammography Experience," *Journal of the American Board of Family Practice* 6 (1993): 546–55.
63. M. A. Helvie, D. R. Pennes, et al., "Mammographic Follow-up of Low-Suspicion Lesions: Compliance Rate and Diagnostic Yield," *Radiology* 178 (1991): 155–58.
64. Moskowitz, "Breast Cancer."
65. J. A. Harvey, L. L. Fajardo, et al., "Previous Mammograms in Patients

with Impalpable Breast Carcinoma: Retrospective vs Blinded Interpretation," 1993 American Roentgen Ray Society President's Award, *American Journal of Roentgenology* 161 (1993): 1167–72.

66. W. A. Berg, N. D. Anderson, et al., "MR Imaging of the Breast in Patients with Silicone Breast Implants: Normal Postoperative Variants and Diagnostic Pitfalls," *American Journal of Roentgenology* 163 (1994): 575–78.

67. D. L. Monticciolo, R. C. Nelson, et al., "MR Detection of Leakage from Silicone Breast Implants: Value of a Silicone-Selective Pulse Sequence," *American Journal of Roentgenology* 163 (1994): 51–56.

CHAPTER 4: NEW BIOPSY OPTIONS

1. L. J. Layfield, E. A. Chrischilles, et al., "The Palpable Breast Nodule. A Cost-Effectiveness Analysis of Alternate Diagnostic Approaches," *Cancer* 72 (1993): 1642–51.

2. Ibid.

3. W. H. Hindle, P. A. Payne, et al., "The Use of Fine-Needle Aspiration in the Evaluation of Persistent Palpable Dominant Breast Masses," *American Journal of Obstetrics and Gynecology* 168 (1993): 1814–18.

4. J. S. Mitnick, M. F. Vasquez, et al., "Stereotactic Localization for Fine Needle Aspiration Biopsy Inpatients with Augmentation Prostheses," *Annals of Plastic Surgery* 29 (1992): 31–35.

5. S. H. Parker, W. E. Jobe, et al., "US-Guided Automated Large Core Breast Biopsy," *Radiology* 187 (1993): 507–511.

CHAPTER 5: BREAST SELF-EXAMINATION

1. M. S. O'Malley and S. W. Fletcher. "Screening for Breast Cancer with Breast Self-Examination: A Critical Review," *Journal of the American Medical Association* 257 (16) (1987): 2197–203.

2. K. Grady, "The Efficacy of Breast Self-Examination," *The Journals of Gerontology* 47 (special issue) (1992): 69–74.

3. S. S. Kegeles, "Education for Breast Self-Examination: Why, Who, What, and How?" *Preventive Medicine* 14 (1985): 702–720.

4. *Breast Cancer Action* (San Francisco, 1994).

5. V. F. Semiglazov et al., "Study of the Role of Breast Self-Examination in the Reduction of Mortality from Breast Cancer," *European Journal of Cancer* 29A (14) (1993): 2039–46.

6. NABCO, *Facts About Breast Cancer in the USA* (New York, 1994).

7. L. S. Kaplan, "Breast Cancer Screening Among Older Racial/Ethnic Minorities and Whites: Barriers to Early Detection," *The Journals of Gerontology* 47 (special issue) (1992): 101–110.

8. R. S. Foster, "Clinical Breast Examination and Breast Self-Examination: Past and Present Effect of Breast Cancer Survival," *American Cancer Society Workshop on Guidelines and Screening for Breast Cancer*, Pasadena, California, October 11–13, 1991.

9. S. W. Fletcher et al., "Physicians' Abilities to Detect Lumps in Silicone Breast Models," *Journal of the American Medical Association* 253 (15) (1985): 2224–28.

10. T. C. Jacob and N. Penn, "The Need and Value of Breast Self-Examination," *Journal of the National Medical Association* 80 (7) (1988): 777–87.

11. Ibid.

12. C. J. Baines, "Breast Self-Examination," *American Cancer Society Workshop on Guidelines and Screening for Breast Cancer*, Pasadena, California, October 11–13, 1991.

13. Jacob and Penn, "Need and Value of Breast Self-Examination."

14. Baines, "Breast Self-Examination."

15. C. M. Huguley et al., "Breast Self-Examination and Survival from Breast Cancer," *Cancer* 62 (1988): 1389–96.

16. J. E. Muscat and M. Huncharek, "Breast Self-Examination and Extent of Disease: A Population-Based Study," *Cancer Detection and Prevention* 15 (2) (1991): 155–59.

17. M. Costanza and R. Foster, "Relationship Between Breast Self-Examination and Death from Breast Cancer by Age Groups," *Cancer Detection and Prevention* 7 (1984): 103–108.

18. Jacob and Penn, "Need and Value of Breast Self-Examination."

19. J. Philip et al., "Breast Self-Examination: Clinical Results from a Population-Based Prospective Study," *British Journal of Cancer* 50 (1984): 7–12.

20. V. Koroltchouk et al., "The Control of Breast Cancer: A World Health Organization Perspective," *Cancer* 65 (1990): 2803–2810.

21. Jacob and Penn, "Need and Value of Breast Self-Examination."

22. C. J. Baines, "Some Thoughts on Why Women Don't Do Breast Self-Examination," *Cancer Medical Association* 128 (1983): 255–56.

23. D. N. Rutledge, "Factors Related to Women's Practice of Breast Self-Examination," *Nursing Research* 36 (2) (1987): 117–21.

24. V. Champion, "Breast Self-Examination in Women 65 and Older," *The Journals of Gerontology* 47 (special issue) (1992): 75–79.

25. T. C. Jacob et al., "Effects of Cognitive Style and Maintenance Strategies on Breast Self-Examination (BSE) Practice by African American Women," *Journal of Behavioral Medicine* 15 (6) (1992): 589–609.

26. M. E. Costanza, "Breast Cancer Screening in Older Women: Overview,"*The Journals of Gerontology* 47 (special issue) (1992): 1–3.

27. L. S. Caplan et al., "Breast Cancer Screening Among Older Racial/Ethnic Minorities and Whites: Barriers to Early Detection," *The Journals of Gerontology* 47 (special issue) (1992): 101–110.

28. Champion, "Breast Self-Examination."
29. Baines, "Some Thoughts on Why Women."
30. O'Malley and Fletcher, "Screening for Breast Cancer."
31. R. L. Olson and E. S. Mitchell, "Self-Confidence as a Critical Factor in Breast Self-Examination" (November/December 1989): 476–81.
32. B. Nettles-Carlson, "Detection of Breast Cancer," *Journal of Obstetrics, Gynecologic, and Neonatal Nursing* (September/October 1989): 373–81.
33. Caplan, et al., "Breast Cancer Screening."
34. D. D. Celentano and D. Holtzman, "Breast Self-Examination Competency: An Analysis of Self-Reported Practice and Associated Characteristics," *American Journal of Public Health* 73 (11) (1983): 1321–23.
35. Jacob and Penn, "Need and Value of Breast Self-Examination."
36. D. D. Celentano, op. cit. (1983).
37. S. W. Alagna and D. M. Reddy, "Predictors of Proficient Technique and Successful Lesion Detection in Breast Self-Examination," *Health Psychology* 3 (2) (1984): 113–27.
38. Olson and Mitchell, "Self-Confidence."
39. Kegeles, "Education for Breast Self-Examination."
40. C. M. Huguley and R. L. Brown, "The Value of Breast Self-Examination," *Cancer* 47 (1981): 989–95.
41. Nettles-Carlson, "Detection of Breast Cancer."
42. O'Malley and Fletcher, "Screening for Breast Cancer."
43. Baines, "Some Thoughts on Why Women."
44. American Cancer Society, *How to Examine Your Breasts* (1992).
45. Baines, "Breast Self-Examination."
46. Susan Love, *Dr. Susan Love's Breast Book* (Reading, Mass.: Addison-Wesley, 1990).
47. American Cancer Society Facts and Figures (1986).
48. Love, p. 29. (1990).
49. *The Wall Street Journal,* April 12, 1994.
50. Ibid.

CHAPTER 6: ESTROGEN: THE REAL STORY

1. R. J. King, "William L. McGuire Memorial Symposium. Estrogen and Progestin Effects in Human Breast Carcinogenesis," *Breast Cancer Research and Treatment* 17 (1993): 3–15.
2. K. A. Fackelmann, "Motherhood and Cancer," *Science News* 142 (1992): 298–300.
3. L. Bernstein and R. K. Ross, "Endogenous Hormones and Breast Cancer Risk," *Epidemiologic Reviews* 15 (1993): 48–65.
4. R. Ballard-Barbash, "Anthropometry and Breast Cancer. Body Size—a Moving Target," *Cancer* 74 (1994): 1090–1100.

5. B. E. Henderson, R. K. Ross, et al., "Endogenous Hormones as a Major Factor in Human Cancer," *Cancer Research* 42 (1982): 3232–37.

6. B. A. Stoll, L. J. Vatten, et al., "Does Physical Maturity Influence Breast Cancer Risk?" *Acta Oncologica* 33 (1994): 171–76.

7. H. M. Lemon, H. H. Wotiz, et al., "Reduced Estriol Excretion in Patients with Breast Cancer Prior to Endocrine Therapy," *Journal of the American Medical Association* 196 (1966): 112–20.

8. H. Adlercreutz, S. L. Gorbach, et al., "Estrogen Metabolism and Excretion in Oriental and Caucasian Women," *Journal of the National Cancer Institute* 86 (1994): 1076–82.

9. H. M. Lemon, J. W. Heidel, et al., "Increased Catechol Estrogen Metabolism as a Risk Factor for Nonfamilial Breast Cancer," *Cancer* 69 (1992): 457–65.

10. H. L. Bradlow, J. J. Michnovicz, et al., "Effects of Dietary Indole-3-Carbinol on Estradiol Metabolism and Spontaneous Mammary Tumors in Mice," *Carcinogenesis* 12 (1991): 1571–74.

11. C. P. Martucci and J. Fishman, "P450 Enzymes of Estrogen Metabolism," *Pharmacology Therapeutics* 57 (1993): 237–57.

12. Bradlow, Michnovicz, et al., "Effects of Dietary Indole-3-Carbinol."

13. Ibid.

14. V. L. Ernster, M. R. Wrensch, et al., "Benign and Malignant Breast Disease: Initial Study Results of Serum and Breast Fluid Analyses of Endogenous Estrogens," *Journal of the National Cancer Institute* 79 (1987): 949–60.

15. Ibid.

16. N. L. Petrakis, M. R. Wrensch, et al., "Influence of Pregnancy and Lactation on Serum and Breast Fluid Estrogen Levels: Implications for Breast Cancer Risk," *International Journal of Cancer* 40 (1987): 587–91.

17. L. Bernstein, R. K. Ross, et al., "The Effects of Moderate Physical Activity on Menstrual Cycle Patterns in Adolescence: Implications for Breast Cancer Prevention," *British Journal of Cancer* 55 (1987): 681–85.

18. D. Apter and R. Vihko, "Early Menarche, a Risk Factor for Breast Cancer, Indicates Early Onset of Ovulatory Cycles," *Journal of Clinical Endocrinology and Metabolism* 57 (1983): 82–86.

19. H. J. Thompson, "Effect of Exercise Intensity and Duration on the Induction of Mammary Carcinogenesis," *Cancer Research* 54 (1994): 1960–63.

20. L. Bernstein, B. E. Henderson, et al., "Physical Exercise and Reduced Risk of Breast Cancer in Young Women," *Journal of the National Cancer Institute* 86 (1994): 1403–1408.

21. S. N. Blair, H. W. Kihl, et al., "Physical Fitness and All-Cause Mortality: A Prospective Study of Healthy Men and Women," *Journal of the American Medical Association* 262 (1989): 2395–401.

22. M. E. Reichman, J. T. Judd, et al., "Effects of Alcohol Consumption on Plasma and Urinary Hormone Concentrations in Premenopausal Women," *Journal of the National Cancer Institute* 85 (1993): 722–27.
23. V. C. Jordan, M. H. Jeng, et al., "The Estrogenic Activity of Synthetic Progestins Used in Oral Contraceptives," Cancer 71 (1993): 1501–1505.
24. J. L. Stanford and D. B. Thomas, "Exogenous Progestins and Breast Cancer," *Epidemiologic Reviews* 15 (1993): 98–107.
25. G. Plu-Bureau, M. G. L"e, [??], et al., "Progestogen Use and Decreased Risk of Breast Cancer in a Cohort Study of Premenopausal Women with Benign Breast Disease," *British Journal of Cancer* 70 (1994): 270–77.
26. C. E. Chilvers and S. J. Smith, "The Effects of Patterns of Oral Contraceptive Use on Breast Cancer Risk in Young Women. The UK National Case-Control Study Group," *British Journal of Cancer* 69 (1994): 922–23.
27. E. White, K. E. Malone, et al., "Breast Cancer Among Young U.S. Women in Relation to Oral Contraceptive Users," *Journal of the National Cancer Institute* 86 (1994): 505–514.
28. Stanford and Thomas, "Exogenous Progestins and Breast Cancer."
29. L. B. Tyrer, "Current Controversies and Future Direction of Oral Contraception," *Current Opinion in Obstetrics and Gynecology* 5 (1993): 833–38.
30. M. Thorogood and L. Villard-Mackintosh, "Combined Oral Contraceptives: Risks and Benefits," *British Medical Bulletin* 49 (1993): 124–39.
31. M. P. Vessey, "Benefits and Risks of Oral Contraceptives," *Methods of Information Medicine* 32 (3) (1993): 222–24.
32. M. A. Stenchever, "Risks of Oral Contraceptive Use in Women Over 35," *Journal of Reproductive Medicine* 38 (1993): 1030–35.
33. W. Hawley, J. Nuovo, et al., "Do Oral Contraceptive Agents Affect the Risk of Breast Cancer? A Meta-analysis of the Case-Control Reports," *Journal of the American Family Practice* 6 (1993): 123–35.
34. P. A. Wingo, N. C. Lee, et al., "Age-Specific Differences in the Relationship Between Oral Contraceptive Use and Breast Cancer," *Cancer* 71 (1993): 1506–1517.
35. D. V. Spicer and M. C. Pike, "The Prevention of Breast Cancer Through Reduced Ovarian Steroid Exposure," *Acta Oncologica* 31 (1992): 167–74.
36. D. V. Spicer and M. C. Pike, "Breast Cancer Prevention Through Modulation of Endogenous Hormones," *Breast Cancer Research and Treatment* 28 (1993): 179–93.
37. C. Chilvers, "Breast Cancer and Depo-medroxyprogesterone Acetate: A Review," *Contraception* 49 (1994): 211–22.
38. Stanford and Thomas, "Exogenous Progestins and Breast Cancer."
39. E. Barrett-Conner, "Epidemiology and the Menopause: A Global Overview," *International Journal of Fertility and Menopausal Studies* 38 (1993): 6–14.

40. D. J. Marchant, "Supplemental Estrogen Replacement," *Cancer* 74 (1994): 512–17.

41. R. Vassilopoulou-Sellin, "Estrogen Therapy in Women at Increased Risk for Breast Cancer," *Breast Cancer Research and Treatment* 28 (1993): 167–77.

42. L. C. Harlan, R. J. Coates, et al., "Estrogen Receptor Status and Dietary Intakes in Breast Cancer Patients," *Epidemiology* 4 (1993): 25–31.

43. Ibid.

44. D. P. Rose, A. P. Boyar, et al., "Effect of a Low-Fat Diet on Hormone Levels in Women with Cystic Breast Disease, I. Serum Steroids and Gonadotropins," *Journal of the National Cancer Institute* 78 (1987): 623–26.

45. C. Longcope, S. Gorbach, et al., "The Effect of a Low-Fat Diet on Estrogen Metabolism," *Journal of Clinical Endocrinology and Metabolism* 64 (1987): 1246–50.

CHAPTER 7: THE PROS AND CONS OF HORMONE REPLACEMENT THERAPY

1. Penny Wise Budoff, *No More Hot Flashes and Other Good News* (New York: Putnam, 1983).

2. Rod R. Seeley, Trent D. Stephens, and Philip Tate, *Essentials of Anatomy and Physiology* (St. Louis: Mosby, 1991).

3. E. Barrett-Connor and T. L. Bush, "Estrogen and Coronary Heart Disease in Women," *Journal of the American Medical Association* 249 (1983): 359–61.

4. F. Albright et al., "Postmenopausal Osteoporosis: Its Clinical Features," *Journal of the American Medical Association* 116 (1941): 2465–74.

5. A. Paganini-Hill and R. Ross, "Endometrial Cancer and Patterns of Use of Oestrogen Replacement Therapy: A Cohort Study," *British Journal of Cancer* 59 (1989): 445–47.

6. I. Persson et al., "Risk of Endometrial Cancer After Treatment with Oestrogens Alone or in Conjunction with Progestogens: Results of a Prospective Study," *British Medical Journal* 298 (1989): 147–51.

7. B. Zumoff, "Biological and Endocrinological Insights into the Possible Breast Cancer Risk from Menopausal Estrogen Replacement Therapy," *Steroids* 58 (1993): 196–204.

8. K. K. Steinberg et al., "A Meta-analysis of the Effect of Estrogen Replacement Therapy on the Risk of Breast Cancer," *Journal of the American Medical Association* 265 (1991): 1985–90.

9. W. D. Dupont and D. L. Page, "Therapy and Breast Cancer," *Archives of Internal Medicine* 151 (1991): 67–72.

10. B. K. Armstrong, "Oestrogen Therapy after the Menopause—Boon or Bane?" *Medical Journal of Australia* 148 (1988): 213–14.

11. D. Grady and V. Ernster, "Invited Commentary: Does Postmenopausal Hormone Therapy Cause Breast Cancer?" *American Journal of Epidemiology* 134 (1991): 1396–1400.

12. G. A. Colditz et al., "Hormone Replacement Therapy and Risk of Breast Cancer: Results from Epidemiologic Studies," *American Journal of Obstetrics and Gynecology* 168 (5) (1993): 1473–80.

13. Grady and Ernster, "Invited Commentary."

14. R. D. Gambrell et al., "Decreased Incidence of Breast Cancer in Postmenopausal Estrogen-Progestogen Users," *Obstetrics & Gynecology* 62 (4) (1983): 435–43.

15. Leif Bergkvist et al., "The Risk of Breast Cancer After Estrogen and Estrogen-Progestin Replacement," *New England Journal of Medicine* 321 (5) (1989): 293–97.

16. John R. Lee, *Natural Progesterone* (Sebastopol, Calif.: BLL Publishing, 1993).

17. T.K.A. Key and M. C. Pike, "The Role of Oestrogens and Progestogens in the Epidemiology and Prevention of Breast Cancer," *European Journal of Cancer & Clinical Oncology* 24 (1) (1988): 29–43.

18. R. Grattarola, "The Premenstrual Endometrial Pattern of Women with Breast Cancer," *Cancer* 17 (1964): 1119–22.

19. L. D. Cowan et al., "Breast Cancer Incidence in Women with a History of Progesterone Deficiency," *American Journal of Epidemiology* 114 (1981): 209–217.

20. C. B. Coulam et al., "Chronic Anovulation Syndrome and Associated Neoplasia," *Obstetrics & Gynecology* 61 (1983): 403–407.

21. R. E. Lunenfeld et al., "Cancer Incidence in a Cohort of Infertile Women," *American Journal of Epidemiology* 125 (1987): 780–90.

22. Cowan et al., "Breast Cancer Incidence."

23. Package insert for Provera brand of medroxyprogesterone acetate, Upjohn Company, Kalamazoo, Michigan.

24. Samuel S. Epstein, *The Politics of Cancer* (Garden City, N.Y.: Anchor/Doubleday, 1979).

25. Code of Federal Regulations, Title 21, Section 556.240.

26. Lee, *Natural Progesterone.*

27. V. A. Tzingounis et al., "Estriol in the Management of the Menopause," *Journal of the American Medical Association* 239 (16) (1978): 1638–41.

28. C. Lauritzen, "Results of a 5 Year Prospective Study of Estriol Succinate Treatment in Patients with Climacteric Complaints," *Hormone Metabolism Research* 19 (1987): 579–84.

29. *Chain Drug Review,* August 29, 1994, p. 14.

30. Sidney Rosenberg, "Early Menopause and the Risk of Myocardial Infarction," *American Journal of Obstetrics and Gynecology* 139 (1981): 47.

31. R. K. Ross et al., "Menopausal Oestrogen Therapy and Protection from

Death from Ischemic Heart Disease," *Lancet* 1 (April 18, 1981): 1 (8225) 858–60.

32. Trudy L. Bush, et al., "Estrogen Uses and All-Cause Mortality," *Journal of the American Medical Association* 249 (1983): 903–11.

33. Erkki Hirvonen et al., "Effects of Different Progestogens on Lipoproteins During Postmenopausal Replacement Therapy," *New England Journal of Medicine* 304 (1981): 560–62.

34. V. L. Ernster et al., "Clinical Perspectives: Benefits and Risks of Menopausal Estrogen and/or Progestin Hormone Use," *Preventive Medicine* 17 (1989): 201.

35. Hirvonen et al, "Effects of Different Progestogens."

36. B. L. Riggs and L. J. Melton III, "Involutional Osteoporosis," *New England Journal of Medicine* 314 (1986): 1676–86.

37. B. Ettinger and D. Grady, "The Waning Effect of Postmenopausal Estrogen Therapy on Osteoporosis," *New England Journal of Medicine* 329 (16) (1993): 1192–93.

38. J. R. Lee, "Osteoporosis Reversal: The Role of Progesterone," *International Clinical Nutrition Review* 10 (3) (1990): 384–91.

39. Henry M. Lemon et al., "Increased Catechol Estrogen Metabolism as a Risk Factor for Nonfamilial Breast Cancer," *Cancer* 69 (2) (1992): 457–64.

40. Henry M. Lemon et al., "Reduced Estriol Excretion in Patients with Breast Cancer Prior to Endocrine Therapy," *Journal of the American Medical Association* 196 (1966): 1128–36.

CHAPTER 8: DIET: EAT RIGHT FOR LIFE

1. U.S. Senate Report, *Dietary Goals for the United States* (Washington, D.C.: U.S. Government Printing Office, 1977).

2. T. Hirayama, "Epidemiology of Breast Cancer with Special Reference to the Role of Diet," *Preventive Medicine* 7 (1978): 173–95.

3. K. K. Carroll, "Experimental Evidence of Dietary Factors and Hormone-Dependent Cancers," *Cancer Research* 35 (1975): 3374–83.

4. W. C. Willett et al., "Dietary Fat and Fiber in Relation to Risk of Breast Cancer," *Journal of the American Medical Association* 268 (1992): 2037–44.

5. Robert M. Kradjian, *Save Yourself from Breast Cancer* (New York: Berkeley, 1994).

6. H. Adlercreutz and F. Martin, "Biliary Excretion and Intestinal Metabolism of Progesterone and Estrogens in Man," *Journal of Steroid Biochemistry* 13 (1980): 231–44.

7. B. R. Goldin et al., "Estrogen Excretion Patterns and Plasma Levels in Vegetarian and Omnivorous Women," *New England Journal of Medicine* 307 (1982): 1542–47.

8. D. P. Rose, "Dietary Fiber, Phytoestrogens, and Breast Cancer," *Nutrition* 8 (1) (1992): 47–51.

9. N. L. Petrakis and E. B. King, "Cytological Abnormalities in Nipple Aspirates of Breast Fluid from Women with Severe Constipation," *Lancet* 2 (1981): 1203–1204.

10. W. Arbuthnot Lane, "Chronic Intestinal Stasis," *British Medical Journal* 1 (1912): 989–93.

11. William S. Bainbridge, "Benign Mammary Tumors and Intestinal Toxemia," *American Journal of Obstetrics and Gynecology* 1 (1920): 465–75.

12. Petrakis and King, "Cytological Abnormalities."

13. B. R. Goldin et al., "Estrogen Excretion Patterns and Plasma Levels in Vegetarian and Omnivorous women," *New England Journal of Medicine* 307 (1982): 1542–47.

14. D. P. Rose et al., "High-Fiber Diet Reduces Serum Estrogen Concentrations in Premenopausal Women," *American Journal of Clinical Nutrition* 54 (1991): 520–25.

15. J. J. Michnovicz and H. L. Bradlow, "Altered Estrogen Metabolism in Humans Following Consumption of Indole-3-Carbinol," *Nutrition and Cancer* 16 (1991): 56–66.

16. Y. Zhang et al., "A Mayor Inducer of Anticarcinogenic Protective Enzymes from Broccoli: Isolation and Elucidation of Structure," *Proceedings of the National Academy of Science* 89 (1992): 2399–403.

17. Ibid.

18. S. Seely, "Diet and Breast Cancer: The Possible Connection with Sugar Consumption," *Medical Hypotheses* 11 (1983): 319–27.

19. M. Lender et al., "Diabetes Autoimmune Thyroid Disease and Breast Cancer," *Lancet* 19 (May 21, 1977) 1 (8021): 1110.

20. G. Block et al., "Fruit, Vegetables, and Cancer Prevention: A Review of the Epidemiological Evidence, *Nutrition and Cancer* 18 (1) (1992): 3–4.

21. *Medical World News*, vol. 34, no. 1, January 1993.

22. S. Harris, "Organochlorine Contamination of Breast Milk" (Washington, D.C.: Environmental Defense Fund, November 7, 1979).

23. Lewis Regenstein, *How to Survive America the Poisoned* (Washington D.C.: Acropolis Books, 1986) p. 273.

24. Frances Moore Lappé, *Diet for a Small Planet* (New York: Ballantine, 1982).

25. Bob L. Smith, "Organic Foods vs. Supermarket Foods: Element Levels," *Journal of Applied Nutrition* 45 (1) (1993): 35–39.

CHAPTER 9: ANTIOXIDANTS: THE FIRST LINE OF DEFENSE

1. D. Harman, "Free Radical Theory of Aging: The 'Free Radical' Diseases," *Journal of the American Aging Association* 7 (4) (1984): 111–31.

2. T. K. Basu et al., "Serum Vitamins A and E, Beta-carotene, and Selenium in Patients with Breast Cancer," *Journal of the American College of Nutrition* 8 (6) (1989): 524–28.

3. J. Chen et al., "Antioxidant Status and Cancer Mortality in China," *International Journal of Epidemiology* 21 (4) (1992): 625–35.

4. Linus Pauling, "Ascorbic Acid: Biological Functions and Relation to Cancer," NCI Symposium, April 1989.

5. Balz Frei, "Ascorbic Acid: Biological Functions and Relation to Cancer," NCI Symposium, April 1989.

6. G. Block, "Vitamin C and Cancer Prevention: The Epidemiologic Evidence," *American Journal of Clinical Nutrition* 53 (1991): 270S–82S.

7. G. R. Howe et al., "Dietary Factors and Risk of Breast Cancer: Combined Analysis of 12 Case-Controlled Studies," *Journal of the National Cancer Institute* 82 (1990): 561–69.

8. J. E. Enstrom et al., "Vitamin C Intake and Mortality Among a Sample of the United States Population," *Epidemiology* 3 (3) (1992): 194–202.

9. J. E. Packer et al., "Direct Observation of a Free Radical Interaction Between Vitamin E and Vitamin C," *Nature* 278 (1979): 737–38.

10. E. Niki et al., "Regeneration of Vitamin E from Alpha-Chromanoxyl Radical by Glutathione and Vitamin C," *Chemistry Letters* 6 (1982): 789–92.

11. D. Harman, "Dimethylbenzanthracene Induced Cancer. Alpha-tocopherol as a Potential Modifier of Daunomycin Carcinogenicity on Sprague Dawley Rats," *Clinical Research* 17 (1969): 125.

12. C. Lee and C. Chen, "Enhancement of Tumorigenesis in Rats by Vitamin E Efficiency," *Proceedings of the American Association of Cancer Research, Annual Meeting of the American Society of Clinical Oncologists* 20: 132, Abstract 531 (1979).

13. C. Ip, "Dietary Vitamin E Intake and Mammary Carcinogenesis in Rats," *Carcinogenesis* 3 (1982): 1453–56.

14. P. M. Horvath and C. Ip, "Synergistic Effect of Vitamin E and Selenium in the Chemoprevention of Mammary Carcinogenesis in Rats," *Cancer Research* 43 (1983): 5335–41.

15. P. Knekt, "Serum Vitamin E Level and Risk of Female Cancers," *International Journal of Epidemiology* 17 (2) (1988): 281–86.

16. N. J. Wald et al., "Plasma Retinol, B-carotene and Vitamin E Levels in Relation to Future Risk of Breast Cancer," *British Journal of Cancer* 49 (1984): 321–24.

17. L. A. McKeown, "Vitamin E May Cut Heart Risk," *Medical Tribune* 33 (1992): 1.

18. C. H. Hennekens et al., "Vitamin A, Carotenoids and Retinoids," *Cancer* 58 (1986): 1837–41.

19. G. W. Burton and K. U. Ingold, "Beta-carotene: An Unusual Type of Lipid Antioxidant," *Science* 224 (1984): 569–73.

20. N. I. Krinsky and S.S.M. Deneke, "Interaction of Oxygen and Oxy-radicals with Carotenoids," *Journal of the National Cancer Institute* 69 (1982): 205–210.

21. Hennekens et al., "Vitamin A, Carotenoids and Retinoids."

22. C. La Vecchia et al., "Dietary Factors and the Risk of Breast Cancer," *Nutrition and Cancer* 10 (1987): 205–214.

23. K. Katsouyanni et al., "Risk of Breast Cancer Among Greek Women in Relation to Nutrient Intake," *Cancer* 61 (1988): 181–85.

24. T. E. Rohan et al., "A Population-Based Case-Control Study of Diet and Breast Cancer in Australia," *American Journal of Epidemiology* 128 (3) (1988): 478–89.

25. Alpha-Tocopherol, Beta-Carotene Cancer Prevention Study Group, "The Effect of Vitamin E and beta carotene on the Incidence of Lung Cancer and Other Cancers in Male Smokers," *New England Journal of Medicine* 330 (15) (1994): 1029–35.

26. G. N. Schrauzer and D. Ishmael, "Effects of Selenium and of Arsenic on the Genesis of Spontaneous Mammary Tumors in Inbred C3H Mice," *Annals of Clinical Laboratory Science* 4 (1974): 441.

27. C. Ip, "Prophylaxis of Mammary Neoplasia by Selenium Supplementation in the Initiation and Promotion Phases of Carcinogenesis," *Cancer Research* 41 (1981): 4386.

28. G. N. Schrauzer, "Selenium: Mechanistic Aspects of Anticarcinogenic Action," *Biological Trace Element Research* 33 (1992): 51–62.

29. G. N. Schrauzer, "Selenium in Nutritional Cancer Prophylaxis: An Update," in *Vitamins, Nutrition, and Cancer,* ed. A. S. Prasad (Basel, Switzerland: Kraager, 1984), pp. 240–50.

30. J. L. Martin and J. S. Spallholz, "Selenium in the Immune Response," *Proceedings of the Symposium on Selenium-Tellurium in the Environment, Notre Dame, 1976* (Pittsburgh: Industrial Health Foundation, 1976), pp. 204–209.

31. R. J. Shamberger et al., "Antioxidants and Cancer. Part VI. Selenium and Age-Adjusted Human Cancer Mortality," *Archives of Environmental Health* 31 (1976): 231.

32. G. N. Schrauzer et al., "Cancer Mortality Correlation Studies—III: Statistical Associations with Dietary Selenium Intakes," *Bioinorganic Chemistry* 7 (1977): 23.

33. W. C. Willett et al., "Prediagnostic Serum Selenium and Risk of Cancer," *Lancet* 2 (1983): 130.

34. R. J. Shamberger, "Relationship of Selenium to Cancer. Inhibitory Effect of Selenium on Carcinogenesis," *Journal of the National Cancer Institute* 44 (1970): 931–41.

35. G. N. Schrauzer, "Selenium and Cancer: A Review," *Bioinorganic Chemistry* 5 (1976): 275–81.

36. K. McConnell et al., "The Relationship of Dietary Selenium and Breast Cancer," *Journal of Surgical Oncology* 15 (1980): 67–70.
37. G. N. Schrauzer et al., "Selenium in the Blood of Japanese and American Women with and without Breast Cancer and Fibrocystic Disease," *Japanese Journal of Cancer Research* 76 (1985): 374–77.
38. Schrauzer, "Selenium and Cancer."
39. L. Hardell et al., "Levels of Selenium in Plasma and Glutathione Peroxidase in Erythrocytes and the Risk of Breast Cancer," *Biological Trace Element Research* 36 (1993): 99–108.
40. G. Yang et al., "Studies of Maximal and Minimal Safe Intake and Requirement of Selenium," The Fourth International Symposium on Selenium in Biology and Medicine, Tubingen, Germany, 1988.

CHAPTER 10: DIETARY FAT: THE 20 PERCENT SOLUTION

1. Committee on Diet, Nutrition and Cancer, National Research Council, National Academy of Sciences, *Diet, Nutrition and Cancer* (Washington, D.C.: National Academy Press, 1982).
2. D. J. Hunter and W. C. Willett, "Diet, Body Size, and Breast Cancer," *Epidemiologic Reviews* 15 (1993): 110–32.
3. P. J. Goodwin and N. F. Boyd, "Critical Appraisal of the Evidence That Dietary Fat Intake Is Related to Breast Cancer Risk in Humans," *Journal of the National Cancer Institute* 79 (1987): 473–85.
4. G. R. Howe, "Dietary Fat and Breast Cancer Risks. An Epidemiologic Perspective," *Cancer* 74 (1994): 1078–84.
5. E. L. Wynder et al., "Contribution of the Environment to Cancer Incidence: An Epidemiologic Exercise," *Journal of the National Cancer Institute* 58 (1977): 825–32.
6. B. Armstrong and R. Doll, "Environmental Factors and Cancer Incidence and Mortality in Different Countries, with Special Reference to Dietary Practice," *International Journal of Cancer* 15 (1975): 617–31.
7. D. P. Rose, A. P. Boyar, et al., "International Comparisons of Mortality Rates for Cancer of the Breast, Ovary, Prostate, Womb, and Per Capita Food Consumption," *Cancer* 58 (1986): 2363–71.
8. J. Staszewsky and W. Haenszel, "Cancer Mortality Among Polish Born in the United States," *Journal of the National Cancer Institute* 35 (1965): 292–97.
9. W. Haenzsal, "Cancer Mortality Among the Foreign-Born in the United States," *Journal of the National Cancer Institute* 26 (1961): 37–132.
10. P. Buell, "Changing Incidence of Breast Cancer in Japanese-American Women," *Journal of National Cancer Institute* 51 (1973): 1479–83.
11. H. King and F. B. Locke, "Cancer Mortality Among Chinese in the United States," *Journal of the National Cancer Institute* 65 (1980): 1141–48.

12. K. K. Carroll, "Dietary Fat and Breast Cancer," *Lipids* 27 (1992): 793–97.
13. W. C. Willett, D. J. Hunter, et al., "Dietary Fat and Fiber in Relation to Risk of Breast Cancer," *Journal of the American Medical Association* 268 (1992): 2037–44.
14. N. Boyd, "Nutrition and Breast Cancer" [editorial], *Journal of the National Cancer Institute* 85 (1993): 6–7.
15. M. Ewertz and C. Gill, "Dietary Factors and Breast-Cancer Risk in Denmark," *International Journal of Cancer* 46 (1990): 779–84.
16. S. Richardson, M. Gerber, et al., "The Role of Fat, Animal Protein and Some Vitamin Consumption in Breast Cancer: A Case Control Study in Southern France," *International Journal of Cancer* 48 (1991): 1–9.
17. Y. Shun-Zhang, L. Rui-Fang, et al., "A Case-Control Study of Dietary and Nondietary Risk Factors for Breast Cancer in Shanghai," *Cancer Research* 50 (1990): 5017–21.
18. E. Barrett-Connor and N. J. Freidlander, "Dietary Fat, Calories, and the Risk of Breast Cancer in Postmenopausal Women: A Prospective Population-Based Study," *Journal of the American College of Nutrition* 12 (1993): 390–99.
19. H. Merzensch, H. Boeing, et al., "Dietary Fat and Sports Activity as Determinants for Age at Menarche," *American Journal of Epidemiology* 138 (1993): 217–24.
20. A. P. Boyar, D. P. Rose, et al., "Recommendations for the Prevention of Chronic Disease: The Application for Breast Disease," *American Journal of Clinical Nutrition* 48 (1988): 896–900.
21. B. R. Goldin, H. Adlercreutz, et al., "Estrogen Excretion Patterns and Plasma Levels in Vegetarian and Omnivorous Women," *New England Journal of Medicine* 307 (1982): 1542–47.
22. E. Nordevang, E. Azavedo, et al., "Dietary Habits and Mammographic Patterns in Patients with Breast Cancer," *Breast Cancer Research and Treatment* 26 (1993): 207–215.
23. M. J. Hill, J. S. Crowther, et al., "Bacteria and Aetiology of Cancer of Large Bowel," *Lancet* 1 (1971): 95–100.
24. Goldin, Adlercreutz, et al., "Estrogen Excretion Patterns."
25. L. Holmberg, E. M. Ohlander, et al., "Diet and Breast Cancer Risk. Results from a Population-Based, Case-Control Study in Sweden," *Archives of Internal Medicine* 154 (1994): 1805–1811.
26. C. W. Welsch, "Relationship Between Dietary Fat and Experimental Mammary Tumorigenesis: A Review and Critique," *Cancer Research* 52 (1992): 2040s–48s.
27. G. A. Boissonneault, C. E. Elson, et al., "Net Energy Effects of Dietary Fat on Chemically Induced Carcinogenesis in F-344 Rats," *Journal of the National Cancer Institute* 76 (1986): 335–38.

28. A. Tannenbaum, "The Genesis and Growth of Tumors. II: Effects of Caloric Restriction Per Se," *Cancer Research* 2 (1942): 460–67.
29. A. Tannenbaum and H. Silverstone, "Nutrition in Relation to Cancer," *Advanced Cancer Research* 1 (1953): 451–501.
30. K. K. Carroll and L. M. Braden, "Dietary Fat and Mammary Carcinogenesis," *Nutrition and Cancer* 6 (1985): 254–59.
31. S. L. Selenskas, M. M. Ip, et al., "Similarity Between Trans Fat and Saturated Fat in the Modification of Rat Mammary Carcinogenesis," *Cancer Research* 44 (1984): 1321–26.
32. S. J. London, F. M. Sacks, et al., "Fatty Acid Composition of the Subcutaneous Adipose Tissue and Risk of Proliferative Benign Breast Disease and Breast Cancer," *Journal of the National Cancer Institute* 85 (1993): 785–93.
33. S. I. Grammatikos, P. V. Subbaiah, et al., "N-3 and N-6 Fatty Acid Processing and Growth Effects in Neoplastic and Non-cancerous Human Mammary Epithelial Cell Lines," *British Journal of Cancer* 70 (1994): 219–27.
34. R. A. Karmali, "N-3 Fatty Acids and Cancer," *Journal of Internal Medicine* 225 (1989): 197–200.
35. D. P. Rose and J. M. Connolly, "Effects of Fatty Acids and Inhibitors of Eicosanoid Synthesis on the Growth of a Human Breast Cancer Cell Line in Culture," *Cancer Research* 50 (1990): 7139–44.
36. L. Kaizer, N. F. Boyd, et al., "Fish Consumption and Breast Cancer Risk: An Ecological Study," *Nutrition and Cancer* 12 (1989): 61–68.
37. A. Trichopoulou, K. Katsouyanni, et al., "Consumption of Olive Oil and Specific Food Groups in Relation to Breast Cancer Risk in Greece," *Journal of the National Cancer Institute* 87 (1995): 110–6.
38. D. P. Rose and J. M. Connolly, "Dietary Prevention of Breast Cancer," *Medical Oncology & Tumor Pharmacotherapy* 7 (2/3) (1990): 121–30.
39. V. W. Pinn, "The Role of the NIH's Office of Research on Women's Health," *Academic Medicine* 69 (1994): 698–702.
40. N. B. Cummings, "Women's Health and Nutrition Research: US Governmental Concerns," *Journal of the American College of Nutrition* 12 (1993): 329–36.
41. E. Marshall, "Women's Health Initiative Draws Flak," *Science* 262 (1993): 838.
42. M. Jain, A. B. Miller, et al., "Premorbid Diet and the Prognosis of Women with Breast Cancer," *Journal of the National Cancer Institute* 86 (1994): 1390–97.
43. R. Verreault, J. Brisson, et al., "Dietary Fat in Relation to Prognostic Factors in Breast Cancer," *Journal of the National Cancer Institute* 80 (1988): 819–25.
44. R. T. Chlebowski, G. L. Blackburn, et al., "Adherence to a Dietary Fat Intake Reduction Program in Postmenopausal Women Receiving Therapy

for Early Breast Cancer. The Woman's Intervention Nutrition Study," *Journal of Clinical Oncology* 11 (1993): 2072–80.

45. L. E. Holm, E. Nordevang, et al., "Treatment Failure and Dietary Habits in Women with Breast Cancer," *Journal of the National Cancer Institute* 85 (1993): 32–36.

46. D. P. Rose, J. M. Connolly, et al., "The Effects of a Low-Fat Diet Intervention and Tamoxifen Adjuvant Therapy on the Serum Estrogen and Sex Hormone-Binding Globulin Concentrations of Postmenopausal Breast Cancer Patients," *Breast Cancer Research and Treatment* 27 (1993): 253–62.

47. L. C. Harlan, R. J. Coates, et al., "Estrogen Receptor Status and Dietary Intakes in Breast Cancer Patients," *Epidemiology* 4 (1993): 25–31.

48. D. P. Rose and M. A. Hatala, "Dietary Fatty Acids and Breast Cancer Invasion and Metastasis," *Nutrition and Cancer* 21 (1994): 103–111.

49. D. P. Rose and J. M. Connolly, "Effects of Dietary Omega-3 Fatty Acids on Human Breast Cancer Growth and Metastasis in Nude Mice," *Journal of the National Cancer Institute* 85 (1993): 1743–47.

50. L. A. Cohen, D. P. Rose, et al., "A Rationale for Dietary Intervention in Postmenopausal Breast Cancer Patients: An Update," *Nutrition and Cancer* 19 (1993): 1–10.

51. R. T. Chlebowski, D. Rose, et al., "Adjuvant Dietary Fat Intake Reduction in Postmenopausal Breast Cancer Patient Management. The Women's Intervention Nutrition Study (WINS)," *Breast Cancer Research and Treatment* 20 (1992): 73–84.

52. K. Heber, J. M. Ashley, et al., "Assessment of Adherence to a Low-Fat Diet for Breast Cancer Prevention," *Preventive Medicine* 21 (1992): 218–27.

53. Chlebowski, Blackburn, et al., "Adherence to a Dietary Fat Intake Reduction Program."

CHAPTER 11: TAKING NUTRITIONAL SUPPLEMENTS

1. H. E. Sigerist, *The University at the Crossroads* (New York: Shuman, 1946), p. 114.

2. *Myths of Vitamins, FDA Consumer* Vol. 8, No. 2, (1974) p. 4.

3. B. H. Patterson et al., "Fruit and Vegetables in the American Diet: Data from the NHANES II Survey," *American Journal of Public Health* 80 (2) (1990): 1443–49.

4. E. M. Pao and S. J. Mickle, "Problem Nutrients in the United States," *Food Technology* 35 (1981): 58–62.

5. M. C. Fisher and P. A. Lachance, "Nutrition Evaluation of Published Weight-Reducing Diets," *Journal of the American Dietetic Association* 85 (1985): 450–54.

6. A. S. Prasad et al., "Effect of Oral Contraceptive Agents on Nutrients: II. Vitamins," *American Journal of Clinical Nutrition* 28 (1975): 385–91.
7. B. Smith, "Organic Foods vs Supermarket Foods: Element Levels," *Journal of Applied Nutrition* 45 (1) (1993): 35–39.
8. Donald R. Davis, "Nutritional Needs and Biochemical Diversity," in *Medical Applications of Clinical Nutrition,* ed. Jeffrey Bland (New Canaan, Conn.: Keats, 1983).
9. Roger J. Williams, *Biochemical Individuality: The Basis for the Genetotrophic Concept* (New York: Wiley; Austin: Univerity of Texas Press, 1956).
10. *What About Vitamin C? FDA Consumer* Vol. 8, No. 8 (1974) p. 29.
11. *Vitamin E—Miracle or Myth? FDA Consumer* Vol. 7, No. 6 (1973) p. 24.
12. L. A. McKeown, "Vitamin E May Cut Heart Risk," *Medical Tribune* 33 (1992): 1.
13. J. K. Chandra, "Effect of Vitamin and Trace-Element Supplementation on Immune Responses and Infection in Elderly Subjects," *Lancet* 340 (1992): 1124–27.
14. Donald Loomis, "Fatalities from Prescription Drugs, Non-prescription Drugs, and Nutrients," *Townsend Letter for Doctors,* April 1992.
15. Emile G. Bliznakov and Gerald L. Hunt, *The Miracle Nutrient Coenzyme Q10* (New York: Bantam, 1986).
16. Karl Folkers et al., "Partial and Complete Regression of Breast Cancer in Patients in Relation to Dosage of Coenzyme Q10," *Biochemical and Biophysical Research Communications* 199 (3) (1994): 504–508.
17. Ibid.

CHAPTER 12: THE SOY PHENOMENON

1. H. Nagasawa, "Nutrition and Breast Cancer: A Survey of Experimental and Epidemiological Evidence," *International Cancer Research Scientific Report* 8 (1980): 786–91.
2. P. Buell, "Changing Incidence of Breast Cancer in Japanese-American Women," *Journal of the National Cancer Institute* 51 (5) (1973): 1479–83.
3. G. E. Gray et al., "Breast Cancer Incidence and Mortality Rates in Different Countries in Relation to Known Factors and Dietary Practice," *British Journal of Cancer* 39 (1979): 1–7.
4. G. Hems, "The Contribution of Diet and Child Bearing to Breast Cancer Rates," *British Journal of Cancer* 37 (1978): 974–82.
5. J. E. Baggott et al., "Effect of Miso (Japanese Soybean Paste) and NaCl on DMBA-Induced Rat Mammary Tumors," *Nutrition and Cancer* 14 (2) (1990): 103–109.
6. M. Messina and S. Barnes, "The Role of Soy Products in Reducing Risk of Cancer," *Journal of the National Cancer Institute* 83 (8) (1991): 541–46.

7. P. M. Martin et al., "Phytoestrogen Interaction with Estrogen Receptors in Human Breast Cancer Cells," *Endocrinology* 103 (1978): 1860–67.
8. H. P. Lee et al., "Dietary Effects on Breast-Cancer Risk in Singapore," *Lancet* 337 (1991): 1197–1200.
9. H. Adlercreutz et al., "Dietary Phytoestrogens and Cancer: In Vitro and In Vivo Studies," *Journal of Steroid Biochemistry & Molecular Biology* 41 (3–8) (1992): 331–37.
10. K.D.R. Setchell et al, "Nonsteroidal Estrogens of Dietary Origin: Possible Roles in Hormone-Dependent Disease," *American Journal of Clinical Nutrition* 40 (1984): 569–78.
11. E. Meddleton and C. Kandaswami, "Anticancer and Anticarcinogenic Properties of Plant Flavonoids," *Adjuvant Nutrition in Cancer Treatment*, 1992 Symposium Proceedings, Cancer Treatment Research Foundation, Arlington Heights, Illinois.
12. Messina and Barnes, "Role of Soy Products."
13. H. Neurath, "Evolution of Proteolytic Enzymes," *Science* 224 (1984): 350–57.
14. A. R. Kennedy and J. B. Little, "Effects of Protease Inhibitors on Radiation Transformation In Vitro," *Cancer Research* 41 (1981): 2103–08.
15. Messina and Barnes, "Role of Soy Products."
16. Lilian U. Thompson and Lin Zhang, "Phytic Acid and Minerals: Effect on Early Markers of Risk for Mammary and Colon Carcinogenesis," *Carcinogenesis* 12 (11) (1991): 2041–45.
17. R. F. Raicht et al., "Protective Effect of Plant Sterols Against Chemically Induced Colon Tumors in Rats," *Cancer Research* 40 (1980): 403–405.
18. R. Bomford, "Studies on the Cellular Site of Action of the Adjuvant Activity of Saponin for Sheep Erythocytes," *International Archives of Allergy and Applied Immunology* 67 (1982): 127–31.
19. D. Oakenfull, "Saponins in Food—a Review," *Food Chemistry* 6 (1981): 19–40.
20. B. S. Aswal et al., "Screening of Indian Plants for Biological Activity— Part X," *Indian Journal of Experimental Biology* 22 (1984): 312–32.
21. "Soyatech Surveys and Estimates" (Bar Harbor, Maine: Soyatech, 1990).
22. M. Messina and V. Messina, "Increasing Use of Soyfoods and Their Potential Role in Cancer Prevention," *Journal of the American Dietetic Association* 91 (7) (July 1991): 836–40.
23. J. A. Duke, *Handbook of Nuts* (Boca Raton, Fla.: CRC Press, 1989).

CHAPTER 13: THE DANGER OF PESTICIDES

1. M. S. Wolff et al., "Blood Levels of Organochlorine Residues and Risk of Breast Cancer," *Journal of the National Cancer Institute* 85 (8) (1993): 648–52.

2. Rachel Carson, *Silent Spring* (New York: Crest, 1962).

3. M. Wassermann et al., "Organochlorine Compounds in Neoplastic and Adjacent Apparently Normal Breast Tissue," *Bulletin of Environmental Contamination Toxicology* 15 (1976): 478–84.

4. R. Duggan, "Dietary Intake of Pesticide Chemicals in the United States, June 1966–April 1968," *Pesticides Monitoring Journal* 2 (1969): 140.

5. P. E. Cornellussen, "Pesticide Residues in Total Diet," *Pesticides Monitoring Journal* 2 (1969): 152.

6. S. Lustgarder, "Persistent Residues in Produce," *Vegetarian Times*, August 1994, p. 16.

7. Ibid.

8. Ibid.

9. F. Falck, Jr., et al., "Pesticides and Polychlorinated Biphenyl Residues in Human Breast Lipids and Their Relation to Breast Cancer," *Archives of Environmental Health* 47 (2) (1992): 143–46.

10. A. Manz et al., "Cancer Mortality Among Workers in Chemical Plant Contaminated with Dioxin," *Lancet* 338 (1991): 959–64.

11. J. B. Westin and E. Richter, "The Israeli Breast-Cancer Anomaly," *Annals of the New York Academy of Sciences* 609 (1990): 269–79.

12. M. Unger et al., "Organochlorine Compounds in Human Breast Fat from Deceased with and without Breast Cancer and in a Biopsy Material from Newly Diagnosed Patients Undergoing Breast Surgery," *Environmental Research* 34 (1984): 24–28.

13. Greenpeace Report, *Chlorine, Human Health, and the Environment: The Breast Cancer Warning*, October 1993.

14. D. Perlmutter, "Organochlorines, Breast Cancer, and GATT," *Journal of the American Medical Association* 271 (15) (April 20, 1994): 1160–1

15. *Tap Water Blues: Herbicides in Drinking Water*, October 1994. Environmental Working Group, 1718 Connecticut Avenue, N.W., Suite 600, Washington, D.C. 20009.

CHAPTER 14: EXERCISE: FEEL GOOD AND LIVE LONGER

1. L. Bernstein et al., "Physical Exercise and Reduced Risk of Breast Cancer in Young Women," *Journal of the National Cancer Institute* 86 (18) (1994): 1403–1408.

2. R. E. Frisch et al., "Lower Prevalence of Breast Cancer and Cancers of the Reproductive System Among Former College Athletes Compared to Non-athletes," *British Journal of Cancer* 52 (1985): 885–91.

3. J. E. Vena et al., "Occupational Exercise and Risk of Cancer," *American Journal of Clinical Nutrition* 45 (1987): 318–27.

4. V. J. Bihko et al., "Risk of Breast Cancer Among Female Teachers of Physical Education and Languages," *Acta Oncologica* 31 (2) (1992): 201–204.

5. L. Bernstein et al., "The Effects of Moderate Physical Activity on Menstrual Cycle Patterns in Adolescence: Implications for Breast Cancer Prevention," *British Journal of Cancer* 55 (1987): 681–85.

6. B. E. Henderson et al., "Estrogens as a Cause of Human Cancer: The Richard and Hinda Rosenthal Foundation Award Lecture," *Cancer Research* 48 (1988): 246–53.

7. Bernstein et al., "Effects of Moderate Physical Activity."

8. M. C. Pike, et al., "Oral Contraceptive Use and Early Abortion as Risk Factors for Breast Cancer in Young Women," *British Journal of Cancer* 43 (1981): 72–76.

9. D. Apter and R. Vihko, "Early Menarche, a Risk Factor for Breast Cancer, Indicates Early Onset of Ovulatory Cycles," *Journal of Clinical Endocrinology and Metabolism* 57 (1983): 82–86.

10. M. P. Warren, "The Effects of Exercise on Pubertal Progression and Reproductive Function in Girls," *Journal of Clinical Endocrinology and Metabolism* 51 (5) (1980): 1150–54.

11. B. MacMahon, et al., "Etiology of Human Breast Cancer: A Review," *Journal of the National Cancer Institute* 50 (1973): 21–42.

12. Bernstein et al., "Effects of Moderate Physical Activity."

13. Bonen, A. et al., "Profiles of Selected Hormones During Menstrual Cycles of Teenage Athletes," *Journal of Applied Physiology* 50 (1981): 545–51.

14. D. A. Wakat and K. E. Sweeney, "Etiology of Athletic Amenorrhea in Cross-Country Runners," *Medical Science Sports* 11 (1979): 91.

15. D.J.P. Ferguson and T. J. Anderson, "Morphological Evaluation of Cell Turnover in Relation to the Menstrual Cycle in the 'Resting' Human Breast," *British Journal of Cancer* 44 (1981): 177–81.

16. T. A. Longacre and S. A. Bartow, "A Correlative Morphologic Study of Human Breast and Endometrium in the Menstrual Cycle," *American Journal of Surgical Pathology* 10 (1986): 382–93.

17. M. Shangold et al, "The Relationship Between Long-Distance Running, Plasma Progesterone and Luteal Phase Length," *Fertility and Sterility* 31 (1979): 130–33.

18. *New York Running News,* December/January 1994, p. 65.

19. "Participation of High School Students in School Physical Education—United States," *Morbidity and Mortality Weekly Report* 40 (1991): 613–15.

20. "Vigorous Physical Activity Among High School Students—United States," *Morbidity and Mortality Weekly Report* 41 (1992): 33–35.

21. Otto Warburg, "The Prime Cause and Prevention of Cancer with Two

Prefaces on Prevention," revised Lindau Lecture, delivered at the 1966 annual meeting of Nobel Prize winners at Lindau, Germany.

22. William Evans and Irvin H. Rosenberg, *Biomarkers: The 10 Keys to Prolonging Vitality* (New York: Simon & Schuster 1991).

23. Swami Sivananda Radha, *Hatha Yoga: The Hidden Language* (Boston: Shambhala 1989).

24. B.K.S. Iyengar, *Light on Yoga* (New York: Schocken Books 1966).

25. B.K.S. Iyengar, *Light on Yoga*.

26. Lisa G. Hampton, "The Influence of Yoga, Meditation and Walking on Stress and Immune Responses," *Thesis Defense, University of California, San Diego, Department of Physical Education, May 11, 1995*.

27. Bonnie G. Berger and David R. Owen, "Mood Alteration with Yoga and Swimming: Aerobic Exercise May Not Be Necessary," *Perceptual and Motor Skill* 75 (1992): 1331–1343.

28. Paul A. Czubryt, "The Influence of Tai Chi, Meditation and Walking on Stress and Immune Responses," *Thesis Defense, University of California, San Diego, Department of Physical Education, May 11, 1995*.

CHAPTER 15: SMOKING AND BREAST CANCER

1. B. MacMahon et al, "Cigarette Smoking and Urinary Estrogens," *New England Journal of Medicine* 307 (1982): 1062–65.

2. R. A. Hiatt and B. H. Fireman, "Smoking, Menopause, and Breast Cancer," *Journal of the National Cancer Institute* 76 (1986): 833–38.

3. N. L. Petrakis et al, "Mutagenic Activity in Nipple Aspirates of Human Breast Fluid," *Cancer Research* 40 (1980): 188–89.

4. D. R. Shopland, *The Health Consequences of Smoking: Cancer*, a report of the Surgeon General, Office on Smoking and Health, U.S. Public Health Service, 1982, DHHS Publication No. (PHS) 82-50179.

5. M. Ferson et al., "Low Natural Killer–Cell Activity and Immunoglobulin Levels Associated with Smoking in Human Subjects," *International Journal of Cancer* 23 (1979): 603–609.

6. J. Basu et al, "Smoking and the Antioxidant Ascorbic Acid: Plasma, Leucocyte, and Cervicovaginal Cell Concentrations in Normal Healthy Women," *American Journal of Obstetrics and Gynecology* 163 (6 Pt.1) (1990): 1948–52.

7. E. Rimm et al., "Smoking, Alcohol, and Plasma Levels of Carotenes and Vitamin E," *Annals of the New York Academy of Sciences* 686 (1993): 323–33.

8. D. P. Sandler et al., "Cigarette Smoking and Breast Cancer" [letter], *American Journal of Epidemiology* 123 (1986): 370–71.

9. T. Hirayama, "Cancer Mortality in Nonsmoking Women with Smoking

Husbands Based on a Large-Scale Cohort Study in Japan," *Previews in Medicine* 13 (1984): 680–90.

10. A. Wesley Horton, "Indoor Tobacco Smoke Pollution: A Major Risk Factor for Both Breast and Lung Cancer?" *Cancer* 62 (1988): 6–14.

11. Surgeon General's Report, *The Health Consequences of Involuntary Smoking* (Washington, D.C.: U.S. Government Printing Office, 1986).

12. Samuel S. Epstein, *The Politics of Cancer* (Garden City, N.Y.: Anchor, 1979).

13. A. Wesley Horton, "Epidemiologic Evidence for the Role of Indoor Tobacco Smoke as an Initiator of Human Breast Carcino-genesis," *Cancer Detection and Prevention* 16 (2) (1992): 119–27.

14. Surgeon General's Report, *Health Consequences of Involuntary Smoking.*

15. Horton, "Epidemiologic Evidence."

16. Henry M. Lemon, "Re: Breast Cancer and Cigarette Smoking: A Hypothesis," *American Journal of Epidemiology* 135 (10) (1992): 1184–85.

CHAPTER 16: ALCOHOL CONSUMPTION

1. L. Rosenberg et al., "Breast Cancer and Alcoholic-Beverage Consumption," *Lancet* 1 (1982): 267–70.

2. M. E. Reichman et al., "Effects of Alcohol Consumption on Plasma and Urinary Hormone Concentrations in Premenopausal Women," *Journal of the National Cancer Institute* 85 (9) (1993): 722–27.

3. W. C. Willett et al., "Moderate Alcohol Consumption and the Risk of Breast Cancer," *New England Journal of Medicine* 316 (1987): 1174–80.

4. L. Rosenberg et al., "Alcohol Consumption and Risk of Breast Cancer: A Review of the Epidemiologic Evidence," *Epidemiologic Reviews* 15 (1993): 133–44.

5. C. M. Friedenreich et al, "A Cohort Study of Alcohol Consumption and Risk of Breast Cancer," *American Journal of Epidemiology* 137 (5) (1993): 512–20.

6. M. P. Longnecker et al., "A Meta-analysis of Alcohol Consumption in Relation to Risk of Breast Cancer," *Journal of the American Medical Association* 260 (1988): 652–56.

7. M. P. Longnecker et al., "Risk of Breast Cancer in Relation to Past and Recent Alcohol Consumption," *American Journal of Epidemiology* 136 (1992): 1001.

8. G. A. Colditz et al., "Prospective Study of Estrogen Replacement Therapy and Risk of Breast Cancer in Postmenopausal Women," *Journal of the American Medical Association* 264 (1990): 2648–53.

9. S. London, et al., "Alcohol and Other Dietary Factors in Relation to Serum Hormone Concentrations in Women at Climacteric," *American Journal of Clinical Nutrition* 53 (1991): 166–71.

10. H. O. Adami et al., "Alcoholism and Cancer Risk: A Population-Based Cohort Study," *Cancer Causes and Control* 3 (1992): 419–25.

11. Joyce Steinberg and Pamela Goodwin, "Alcohol and Breast Cancer Risk—Putting the Current Controversy into Perspective," *Breast Cancer Research and Treatment* 19 (1991): 221–31.

CHAPTER 17: THE BENEFITS OF MELATONIN

1. A. J. Lewy, "Ordering Sleep," *Audio-Digest Psychiatry* 23 (14) (1994).

2. R. G. Stevens, S. Davis, et al., "Electric Power, Pineal Function, and the Risk of Breast Cancer," *Faseb Journal* 6 (3) (1992): 853–60.

3. R. G. Stevens, "Breast Cancer and Electric Power," *Biomedicine and Pharmacotherapy* 47 (10) (1993): 435–38.

4. R. P. Liburdy, T. R. Sloma, et al., "ELF Magnetic Fields, Breast Cancer, and Melatonin: 60 Hz Fields Block Melatonin's Oncostatic Action on ER + Breast Cancer Cell Proliferation," *Journal of Pineal Research* 14 (2) (1993): 89–97.

5. S. T. Wilson, D. E. Blask, et al., "Melatonin Augments the Sensitivity of MCF-7 Human Breast Cancer Cells to Tamoxifen In Viro," *Journal of Clinical Endocrinology and Metabolism* 75 (2) (1992): 669–70.

6. S. M. Hill, L. L. Spriggs, et al., "The Growth Inhibitory Action of Melatonin on Human Breast Cancer Cells Is Linked to the Estrogen Receptor System," *Cancer Letters* 64 (3) (1992): 249–56.

7. Y. Furuya, K. Yamamoto, et al., "5-Fluorouracil Attenuates an Oncostatic Effect of Melatonin on Estrogen-Sensitive Human Breast Cancer Cells (MCF7)," *Cancer Letters* 81 (1) (1994): 95–98.

8. P. Lissoni, S. Bami, et al., "Neuroimmunotherapy of Advanced Solid Neoplasms with Single Evening Subcutaneous Injection of Low-Dose Interleukin-2 and Melatonin: Preliminary Results," *European Journal of Cancer* 29A (2) (1993): 185–89.

9. L. Tamarkin, D. Danforth, et al., "Decreased Nocturnal Plasma Melatonin Peak in Patients with Estrogen Receptor Positive Breast Cancer," *Science* 216 (1982): 1003–1005.

10. C. Bartsch, H. Bartsch, et al., "Depression of Serum Melatonin in Patients with Primary Breast Cancer Is Not Due to an Increased Peripheral Metabolism," *Cancer* 67 (1991): 1681–84.

11. M. P. Coleman and R. J. Reiter, "Breast Cancer, Blindness and Melatonin," *European Journal of Cancer* 28 (2–3) (1992): 501–503.

12. Lewy, "Ordering Sleep."

CHAPTER 18: ELECTROMAGNETIC FIELDS

1. J. Waterhouse et al., "Cancer Incidence in Five Continents," vol. IV, *International Agency for Research on Cancer Science Publication*, Lyon, France (1982).
2. N. Wertheimer and E. D. Leeper, "Electrical Wiring Configurations and Childhood Cancer," *American Journal of Epidemiology* 109 (1979): 273–84.
3. S. Savitz, "Case-Control Study of Childhood Cancer and Residential Exposure to Electric and Magnetic Fields," report to the New York State Department of Health, Power Lines Project, 1987.
4. M. Feychting and A. Ahlbom, "Magnetic Fields and Cancer in Children Residing Near Swedish High-Voltage Power Lines," *American Journal of Epidemiology* 138 (7) (1993): 467.
5. M. Coleman and V. Beral, "A Review of Epidemiological Studies of Health Effects of Living Near or Working with Electricity Generation and Transmission Equipment," *International Journal of Epidemiology* 17 (1) (1988): 1–13.
6. M. Cohen et al., "Role of the Pineal Gland in the Aetiology and Treatment of Breast Cancer," *Lancet* 2 (1978): 814–16.
7. W. Loscher et al., "Tumor Promotion in a Breast Cancer Model by Exposure to a Weak Alternating Magnetic Field," *Cancer Letters* 71 (1993): 75–81.
8. R. P. Liburdy, T. R. Sloma, et al., "ELF Magnetic Fields, Breast Cancer, and Melatonin: 60 Hz Fields Block Melatonin's Oncostatic Action on ER + Breast Cancer Cell Proliferation," *Journal of Pineal Research* 14 (2) (1993): 89.
9. D. S. Beniashvili et al., "Low-Frequency Electromagnetic Radiation Enhances the Induction of Rat Mammary Tumors by Nitrosomethyl Urea," *Cancer Letters* 61 (1991): 75–79.
10. G. M. Matanoski et al., "Electromagnetic Field Exposure and Male Breast Cancer," *Lancet* 337 (1991): 737.
11. P. A. Demers et al., "Occupational Exposure to Electromagnetic Fields and Breast Cancer in Men," *American Journal of Epidemiology* 134 (1991): 340–47.
12. T. Tynes et al., "Incidence of Cancer in Norwegian Workers Potentially Exposed to Electromagnetic Fields," *American Journal of Epidemiology* 136 (1992): 81–88.
13. D. P. Loomis, "Cancer of Breast Among Men in Electrical Occupations," *Lancet* 339 (1992): 1482–83.
14. D. P. Loomis et al., "Breast Cancer Mortality Among Female Electrical Workers in the United States," *Journal of the National Cancer Institute* 86 (12) (1994): 921–25.

15. "Swedish Officials Acknowledge EMF-Cancer Connection," *Microwave News* XII (5), September/October 1992.
16. J. E. Vena, "Use of Electric Blankets and Risk of Postmenopausal Breast Cancer," *American Journal of Epidemiology* 134 (2) (1991): 180–85.
17. "Understanding EMF: Electric and Magnetic Fields," pamphlet distributed by San Diego Gas and Electric, December 1994.

CHAPTER 19: TAMOXIFEN AND BREAST CANCER TREATMENT

1. H. P. Leis, Jr., "The Role of Tamoxifen in the Prevention and Treatment of Benign and Malignant Breast Lesions: A Chemopreventive," *International Surgery* 78 (1993): 176–82.
2. A. Costa, "Breast Cancer: Chemoprevention," *European Journal of Cancer* 29A (1993): 589–92.
3. K. B. Horitz, "How Do Breast Cancers Become Hormone Resistant?" *Journal of Steroid Biochemistry and Molecular Biology* 49 (1994): 295–302.
4. M. O'Brien and T. J. Powles, "Tamoxifen in the Prevention of Breast Cancer. Are the Risks Likely to Outweigh the Benefits?" *Drug Safety* 10 (1994): 1–4.
5. M. Morrow and V. C. Jordan, "Risk Factors and the Prevention of Breast Cancer with Tamoxifen," *Cancer Surgery* 18 (1993): 211–29.
6. Leis, "Role of Tamoxifen."
7. T. L. Bush and K. J. Helzisouer, "Tamoxifen for the Primary Prevention of Breast Cancer: A Review and Critique of the Concept and Trial," *Epidemiologic Reviews* 15 (1993): 233–43.
8. J. B. Custodio, T. C. Dinis, et al., "Tamoxifen and Hydroxytamoxifen as Intramembranous Inhibitors of Lipid Peroxidation. Evidence for Peroxyl Radical Scavenging Activity," *Biochemical Pharmacology* 47 (1994): 1989–98.
9. M. Thangaraju, T. Vijayalakshmi, et al., "Effect of Tamoxifen on Lipid Peroxide and Antioxidative System in Postmenopausal Women with Breast Cancer," *Cancer* 74 (1994): 78–82.
10. A. Dziewulska-Bokiniec, J. Wojtacki, et al., "The Effect of Tamoxifen Treatment on Serum Cholesterol Fractions in Breast Cancer Women," *Neoplasma* 41 (1994): 13–16.
11. E. Gold, S. Stapley, et al., "Tamoxifen and Norethisterone: Effects on Plasma Cholesterol and Total Body Calcium Content in the Estrogen Deficient Rat," *Hormone Metabolic Research* 26 (1994): 100–103.
12. A. M. Dnistrian, M. K. Schwartz, et al., "Effects of Tamoxifen on Serum Cholesterol and Lipoproteins During Chemohormonal Therapy," *Clinica Chimica Acta* 223 (1993): 43–52.

13. D. A. Shewmon, J. L. Stock, et al., "Tamoxifen Decreases Lipoprotein (a) in Patients with Breast Cancer," *Metabolism* 43 (1994): 531–32.
14. B. Kristensen, B. Ejlertsen, et al., "Tamoxifen and Bone Metabolism in Postmenopausal Low-Risk Breast Cancer Patients: A Randomized Study," *Journal of Clinical Oncology* 12 (1994): 992–97.
15. E. Gold, Stapley, et al., "Tamoxifen and Norethisterone."
16. C. D. Wright et al., "Effect of Long-Term Tamoxifen Therapy on Cancellous Bone Remodeling and Structure in Women with Breast Cancer," *Journal of Bone Mineral Research* 9 (1994): 153–59.
17. A. J. Neal, K. Evans, et al., "Does Long-Term Administration of Tamoxifen Affect Bone Mineral Density?" *European Journal of Cancer* 29A (1993): 1971–73.
18. Leis, "Role of Tamoxifen."
19. T. F. Anelli, A. Anelli, et al., "Tamoxifen Administration Is Associated with a High Rate of Treatment-Limiting Symptoms in Male Breast Cancer Patients," *Cancer* 74 (1994): 74–77.
20. P. Creamer, K. Lim, et al., "Acute Inflammatory Polyarthritis in Association with Tamoxifen," *British Journal of Rheumatology* 33 (1994): 583–85.
21. J. S. Heier, R. A. Dragoo, et al., "Screening for Ocular Toxicity in Asymptomatic Patients Treated with Tamoxifen," *American Journal of Ophthalmology* 117 (1994): 772–75.
22. A. J. Flash, "Clear Evidence That Long-Term, Low-Dose Tamoxifen Treatment Can Induce Ocular Toxicity: A Prospective Study of 63 Patients," *Survey of Ophthalmology* 38 (1994): 392–93.
23. L. M. Sargent, Y. P. Dragan, et al., "Tamoxifen Induces Hepatic Aneuploidy and Mitotic Spindle Disruption After a Single In Vivo Administration to Female Sprague-Dawley Rats," *Cancer Research* 54 (1994): 3357–60.
24. D. N. Pathak and W. J. Bodell, "DNA Adduct Formation by Tamoxifen with Rat and Human Liver Microsomal Activation Systems," *Carcinogenesis* 15 (1994): 529–32.
25. G. A. Potter, R. McCague, et al., "A Mechanistic Hypothesis for DNA Adduct Formation by Tamoxifen Following Hepatic Oxidative Metabolism," *Carcinogenesis* 15 (1994): 439–42.
26. M. A. Seoud, J. Johnson, et al., "Gynecologic Tumors in Tamoxifen-Treated Women with Breast Cancer," *Obstetrics and Gynecology* 82 (1993): 165-R.
27. R. P. Kaedar, T. H. Boume, et al., "Effects of Tamoxifen on Uterus and Ovaries of Postmenopausal Women in a Randomised Breast Cancer Prevention Trial," *Lancet* 343 (1994): 1318–21.
28. B. Fisher, J. P. Costantino, et al, "Endometrial Cancer in Tamoxifen-Treated Breast Cancer Patients: Findings from the National Surgical

Adjuvant Breast and Bowel Project (NASBP) B-14," *Journal of the National Cancer Institute* 86 (1994): 527–37.

29. U. Magriples, F. Naftolin, et al., "High-Grade Endometrial Carcinoma in Tamoxifen-Treated Breast Cancer Patients," *Journal of Clinical Oncology* 11 (1993): 485–90.

30. F. E. van Leeuwen, J. Benraadt, et al., "Risk of Endometrial Cancer After Tamoxifen Treatment of Breast Cancer," *Lancet* 343 (1994): 448–52.

31. H. E. Sonnendecker, K. Cooper, et al., "Primary Fallopian Tube Adenocarcinoma In Situ Associated with Adjuvant Tamoxifen Therapy for Breast Cancer," *Gynecology Oncology* 52 (1994): 402–407.

32. A. H. Ugwumadu and K. Harding, "Uterine Leiomyomata and Endometrial Proliferation in Postmenopausal Women Treated with the Anti-Oestrogen Tamoxifen," *European Journal of Obstetrics, Gynecology and Reproductive Biology* 54 (1994): 153–56.

33. L. Leo, A. Lanza, et al., "Leiomyomas in Patients Receiving Tamoxifen," *Clinical and Experimental Obstetrics and Gynecology* 21 (1994): 94–98.

34. M. A. Morgan, Y. Gincherman, et al., "Endometriosis and Tamoxifen Therapy," *International Journal of Gynaecology and Obstetrics* 45 (1994): 55–57.

35. L. R. Hajjar, W. Kim, et al., "Intestinal and Pelvic Endometriosis Presenting as a Tumor and Associated with Tamoxifen Therapy: Report of a Case," *Obstetrics and Gynecology* 82 (1993): 642–44.

36. S. Lundgren, J. A. Soreide, et al., "Influence of Tamoxifen on the Tumor Content of Steroid Hormone Receptors," *Anticancer Research* 14 (1994): 1313–16.

37. M. E. Bracke, C. Charlier, et al., "Tamoxifen Restores the E-cadherin Function in Human Breast Cancer MCF-7/6 Cells and Suppresses Their Invasive Phenotype," *Cancer Research* 54 (1994): 4607–4609.

38. S. R. Johnston, B. P. Haynes, et al., "Acquired Tamoxifen Resistance in Human Breast Cancer and Reduced Intra-tumoral Drug Concentration," *Lancet* 342 (1993): 1521–22.

39. C. K. Osborne, M. Jarman, et al., "The Importance of Tamoxifen Metabolism in Tamoxifen-Stimulated Breast Tumor Growth," *Cancer Chemotherapy and Pharmacology* 34 (1994): 89–95.

40. C. K. Osborne, "Mechanisms for Tamoxifen Resistance in Breast Cancer: Possible Role of Tamoxifen Metabolism," *Journal of Steroid Biochemistry and Molecular Biology* 47 (1993): 83–99.

41. D. M. Wolf and V. C. Jordan, William L. McGuire Memorial Symposium, "Drug Resistance to Tamoxifen During Breast Cancer Therapy," *Breast Cancer Research and Treatment* 27 (1993): 27–40.

42. P. E. Sipila, V. J. Wiebe, et al., "Prolonged Tamoxifen Exposure Selects a Breast Cancer Cell Clone That Is Stable In Vitro and In Vivo," *European Journal of Cancer* 29A (1993): 2138–44.

43. K. B. Horitz, "How Do Breast Cancers Become Hormone Resistant?" *Journal of Steroid Biochemistry and Molecular Biology* 49 (1994): 295–302.
44. I. C. Henderson, "Adjuvant Systemic Therapy for Early Breast Cancer," *Cancer* 74 (1994): 401–409.
45. G. Martelli, D. Moglia, et al., "Surgical Resection Plus Tamoxifen as Treatment of Breast Cancer in Elderly Patients: A Retrospective Study," *European Journal of Cancer* 29A (1993): 2080–82.
46. M. Morrow, "Breast Disease in Elderly Women," *Surgery in Clinics of North America* 74 (1994): 145–61.
47. P. P. Rosen, "Proliferative Breast 'Disease,'" *Cancer* 71 (1993): 3798–807.

CHAPTER 20: TREATMENT FOR EARLY BREAST CANCER

1. D. A. August, L. C. Carpenter, et al., "Benefits of a Multidisciplinary Approach to Breast Care," *Journal of Surgical Oncology* 53 (1993): 161–67.
2. C. M. Balch, S. E. Singlerary, et al., "Clinical Decision-making in Early Breast Cancer," *Annals of Surgery* 217 (1993): 207–225.
3. T. M. Pisansky, M. Y. Halyard, et al., "Breast Conservation Therapy for Invasive Breast Cancer: A Review of Prior Trials and the Mayo Clinic Experience," *Mayo Clinic Proceedings* 69 (1994): 515–24.
4. August, Carpenter, et al., "Benefits."
5. S. G. Nayfield, G. C. Bongiovanni, et al., "Statutory Requirements for Disclosure of Breast Cancer Treatment Alternatives," *Journal of the National Cancer Institute* 86 (1994): 1202–1208.
6. P. M. Ravdin, "A Practical View of Prognostic Factors for Staging, Adjuvant Treatment and as Baseline Studies for Possible Future Therapy," *Hematology/Oncology Clinics of North America* 8 (1994): 197–211.
7. E. G. Mansour, P. M. Ravdin, et al., "Prognostic Factors in Early Breast Carcinoma," *Cancer* 74 (1994): 381–400.
8. J. S. Abrams, T. D. Moore, et al., "New Chemotherapeutic Agents for Breast Cancer," *Cancer* 74 (1994): 1164–76.
9. S. G. Arbuck, A. Dorr, et al., "Paclitaxel (Taxol) in Breast Cancer," *Hematology/Oncology Clinics of North America* 8 (1994): 121–40.
10. M. A. Friedman, "New Directions for Breast Cancer Therapeutic Research," *Hematology/Oncology Clinics of North America* 8 (1994): 101–112.
11. A. Sulkes, U. Beller, et al., "Taxol: Initial Israeli Experience with a Novel Anticancer Agent," *Israel Journal of Medical Science* 30 (1994): 70–78.
12. L. E. Holm, E. Nordevang, et al., "Treatment Failure and Dietary Habits in Women with Breast Cancer," *Journal of the National Cancer Institute* 85 (1993): 32–36.
13. U. Veronesi, S. Luini, et al., "Effect of Menstrual Phase on Surgical Treatment of Breast Cancer," *Lancet* 343 (1994): 1545–47.

14. A. P. Corder, M. Cross, et al., "The Timing of Breast Cancer Surgery within the Menstrual Cycle," *Postgraduate Medical Journal* 70 (1994): 281–84.

15. F. E. Gump, "Lobular Carcinoma In Situ (LCIS): Pathology and Treatment," *Journal of Cellular Biochemistry Supplement* 17 (1993): 53–58.

16. B. Fisher and S. Anderson, "Conservative Surgery for the Management of Invasive and Noninvasive Carcinoma of the Breast: NSABP Trials," *World Journal of Surgery* 18 (1994): 63–69.

17. B. Fisher, J. Costantino, et al., "Lumpectomy Compared with Lumpectomy and Radiation Therapy for the Treatment of Intraductal Breast Cancer," *New England Journal of Medicine* 328 (1993): 1581–86.

18. Fisher and Anderson, "Conservative Surgery."

19. T. M. Pisansky, M. Y. Halyard, et al., "Breast Conservation Therapy for Invasive Breast Cancer.

20. L. G. Arnesson, S. Smeds, et al., "Recurrence-Free Survival in Patients with Small Breast Cancer. An analysis of Cancers 10 mm or Less Detected Clinically and by Screening," *European Journal of Surgery* 160 (1994): 271–76.

21. T. M. Pisansky, M.Y. Halyard, et al., "Breast Conservation Therapy for Invasive Breast Cancer.

22. L. E. Rutqvist, "Radiation Therapies for Breast Cancer: Current Knowledge on Advantages and Disadvantages," *Recent Results in Cancer Research* 127 (1993): 119–27.

23. G. Liljegren, L. Holmberg, et al., "Sector Resection with or without Postoperative Radiotherapy for Stage I Breast Cancer: Five-year Results of a Randomized Trial. Uppsala-Orebro Breast Cancer Study Group," *Journal of the National Cancer Institute* 86 (1994): 717–22.

24. L. E. Rutqvist, D. Pettersson, et al., "Adjuvant Radiation Therapy versus Surgery Alone in Operable Breast Cancer: Long-Term Follow-up of a Randomized Clinical Trial," *Radiotherapy and Oncology* 26 (1993): 104–110.

25. S. H. Levitt, "The Importance of Locoregional Control in the Treatment of Breast Cancer and Its Impact on Survival," *Cancer* 74 (1994): 1840–46.

26. M. C. Posner and N. Wolmark, "Indications for Breast-Preserving Surgery and Adjuvant Therapy in Early Breast Cancer," *International Surgery* 79 (1994): 43–47.

27. T. J. Smith and B. E. Hillner, "The Efficacy and Cost-Effectiveness of Adjuvant Therapy of Early Breast Cancer in Premenopausal Women," *Journal of Clinical Oncology* 11 (1993): 771–76.

28. J. F. Forbes, "Surgery of Early Breast Cancer," *Current Opinion in Oncology* 5 (1993): 966–75.

29. Arnesson, Smeds, et al., "Recurrence-Free Survival."

30. W. C. Wood, "Integration of Risk Factors to Allow Patient Selection for

Adjuvant Systemic Therapy in Lymph Node–Negative Breast Cancer Patients," *World Journal of Surgery* 18 (1994): 39–44.

31. D. W. Kinne, "Controversies in Primary Breast Cancer Management," *American Journal of Surgery* 166 (1993): 502–508.

32. K. K. Hughes, "Psychosocial and Functional Status of Breast Cancer Patient. The Influence of Diagnosis and Treatment of Choice," *Cancer Nursing* 16 (1993): 222–29.

33. M. Blichert-Toft, "Breast Conserving Therapy for Mammary Carcinoma: Psychosocial Indications and Limitations," *Annals of Medicine* 24 (1992): 445–51.

34. P. A. Newcomb and P. M. Lantz, "Recent Trends in Breast Cancer Incidence, Mortality and Mammography," *Breast Cancer Research and Treatment* 28 (1993): 97–106.

35. National Cancer Institute briefing materials, background paper: "Revisions to the National Cancer Institute Breast Cancer Screening Guidelines," September 13, 1993.

CHAPTER 21: BREAST IMPLANTS: AN INCREASED RISK?

1. W. A. Berg, N. D. Anderson, et al., "MR Imaging of the Breast in Patients with Silicone Breast Implants: Normal Postoperative Variants and Diagnostic Pitfalls," *American Journal of Roentgenology* 163 (1994): 575–78.

2. D. L. Monticciolo, R. C. Nelson, et al., "MR Detection of Leakage from Silicone Breast Implants: Value of a Silicone-Selective Pulse Sequence," *American Journal of Roentgenology* 163 (1994): 51–56.

3. L. G. Dodd, N. Sneige, et al., "Fine-Needle Aspiration Cytology of Silicone Granulomas in the Augmented Breast," *Diagnosis of Cytopathology* 9 (1993): 498–502.

4. J. S. Mitnick, M. F. Vasquez, et al., "Fine Needle Aspiration Biopsy in Patients with Augmentation Protheses and a Palpable Mass," *Annals of Plastic Surgery* 31 (1993): 241–44.

5. G. R. Evans, S. Slezak, et al., "Silicon Tissue Assays in Nonaugmented Cadaveric Patients: Is There a Baseline Level?" *Plastic and Reconstructive Surgery* 93 (1994): 1117–22.

6. R. N. Silver, E. E. Sahn, et al., "Demonstration of Silicon in Sites of Connective-Tissue Disease in Patients with Silicone-Gel Breast Implants," *Archives of Dermatology* 129 (1993): 63–68.

7. M. Copeland, A. Kressel, et al., "Systemic Inflammatory Disorder Related to Fibrous Breast Capsules After Silicone Implant Removal," *Plastic and Reconstructive Surgery* 92 (1993): 1179–81.

8. N. Kossovsky and C. J. Freiman, "Silicone Breast Implant Pathology. Clinical Data and Immunologic Consequences," *Archives of Pathology and Laboratory Medicine* 118 (1994): 686–93.

9. S. H. Yoshida, C. C. Chang, et al., "Silicon and Silicone: Theoretical and Clinical Implications of Breast Implants," Regulatory Toxicology and Pharmacology 17 (1993): 3–18.
10. A. J. Bridges and F. B. Vasey, "Silicone Breast Implants. History, Safety, and Potential Complications," Archives of Internal Medicine 153 (1993): 2638–44.
11. W. Peters, E. Keystone, et al., "Is There a Relationship Between Antibodies and Silicone-Gel Implants?" Annals of Plastic Surgery 32 (1994): 1–5.
12. A. J. Park, R. J. Black, et al., "Silicone Gel Breast Implants, Breast Cancer and Connective Tissue Disorders," British Journal of Surgery 80 (1993): 1097–1100.
13. R. F. Spiera, A. Gibofsky, et al., "Silicone Gel Filled Breast Implants and Connective Tissue Disease: An Overview," Journal of Rheumatology 21 (1994): 239–45.
14. S. E. Gabriel, W. O'Fallon, et al., "Risk of Connective-Tissue Diseases and Other Disorders After Breast Implantation," New England Journal of Medicine 330 (1994): 1697–1702.
15. M. J. Duffy and J. E. Woods, "Health Risks of Failed Silicone Gel Breast Implants: A 30-Year Clinical Experience," Plastic and Reconstructive Surgery 94 (1994): 295–99.
16. S. S. Teuber, M. J. Rowley, et al., "Anti-Collagen Autoantibodies Are Found in Women with Silicone Breast Implants," Journal of Autoimmunology 6 (1993): 367–77.
17. A. R. Shons and W. Schubert, "Silicone Breast Implants and Immune Disease," Annals of Plastic Surgery 28 (1992): 491–99.
18. A. Campbell et al., "Suppression of Natural Killer Cell Activity in Patients with Silicone Breast Implants: Reversal upon Explanation," Toxicology and Industrial Health 10 (1994): 149–54.
19. B. G. Steinbach, N. S. Hardt, et al, "Mammography: Breast Implants—Types, Complications, and Adjacent Breast Pathology," Current Problems in Diagnostic Radiology 22 (1993): 39–86.
20. M. A. Ganott, K. M. Harris, et al., "Augmentation Mammoplasty: Normal and Abnormal Findings with Mammography and US," Radiographics 12 (1992): 281–95.
21. A. J. Liebman and B. D. Kruse, "Imaging of Breast Cancer After Augmentation Mammoplasty," Annals of Plastic Surgery 30 (1993): 111–15.
22. B. G. Steinbach, N. S. Hardt, et al., "Breast Implants, Common Complications, and Concurrent Breast Disease," Radiographics 13 (1993): 95–118.
23. D. C. Birdsell, H. Jenkins, et al., "Breast Cancer Diagnosis and Survival in Women with and without Breast Implants," Plastic and Reconstructive Surgery 92 (1993): 795–800.
24. E. P. Winer, K. Fee-Fulkerson, et al., "Silicone Controversy: A Survey of Women with Breast Cancer and Silicone Implants," Journal of the National Cancer Institute 85 (1993): 1407–11.

CHAPTER 22: THE LATEST ON NONSEXUAL BREAST MASSAGE

1. T.G.C. Murrell, "Epidemiological and Biochemical Support for a Theory on the Cause and Prevention of Breast Cancer," *Medical Hypotheses* 36 (1991): 389–96.
2. M. L'Hermite and M. L'Hermite-Baleriaux, "Prolactin and Breast Cancer," *European Journal of Cancer and Clinical Oncology* 24 (6) (1988): 955–58.
3. P. A. Baghurst, "Diet, Prolactin, and Breast Cancer," *American Journal of Clinical Nutrition* 56 (1992): 943–49.
4. R. C. Kolodny et al., "Mammary Stimulation Causes Prolactin Secretion in Nonlactating Women," *Nature* 238: 284–85.
5. J. Amico and B. E. Finley, "Breast Stimulation in Cycling Women, Pregnant Women and a Woman with Induced Lactation: Pattern of Release of Oxytocin, Prolactin and Luteinizing Hormone," *Clinical Endocrinology* 25 (1986): 97–106.
6. D. Curties, *Therapeutic Massage: Concepts for Clinical Practice* (Hanover, MD: Mosbey), book release pending.
7. D. Curties, "Breast Massage: Discussion Paper and Suggested Guidelines," *Journal of Soft Tissue Manipulation* June/July (1993): 4–6.
8. D. Curties, "Breast Massage."
9. Anderson, Mark. "Wearing Too-tight Bras May Lead To Breast Cancer." *Valley Advocate Newspaper*, May 4, 1995.
10. Grismaijer, Soma and Sydney Ross Singer. *Dressed to Kill: The Link Between Breast Cancer and Bras.* (Long Island, NY: Avery).
11. G. Wittlinger and H. Wittlinger, *Introduction to Dr. Vodder's Manual Lymph Drainage* (Heidelberg: Haug 1982).
12. D. Wyrick, "European Manual Lymph Drainage," *Body Therapy*, October/November (1994): 17–18.
13. J.P. Cooke, "Lymphatic Disorders," *Vascular Medicine: A Textbook of Vascular Biology and Diseases,* Joseph Loscalzo et al. editors (Little, Brown and Company: Boston 1988).
14. S. Passik, "Psychological Aspects of Lymphedema after Breast Cancer Treatment," *National Lymphedema Network Newsletter,* Vol. 4, No. 4. p. no 1.
15. S. Passik, "Psychological Aspects of Lymphadema after Breast Cancer Treatment."
16. D. Wyrick, "European Manual Lymph Drainage."
17 Norman Cousins, *The Healing Heart* (New York: Avon Books 1983).
18. D. Curties, *Therapeutic: Concepts for Clinical Practice.*
19. D. Curties, *Therapeutic: Concepts for Clinical Practice.*

CHAPTER 23: THE MIND/BODY CONNECTION

1. Larry Dossey, *Meaning & Medicine* (New York: Bantam, 1991).
2. L. T. Vollhardt, "Psychoneuroimmunology: A Literature Review," *American Orthopsychiatric Association* 6 (1) (1991): 35–47.
3. C. B. Pert, "The Wisdom of the Receptors: Neuropeptides, the Emotions and Bodymind," *Advances* 3 (3) (1986): 8–16.
4. J. E. Blalack, "The Immune System as a Sensory Organ," *Journal of Immunology* 132 (1984): 1067–70.
5. S. S. Hall, "A Molecular Code Links Emotions, Mind and Health," *Smithsonian*, June 1989, 62–71.
6. Lawrence L. LeShan, *You Can Fight for Your Life: Emotional Factors in the Causation of Cancer* (New York: M. Evans, 1977).
7. S. Greer and M. Watson, "Towards a Psychobiological Model of Cancer: Psychological Considerations," *Social Science Medicine* 20 (8) (1985): 773–77.
8. L. Temoshok, "Personality, Coping Style, Emotion and Cancer: Towards an Integrated Model," *Cancer Surveys* 6 (3) (1987): 545–67.
9. C. L. Cooper and E. Faragher, "Coping Strategies and Breast Disorder/Cancer," *Psychological Medicine* 22 (1992): 447–55.
10. Greer and Watson, "Towards a Psychobiological Model of Cancer."
11. S. Greer and T. Morris, "Psychological Attributes of Women Who Develop Breast Cancer: A Controlled Study," *Journal of Psychosomatic Research* 19 (1975): 147–53.
12. M. Watson and S. Greer, "Relationship Between Emotional Control, Adjustment to Cancer and Depression and Anxiety in Breast Cancer Patients," *Psychological Medicine* 21 (1991): 51–57.
13. F. Vrazo, "They Blame Selves for Breast Cancer," *San Diego Union*, October 31, 1994.
14. A. O'Leary, "Stress, Emotion, and Human Immune Function," *Psychological Bulletin* 108 (3) (1990): 363–82.
15. Vollhardt, "Psychoneuroimmunology."
16. F. M. Burnet, "The Concept of Immunological Surveillance," *Progress in Experimental Tumor Research* 13 (1970): 1–27.
17. M. L. Kripke, "Immunoregulation of Carcinogenesis: Past, Present, and Future," *Journal of the National Cancer Institute* 80 (1988): 722–27.
18. K. W. Pettingale, "Towards a Psychobiological Model of Cancer: Biological Considerations," *Social Science Medicine* 20 (8) (1985): 779–87.
19. Kripke, "Immunoregulation."
20. Pettingale, "Towards a Psychobiological Model."
21. W. H. Redd et al., "Physiologic and Psychobehavioral Research in Oncology," *Cancer* 67 (1991): 813–22.
22. C. L. Cooper and E. B. Faragher, "Psychosocial Stress and Breast Can-

cer: The Inter-relationship Between Stress Events, Coping Strategies and Personality," *Psychological Medicine* 23 (1993): 653–62.

23. C. L. Cooper et al., "Incidence and Perception of Psychosocial Stress: The Relationship with Breast Cancer," *Psychological Medicine* 19 (1989): 415–22.

24. J. R. Edwards et al., "The Relationship Between Psychological Factors and Breast Cancer: Some Unexpected Results," *Behavioral Medicine*, Spring (1990): 5–14.

25. A. Forsen, "Psychosocial Stress as a Risk for Breast Cancer," *Psychotherapy and Psychosomatics* 55 (1991): 176–85.

26. R. Herberman, ed., *NK Cells and Other Natural Effector Cells* (New York: Academic, 1982).

27. R. Herberman and J. Ortaldo, "Natural Killer Cells: Their Role in Defenses Against Disease," *Science* 214 (1981): 24–30.

28. S. M. Levy and R. B. Herberman, "Prognostic Risk Assessment in Primary Breast Cancer by Behavioral and Immunological Parameters," *Health Psychology* 4 (2) (1985): 99–113.

29. S. M. Levy, et al., "Perceived Social Support and Tumor Estrogen/Progesterone Receptor Status as Predictors of Natural Killer Cell Activity in Breast Cancer Patients," *Psychosomatic Medicine* 52 (1990): 73–85.

30. C. S. Weisse, "Depression and Immunocompetence: A Review of the Literature," *Psychological Bulletin* 111 (3) (1992): 475–89.

31. M. Irwin et al., "Plasma Cortisol and Natural Killer Cell Activity During Bereavement," *Biological Psychiatry* 24 (1988): 173–78.

32. O'Leary, "Stress, Emotion."

33. M. Irwin et al., "Reduction of Immune Function in Life Stress and Depression," *Biological Psychiatry* 27 (1990): 22–30.

34. S. Levy et al., "Correlation of Stress Factors with Sustained Depression of Natural Killer Cell Activity and Predicted Prognosis in Patients with Breast Cancer," *Journal of Clinical Oncology* 5 (3) (1987): 348–53.

35. L. Derogatis et al., "Psychological Coping Mechanisms and Survival Time in Metastatic Breast Cancer," *Journal of the American Medical Association* 242 (1979): 1504–1509.

36. S. Greer et al., "Mental Attitudes to Cancer: An Additional Prognostic Factor," *Lancet* 1 (8431) (1985): 750.

37. Levy and Herberman, "Prognostic Risk Assessment."

38. Levy et al., "Correlation of Stress Factors."

39. S. Levy et al., "Survival Hazards Analysis in First Recurrent Breast Cancer Patients: Seven-Year Follow-up," *Psychosomatic Medicine* 50 (1988): 520–28.

40. B. Wise, "Comparison of Immune Response to Mirth and Distress in Women at Risk for Recurrent Breast Cancer," Ph.D. dissertation, University of Pittsburgh Psychology Department, 1987.

41. A. J. Ramirez et al., "Stress and Relapse of Breast Cancer," *British Medical Journal* 298 (6669) (1989): 291–93.

42. S. Greer, "Psychological Response to Cancer and Survival," *Psychological Medicine* 21 (1991): 43–49.

43. O. C. Simonton et al., *Getting Well Again* (New York: Bantam, 1978).

44. Bernie Siegel, *Love, Medicine and Miracles: Lessons Learned About Self-Healing from a Surgeon's Experience with Exceptional Patients* (New York: Harper & Row, 1986).

45. Bernie Siegel, *Peace, Love and Healing* (New York: Harper & Row, 1989).

46. Herbert Benson, "The Relaxation Response," in *Mind/Body Medicine*, eds. D. Goleman and J. Gurin (New York: Consumer Reports Books, 1993).

47. A. Meares, "Stress, Meditation and the Regression of Cancer," *Practitioner* 226 (1371) (1982): 1607–1609.

48. B. L. Gruber et al., "Immunological Responses of Breast Cancer Patients to Behavioral Interventions," *Biofeedback and Self-Regulation* 18 (1) (1993): 1–22.

49. S. Greer et al., "Evaluation of Adjuvant Psychological Therapy for Clinically Referred Cancer Patients," *British Journal of Cancer* 63 (2) (1991): 257–60.

50. S. Greet et al., "Adjuvant Psychological Therapy for Patients with Cancer: A Prospective Randomised Trial," *British Medical Journal* 304 (1992): 675–80.

51. J. S. Goodman, et al., "The Effect of Marital Status on Stage, Treatment, and Survival of Cancer Patients," *Journal of the American Medical Association* 258 (1987): 3125–30.

52. D. Spiegel, "Social Support: How Friends, Family, and Groups Can Help," in *Mind/Body Medicine* eds. D. Goleman and J. Gurin (New York: Consumer Reports Books, 1993).

53. L. F. Berkman and S. L. Syme, "Social Networks, Host Resistance, and Mortality: A Nine-Year Follow-up Study of Alameda County Residents," *American Journal of Epidemiology* 109 (1979): 186–204.

54. "Social Connections and Risk for Cancer: Prospective Evidence from the Alameda County Study," *Behavioral Medicine* 16 (3) (1990): 101–110.

55. Spiegel, in *Mind/Body Medicine*, p. 334.

56. Congress of the U.S. Office of Technology Assessment, *Unconventional Cancer Treatments* (Washington, D.C.: U.S. Government Printing Office, 1990).

57. Ibid.

58. D. Spiegel, "Effect of Psychosocial Treatment on Survival of Patients with Metastatic Breast Cancer," *Lancet* 2 (1989): 2 (8668) 888–91.

59. R. N. Remen, "Spirit: Resource for Healing," *Noetic Sciences Collection* (Sausalito, Calif.: Institute of Noetic Sciences, 1991).

60. C. Kuhn, "A Spiritual Inventory of the Medically Ill Patient," *Psychiatric Medicine* 6 (1988): 87–89.
61. D.J. Benor and R. Benor, "Spiritual Healing, Assuming the Spiritual Is Real," *Advances* 9 (4) (1993): 22–30.
62. D. B. Larson et al., "A Paradigm Shift in Medicine Toward Spirituality?" *Advances* 9 (4) (1993): 39–49.
63. G. L. Klerman and M. N. Weissman, "Increasing Rates of Depression," *Journal of the American Medical Association* 261 (1989): 2229–35.
64. Benor and Benor, "Spiritual Healing," p. 25.
65. E. Leskowitz, "Spiritual Healing, Modern Medicine, and Energy," *Advances* 9 (4) (1993): 50–53.
66. Benor and Benor, "Spiritual Healing," p. 26.
67. D. B. Larson, et al., "Paradigm Shift," p. 44.
68. D. Aldridge, "Is There Evidence for Spiritual Healing?" *Advances* 9 (4) (1993): 4–21.
69. J. B. Ellis and P. C. Smith, "Spiritual Well-Being, Social Desirability and Reasons for Living: Is There a Connection?" *International Journal of Social Psychiatry* 37 (1991): 57–63.
70. D. J. Benor, "Survey of Spiritual Healing Research," *Complementary Medical Research* 4 (1990): 9–33.
71. Dossey, *Meaning & Medicine*, p. 163.
72. D. P. Wirth, "Implementing Spiritual Healing in Modern Medical Practice," *Advances* 9 (4) (1993): 69–81.
73. Benor and Benor, "Spiritual Healing," p. 28.
74. Ibid., p. 27.
75. D. P. Wirth, "The Effect of Noncontact Therapeutic Touch on the Healing Rate of Full Thickness Dermal Wounds," *Subtle Energy* 1 (1) (1990): 1–20.
76. R. C. Byrd, "Positive Therapeutic Effects of Intercessory Prayer in a Coronary Unit Population," *Southern Medical Journal* 81 (7) (1988): 826–29.
77. Benor and Benor, "Spiritual Healing," p. 28.
78. Larson, et al., "Paradigm Shift," p. 40.

CHAPTER 24: ON HEALTH, HEALING, AND EMPOWERMENT

1. Larry Dossey, *Beyond Illness* (Boulder, Colo.: Shambhala, 1984).
2. Anne E. Frahm, *A Cancer Battle Plan* (Colorado Springs, Colo.: Pinon, 1992).
3. Harriet Goldhor Lerner, *The Dance of Anger: A Woman's Guide to Changing the Patterns of Intimate Relationships* (New York: Harper & Row, 1985).

4. Marianne Williamson, *A Woman's Worth* (New York: Random House, 1993).
5. Jean Shinoda Bolen, "Cancer as a Turning Point: From Surviving to Thriving," speech presented at "The Power of Myth and Truth in Healing: Cancer as a Turning Point for the Soul" conference, San Diego, California, October 22, 1994.
6. Lawrence L. LeShan, *Cancer as a Turning Point* (New York: Dutton, 1989).
7. Williamson.
8. Gloria Steinem, *Revolution from Within* (Boston: Little, Brown, 1992).
9. Joan Borysenko, *Minding the Body, Mending the Mind* (New York: Bantam, 1988).
10. Shinoda Bolen.
11. Elaine St. James, *Simplify Your Life* (New York: Hyperion, 1994).
12. —— *Inner Simplicity* (New York: Hyperion, 1995).

Index

acid rain, 143
adjuvant agents, definition of, 232
adjuvant chemotherapy, 93, 246,
   247
adolescence, 146, 162, 208–9
aerobic exercise, 87–88, 197
African-American women, 14, 67,
   95
age, 208–9
   alcohol and, 212–13
   breast cancer incidence and
      mortality rates and, 45, 67
   estrogen receptors and, 94–95, 96
   exercise and, 195–96
   fibroadenoma and, 28–29
   of first menstruation, 21, 85–86,
      89, 151, 197–98
   free radicals and, 131–32, 133
   mammograms and, 17, 39,
      42–46, 54, 58–59, 67, 257
   melatonin and, 216, 219, 220,
      221
   of menopause, 98
   nutritional supplements and,
      162–63
   radiation sensitivity and, 42–43,
      59

as risk factor, 21
   see also postmenopausal women;
      premenopausal women
Agriculture Department, U.S., 109,
   160, 186, 200
AH (epithelial atypical hyperplasia),
   29–30
AIDS, 17, 18
alcohol, 19–20, 129, 211–14, 290
   estrogen levels and, 89–90, 110,
      212, 213, 214
alpha-BHC, 188
Alternatives in Cancer Therapy
   (Pelton), 248–49, 259
alveoli, 26
amenorrhea, 89
American Cancer Society, 13, 21,
   43, 71, 74, 80, 151
American College of Obstetrics and
   Gynecology, 43
American College of Radiology
   (ACR), 43, 46
amino acids, 127, 168, 215–16
angiogenesis, 176
animal cancer studies, 136, 152–53,
   157, 177, 234, 236
animal husbandry, 146

Merck, Sharpe and Dohme, 170
metastasis, 23, 33, 83, 217
  in clinical staging, 36–37
  definition of, 16, 20
  dietary fat and, 155
  mammogram effectiveness re-
    duced by, 16–17
  modes of, 35
Mevacor, 162
milk, 185, 262
  secretion of, 24
  see also lactation
milk products, 128–29
mind/body connection, 267, 273–95
  behavioral medicine and, 275,
    285–89
  cancer personality and, 276–79
  historical perspective on, 274–75
  psychoneuroimmunology and,
    275–76, 281, 282–84, 294
  spirit and, 289–94
mind/body therapy (Hakomi), 10
*Minding the Body, Mending the
  Mind* (Borysenko), 311–12
minerals, 162, 168, 179
Minimum Daily Requirement
  (MDR), 161
miso, 174, 178, 181
monounsaturated fats, 148, 153–54
monounsaturated oils, 129
mortality rates, 13, 14, 15, 21, 23, 66
  age and, 45
  breast self-examinations and,
    68–69
  dietary fat and, 156
  mammograms and, 39, 40
  tamoxifen and, 239–40
MRI (magnetic resonance imaging),
  35, 54
Murrell, T.G.C., 259, 260–62

National Academy of Sciences
  (NAS), 149, 151, 161, 187
National Breast Cancer Coalition, 18
National Cancer Institute (NCI),
  17, 18, 39, 44–45, 115, 124,
  134, 135, 151, 157, 174, 233,
  283

National Health and Nutrition Examination Survey (NHANES
  II), 126, 160
National Institutes of Health, 66,
  154, 155
National Research Council, 143,
  161
natto, 174
natural killer cells, 255, 283, 284
natural progesterone 104–5,
  106–10, 114–15
neuroendocrine system, 273, 275,
  282
neuropeptides, 275–76, 280
nipple discharges or secretions, 29,
  48, 74, 79, 81
nipple retraction, 34
nipple squeezing, in breast self-examinations, 79, 80–81
nipple stimulation, 258, 259,
  260–61, 262
Nixon, Richard M., 13
nonpalpable masses or tumors, 48,
  57, 59
nonsexual breast massage, 258–72
  authors' case for, 262–63
  bras and, 263–64
  breast energetics and, 267–68
  effects of, 258–60
  lymphedema and, 265–66, 268
  lymph system and, 264–65, 268
  Manual Lymph Drainage and,
    264, 266–67, 271
  Murrell's hypothesis on, 260–62
  technique for, 268–71
Norplant, 91–92
Nurses' Health Study, 119, 150, 212
nutrition, 7, 8–9, 10, 21
  see also antioxidants; diet
nutritional supplements, 159–72
  antioxidants, 135, 138–39, 143

obesity, 95
  estrogen and, 86, 88
  rate of, 146
  recurrence and, 156
  as risk factor, 152
oils, 129, 153–54

through diet, 128–30
early detection and, 15–17, 23
through exercise, 195–204
melatonin and, 215–21
nonsexual breast massage and,
258–72
soy and, 173–82
tamoxifen and, 231–40
Twenty-Three-Point Plan for,
315–16
progesterone, 37
effects of deficiency in, 105–6
estrogen and, 108–10
in hormonal contraceptives,
90–91
in hormone replacement therapy, *see* progestin
milk secretion stimulated by, 24
natural, 104–5, 106–10, 114–15
production and function of,
104–5
receptor sites for, 26, 27, 232
progestin (synthetic progesterone),
90, 95, 101, 102–3, 106–10
prognosis, 36–37, 243
progression stage, 20
prolactin, 26, 125, 261–62
proliferation, 141
promotion phase, 19–20, 30, 84, 85,
140, 219
prostate cancer, 154, 222
protease inhibitors, 176–77
protein, 127, 147, 174
Provera, 106
psychoneuroimmunology (PNI),
275–76, 281, 282–84, 294
puberty, 24

radiation, 8, 17, 19, 54
age and sensitivity to, 42–43, 59
see also mammograms
radiation therapy (XRT), 62, 93,
241, 245, 246–47
radiologists, 242
consultations with, 47, 59
selection of, 46–47
stereotactic needle biopsies performed by, 60–64

Recommended Daily Allowance
(RDA) levels, 160–63
of antioxidants, 134
definition of, 160–61
moving beyond, 164–66
of nutritional supplements, 160
rectal cancer, 217
recurrence, 11, 243, 247
dietary fat and, 155–57, 158
Regenstein, Lewis, 126–27
Reichman, Marsha, 212
Remen, Rachel Naomi, 289
REM sleep, 218
research spending, 17–18
Revolution from Within (Steinem),
310
risk factors, 11, 19, 20–22, 27, 28, 37,
281
absence of, 46
alcohol, 211–14
benign breast diseases, 28–31,
60, 88
breast implants, 250–57
controllable, 20, 22
diet, 95, 118–19, 120–23, 125
126–27
dietary fat, 95, 118, 119, 145,
147, 149–54
electromagnetic fields, 222–30
estrogen receptors and, 95
fibrocystic disease, 27–28
hormonal contraceptives, 90–92,
96
hormone replacement therapy,
101–4
lobular carcinoma *in situ,* 33
menstruation, 20, 21, 85–86, 198
obesity, 152
pesticides, 183–94
progesterone deficiency, 105–6
smoking, 205–10
uncontrollable, 20–21, 23
Rosen, Paul P., 240
Rosenberg, Lynn, 212

SAD, *see* seasonal affective disorder; standard American diet
St. James, Elaine, 313